Electrotherapy Explained

Principles and practice

Third edition

John Low BA(Hons), FCSP, DipTP, SRP

Formerly Acting Principal, School of Physiotherapy, Guy's Hospital, London, UK

Ann Reed BA, MCSP, DipTP, SRP

Senior Lecturer, Department of Health Sciences, University of East London, UK

Foreword by

Mary Dyson PhD, MIBiol, CBiol

Director of Tissue Repair Research Unit, UMDS, Guy's Hospital, London

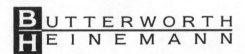
BUTTERWORTH
HEINEMANN

EDINBURGH LONDON NEW YORK OXFORD PHILADELPHIA
ST LOUIS SYDNEY TORONTO 2000

Butterworth-Heinemann
An imprint of Elsevier Limited

First published 1990
Second edition 1994
Third edition 2000
Reprinted 2001 (twice), 2002, 2003, 2004 (twice)

British Library Cataloguing in Publication Data
Low, John
    Electrotherapy explained: principles and practice. – 3rd ed.
    1. Electrotherapeutics
    I. Title   II. Reed, Ann
    615.8´45

Library of Congress in Cataloging in Publication Data
Low, John (John L.)
    Electrotherapy explained: principles and practice/John Low,
    Ann Reed; foreword by Mary Dyson. – 3rd ed.
    p. cm.
    Includes bibliographical references and index.
    ISBN 0 7506 4149 5
    1. Electrotherapeutics   I. Reed, Ann, SRP.   II. Title
    RM871.L69   99–049791
    615.8´45-dc21

ELSEVIER SCIENCE   your source for books,
journals and multimedia
in the health sciences
www.elsevierhealth.com

Typeset by Latimer Trend & Company Ltd, Plymouth
Printed and bound by MPG Books Ltd, Bodmin, Cornwall

Contents

Foreword by Mary Dyson   vii
Preface to the third edition   ix
Preface to the first edition   xi

SECTION I

Chapter 1.   Introduction   1
Chapter 2.   Therapeutic direct current   30
Chapter 3.   Electrical stimulation of nerve and muscle   53
Chapter 4.   Electrophysiological evaluation   141
Chapter 5.   Biofeedback   157

SECTION II

Chapter 6.   Therapeutic ultrasound   172

SECTION III

Chapter 7.   Heat and cold   212
Chapter 8.   Therapeutic conduction heating   241
Chapter 9.   Cold therapy   255

SECTION IV

Chapter 10. Electromagnetic fields: shortwave diathermy, 276
                 pulsed electromagnetic energy and magnetic
                 therapies

SECTION V

Chapter 11. Electromagnetic radiation   315
Chapter 12. Microwave diathermy   327
Chapter 13. Infrared and visible radiations   341
Chapter 14. Laser therapy   356
Chapter 15. Ultraviolet radiation   376

Appendix   413

Index   419

Foreword

Electrotherapy Explained – Principles and Practice was written by John Low and Ann Reed primarily as a textbook for BSc and Diploma students of Physiotherapy. The authors have tried, and in my opinion succeeded, in bridging the gap between theory and practice, and have done so in a manner which is both enlightening and entertaining. The main strength of the book is that it *explains*, as far as possible given the current state of knowledge, both how electrotherapy works, and its value in diagnosis. Principles are stated lucidly and succinctly, the subject matter being arranged in logical groupings to aid understanding and simplify access to the vast body of information that the text contains. The debt owed to the past has not been forgotten, and the development of the various electrotherapeutic agents has been described, putting present-day usage into historical perspective.

The authors have deliberately avoided using a didactic approach, and wherever possible provide all the information required for the practitioner to arrive at an appropriate course of treatment in a logical fashion. The evidence, for the physical and physiological mechanisms proposed, is set out in a comprehensive and constructively critical manner. Where mechanisms are uncertain, this is clearly indicated. I hope that this will focus attention on the urgent need for more research, and will encourage physiotherapists and their colleagues in related disciplines to initiate and take part in it. The book is illustrated with line diagrams which are easy to understand and recall; I anticipate that they will be much used both by students and their tutors. Published work used by the authors in preparing the text is listed at the end of each chapter, making the book a valuable source of references.

John Low and Ann Reed each have over two decades of practical experience as teachers and users of electrotherapy. Their book is a much needed response to the absence of a comprehensive explanatory textbook written at a level suitable for degree-level physiotherapy students. It will also make a welcome and much-consulted addition to any practising physiotherapist's working library, and will be of particular value to those wishing to bring their knowledge of electrotherapy up to date.

In my opinion, *Electrotherapy Explained* lives up to the promise of its title, and I am delighted that the authors have found the time and dedication needed to write this masterly book which will enable them to share their experience as teachers with a wider audience than those privileged to be their pupils.

Mary Dyson, PhD, MIBiol, CBiol, FCSP (Hon.)
London.

Preface to the third edition

The third edition of this book has significant changes in presentation from previous editions, some changes in content but no change in the underlying emphasis on explanation. While the clear text, use of 'summary' and other boxes may make this edition look different from its predecessors the overall structure remains. Thus the grouping of the chapters into electrical, mechanical, thermal and radiation sections is retained.

To enhance clarity new diagrams have been added. There is also much new material, particularly in the realm of recent research. Some material thought to be less useful has been omitted but we have kept most of the pertinent references. We believe this to be helpful since the book is intended as a resource for further study as well as a thorough basic text.

Kipling's (*The Elephant's Child*) has been quoted previously in prefaces to make this particular point.

'I keep six honest serving men,
(They taught me all I knew,)
Their names are What and Why and When,
And How and Where and Who.'

While the concept of 'serving men' may be anachronistic (and perhaps politically incorrect!), the metaphorical expression of the importance of questioning is valid. It must be said that electrotherapy is not a subject of simple certainties and while we have tried to give a reasonable and realistic account it is important to recognize proper scientific uncertainty. It is a great deal better to be informed by the evidence, however contradictory, than to persist with prejudice, or be influenced by fads, fashion or tradition.

No subject can be understood in isolation, and some elementary background in physiology, anatomy and physics is a prerequisite for this text. The latter is covered in a companion book '*Physical Principles Explained*' which is no longer available in a printed version – hence it is not referenced in this text – but is provided as a CD Rom with this book. The links between these two texts will be found to be self-evident. We hope that providing material in this new format will be helpful and acceptable to all.

As in previous editions the valuable work of numerous colleagues will be found noted in the references. Some of these, and others including students, have contributed by freely given discussion, criticism and encouragement. We extend our thanks to them, to our respective families for their support and tolerance, and to Caroline Makepeace and her colleagues at Butterworth-Heinemann for their unstinting help.

John Low and Ann Reed, 1999

Preface to the first edition

Electrotherapy has tended to be a subject confused by traditional naming systems, jargon and didactic statements which have perhaps not always been justified by reason or research. In this book we have attempted to demystify electrotherapy for the physiotherapy student.

We have tried to give a fairly complete coverage of the field describing the most common modalities known to us to be employed by physiotherapists. Our intention is to explain how these modalities work and their effects upon the patient. We have used a different approach to some electrotherapy texts. In the initial chapter of each section we have tried to lay the foundations of the principles of modern electrotherapy, because we feel that a thorough understanding of these principles will ultimately lead to safer and more effective clinical practice. Therefore, the book builds up from the basics without, we hope, sacrificing accuracy to give a description of the types of energy available to the therapist. We have classified treatments of the same kind together so that the book is divided into sections devoted to electrical, mechanical, thermal and radiation energy.

The nature, production, effects and uses on the body tissues of each modality are explained and illustrated with what we hope is a reasonably comprehensive range of references to support the points made. With the very welcome involvement of physiotherapists in research, we hope to give undergraduates access to the vast amount of literature upon which they are encouraged to base their final clinical intervention. For postgraduates and practitioners our aim is to stimulate a vigorous search for answers.

We are well aware of the inherent dangers in explaining 'how things work' and in an attempt to communicate our ideas easily we may have been deliberately less precise than we could have been in some instances. We have tried to use the words that would convey the most meaning in the hope that a thorough understanding of even the more difficult concepts might be reached. Perhaps some of the ideas we offer will ultimately be shown to be too simple or just plain wrong, but we console ourselves that even these explanations can lead to debate and serve as a stepping stone to greater accuracy. Many treatments that have faded from use over the years are now returning in an appropriately modern guise, with new rational explanations. One such example is the use of low-frequency electrical stimulation following the development of the pain gate theory.

Rather than producing a step-by-step guide to technique, we have aimed for a description of the principles, the modalities and practical applications of their use. We believe that if the modality is well understood there can be a wide variation in acceptable technique and treatment within the confines of safe and effective practice.

After many years of teaching electrotherapy we both felt the need to attempt such a book. For our omissions and failings we apologize. However, our sincere hope is that we will have made electrotherapy more comprehensible for some which, in turn, will raise the standards of safe and effective treatment for our patients – the aim of us all.

John Low and Ann Reed, 1990

1 Introduction

The study of any topic is necessarily based on a thorough comprehension of the underlying concepts. Hence a description of the nature of electrical activity in the tissues as well as the normal pattern of repair would seem to provide a proper prologue. Thus, this introductory chapter begins by considering the nature of electrical charges in the human body, looking first at charges within cells and then those acting across cell membranes. The special case of the nerve cell membrane potential as well as the generation and propagation of nerve impulses are considered. The electrical properties of both excitable and non-excitable tissues are then noted.

The healing process is briefly described, including inflammation, proliferation and remodelling. There follows a general overview of the application of physical energy to the body tissues for therapy, with discussion of the effects of applying electric charges to the tissues. To conclude, the basic guidelines for the application of electrotherapy are listed.

At its simplest level electrotherapy can be defined as the treatment of patients by electrical means. By implication this means that electrical forces are applied to the body bringing about physiological changes for therapeutic purposes. However, in addition to these external forces, electrical charges are generated within the body by normal physiological processes. Between these two sets of electrical forces there will be interaction. There will also be interaction between the changes that occur as a result of the body's response to injury and any applied therapeutic agent. Before embarking on the study of external electrical and other forces on the body it is useful to consider the charges that are generated physiologically within the body as well as the response to injury.

ELECTRICAL CHARGES GENERATED BY THE BODY

The body tissues are organized systems of cells which are bathed in fluid. About two-thirds of the body weight is due to water and rather more than half of this is found inside the cells. In order to describe electrical activity in the body tissues and cells two major

Table 1.1 Some size comparisons (all sizes quoted are approximations)

Log scale	Examples
10 – 1 metre	Mean standing height of men = 1.71 m Mean standing height of women = 1.61 m
10^{-2} – 1 centimetre	Mean breadth of hips of women = 37 cm Length of belly of biceps muscle = 10 cm Diameter of aorta = 2.5 cm
10^{-3} – 1 millimetre	Thickness of skin = 1.5–4 mm
10^{-4} – 100 micrometres	Diameter of largest independent cell – amoeba = 100 μm Diameter of muscular arterioles = 50–100 μm
10^{-5} – 10 micrometres	Typical human eukaryote cells diameter = 10–50 μm Diameter of capillary = 8 μm Diameter of cell nucleus = 5–10 μm
10^{-6} – 1 micrometre	Diameter of prokaryote cells (e.g. bacteria) = 1–5 μm Diameter of mitochondria = 1 μm Length of collagen molecule = 0.3 μm Thickness of capillary wall = 0.2 μm
10^{-7} – 100 nanometres	Typical virus diameter = 100 nm
10^{-8} – 10 nanometres	Cell ribosome = 20 nm Typical macromolecules = 4–20 nm Thickness of cell membrane = 5–10 nm Small protein molecule = 4 nm
10^{-9} – 1 nanometre	Diameter of amino acid molecule = 0.5–1 nm Diameter of hydrated sodium ion = 0.5 nm Diameter of oxygen, nitrogen and hydrogen atoms = 0.4 nm Diameter of carbon atom and water molecule = 0.3 nm

distinctions from the familiar way of thinking about electrical phenomena must be recognized.

Firstly, the body tissues formed of eukaryotic cells are essentially 'salt water in lots of leaky little bags'. Electric charges and currents within them are thus due to the presence and movement of ions, i.e. charged atoms. These may be single or linked together as molecules, often macromolecules, and the charges may be single or multiple. Some molecules, e.g. water, are polar with opposite charges at the two ends. The movement of such ions, called convection currents, is much slower than the movement of electrons in the familiar electric circuits of, say, household appliances or electronic apparatus. These electrical circuits with mainly metal conductors depend on the almost instantaneous motion of the nearly massless electron as conduction currents as compared to the much more massive ion. The proton has some 2000 times the mass of the electron so that potassium, for example, with a relative atomic mass of 39 would be 78 000 times the mass of an electron and complex molecules even more massive. Yet the single ion has only the same magnitude of charge as the electron.

Secondly, the size of the electrical pathways involved is very much smaller than commonly encountered electrical circuitry. In order to appreciate the scale of the charge movements which are to be described, Table 1.1 provides some comparisons of sizes. It can be seen that the electric charges within and about the cell are acting in a very small environment, so that when a current is described, for example, as 'crossing the cell membrane' it is through a distance of only a few nanometres. This table is also intended to give information which will help the appreciation of size for other contexts discussed in this book.

The typical patterns of electrical activity in individual cells will be considered first, followed by those of various tissues. It might be expected that electromotive forces generated by single cells would be tiny compared with those of large collections of cells, but the voltages generated by single cells can be astonishingly large. As will be seen later, individual neurons can produce voltage changes across their membranes of about 100 mV, some larger. Typical non-excitable cells have transmembrane potentials of about 80 mV.

In discussing the electrical effects of cells and tissues it must be kept in mind that charges are always relative.

Summary

Electrical activity in the cells of the body:

- is due to the movement of ions – convection currents
- is much slower than that due to electron movement because of the greater mass of the ion
- occurs over very short pathways
- involves relatively constant charges on individual cells of nearly a tenth of a volt
- is described in relative terms.

The arrangement of electric charges in cells

The way in which charges are grouped within and around typical cells has been well described by Charman (1990b) as four concentric zones. The central region of the cell is negative due to the presence of many negatively charged ions, mainly organic molecules particularly proteins and amino acid molecules. The outermost region of the cell is also negatively charged due to the negative charges of molecules at the tips of the glycolipid molecules that project from the cell surface. Between these lie two regions of positive charges on either side and close to the cell membrane. They are both regions in which there are many mobile positive ions, notably sodium, potassium and calcium. It is those regions on either side of the plasma membrane which determine and maintain the electrical behaviour of the cell (Fig. 1.1).

The division between intra- and extracellular fluid is maintained by the cell membrane; this consists of a double layer of lipids in

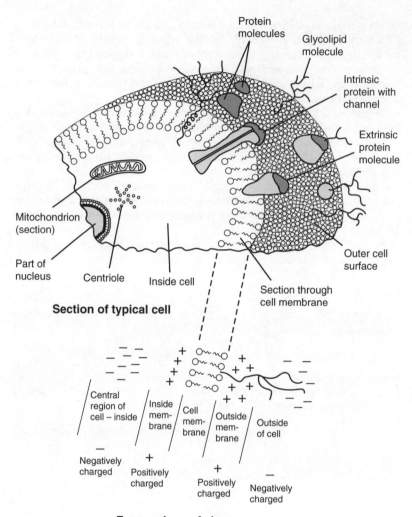

Protein
molecules

Glycolipid
molecule

Intrinsic
protein with
channel

Extrinsic
protein
molecule

Outer cell
surface

Mitochondrion
(section)

Part of
nucleus

Centriole

Inside cell

Section through
cell membrane

Section of typical cell

Central
region of
cell – inside

Inside
mem-
brane

Cell
mem-
brane

Outside
mem-
brane

Outside
of cell

Negatively
charged

Positively
charged

Positively
charged

Negatively
charged

Four regions of charges

Fig. 1.1 Typical cell and electrical regions.

which globular proteins are scattered. The lipid bilayer is arranged so that the hydrophobic (water-hating, hence water-repellent) ends of both layers of lipid molecules face inwards and are thus not in contact with the intra- and extracellular fluid. Some of the globular proteins extend through the thickness of both layers (see Fig. 1.1). It must be understood that the membrane is somewhat oil-like and has a degree of fluidity which varies in different membranes and at different temperatures.

Transport across cell membrane

It may be helpful at this point to outline the major mechanisms by which substances are transported across the cell plasma membrane. There are three mechanisms involved: diffusion, facilitated diffusion and active transport.

Diffusion. This is a process in which small molecules, or ions, move across the membrane from an area of high concentration to one of low concentration. It is the result of Brownian motion of all particles (i.e. heat – the more particle movement, the higher the temperature). The rate of diffusion of a substance through a given distance and area is proportional to the concentration difference and temperature. It is also influenced by the way it crosses the membrane, either through membrane pores or through the lipid molecules. The lipid bilayer is semi-fluid so that some molecules – oxygen, carbon dioxide, fatty acids – can dissolve in the membrane. Water molecules and many ions pass through the membrane pores which are channels in the large transmembrane proteins (see Fig. 1.1). These pores are often of about 0.8 nm diameter. In the case of ions, it is not only the concentration difference that drives their movement across the membrane but also their electrical charge. Thus ions are driven by diffusion down their concentration gradient and by the attraction or repulsion between their charges. The electrochemical potential difference of an ion across a membrane can be described by the Nernst equation. This equation relates the intra- and extracellular concentrations of a given ion with the gas constant, Faraday's constant and temperature.

Facilitated diffusion. Some molecules – e.g. glucose, some other sugars and some amino acids – are linked to a protein carrier molecule which passes them through the membrane more rapidly than simple diffusion would allow. Like simple diffusion, this is an entirely passive process; the molecules are still only moving down their concentration gradients but at a greater rate.

Active transport. This is the process by which ions and molecules are conveyed through the cell membrane against their concentration and electrical gradients. Naturally, energy is needed to drive this process which is derived from adenosine triphosphate (ATP) and involves carrier protein molecules. This process, which is going on all the time, utilizes enormous amounts of energy – it is thought to account for some 30–40% of total energy turnover in humans (Rees and Sternberg, 1984). The movement of sodium, potassium, calcium, hydrogen, iron and chloride ions, as well as various sugars and amino acids, across the cell membrane is effected by this active transport mechanism. Figure 1.2 illustrates these points.

Large molecules are able to enter the cell by a totally different mechanism which does not involve crossing the intact plasma membrane as such.

Pinocytosis (or endocytosis). Small areas of cell membrane invaginate and ultimately pinch themselves off, thus carrying attached macromolecules to the inside of the cell as a vesicle. A similar process involving larger particles or bacteria is familiar as phagocytosis.

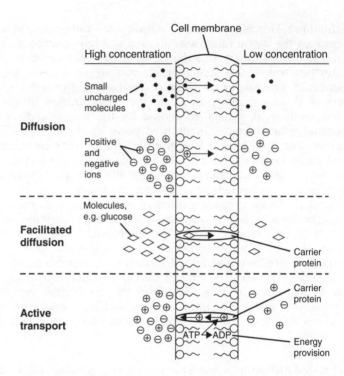

Fig. 1.2 Three mechanisms of transport across the cell membrane.

Summary

Typical cells:

- appear to be relatively stable, negatively charged entities because of the negative charges carried on glycolipid molecules projecting about 20 nm from the plasma membrane
- are negatively charged in their central regions, a charge which is more or less stable
- are surrounded by a cell membrane formed of a semi-lipid bilayer with many scattered proteins
- allow water molecules and some solutes to be passively passed through this membrane
- have active transport mechanisms involving energy use to move other substances against their concentration gradient across the cell membrane
- maintain a variable charge difference across their membranes due to varying numbers of positively charged ions on either side. The inner surface of the membrane remains negative to the outer under most, but not all, circumstances.

All cells have very extensive electrical properties with complex arrangements of charges which are continually varying. The electrical charge across the cell membrane means that it acts as an electrical capacitor. (The typical cell membrane has a capacitance of about $1 \mu F/cm^2$.) Similar charges exist across the membranes surrounding the intracellular organelles, such as the endoplasmic reticulum, Golgi apparatus and nucleus. For an extensive and valuable description of the electrical features of cells and cellular activity, see Charman (1990b,c).

It is the balance of ions that determines the charges found on the surface of cells. All cells tend to maintain high concentrations of potassium ions (K^+) and low concentrations of sodium ions (Na^+) in their intracellular fluid. The extracellular fluid contains plenty of both ions, but more Na^+ than K^+. The cell membrane allows the passage of both these ions to some extent, but has an active transport mechanism that brings K^+ into the cell and expels Na^+. This sodium–potassium (Na^+–K^+) 'pump' uses energy to move these ions against their passive gradients. The passive gradient, as explained above, depends on their relative concentrations across the membrane and on the electrical forces. The Nernst equation will predict the electromotive forces due to any particular concentration of each type of ion separated by a cell membrane.

As already noted, the difference of potential across a normal cell membrane at rest, known as the resting membrane potential, has the inside of the cell negative relative to the outside. The potential varies in the cells of different tissues, being anything between -60 and -90 mV. In nerves and smooth muscle fibres it is usually about -70 mV, for skeletal muscle cells -80 mV and for glial cells -90 mV (Bray *et al.*, 1986). This electrical potential – electrical pressure – across the cell membrane is due to the fact that such membranes are much more permeable to K^+ than to Na^+. Thus K^+ can get out of the cell much more easily than Na^+ can get in. The Na^+–K^+ pump ejects three ions of sodium for every two of potassium that it takes in. The result of both mechanisms is a deficiency of positive charges inside the cell compared to the outside, hence the membrane potential.

As well as the Na^+ and K^+ pump, the concentration of Ca^{2+} outside the cell is maintained at a much higher level than inside by an important Ca^{2+} pump mechanism. Other ions such as H^+ and Cl^- are also moved by an active transport process. In all cases adenosine triphosphate (ATP) is utilized by means of an enzyme (adenosine triphosphatase; ATPase) which is activated by the appropriate ions to supply the energy needed.

The resting membrane potential of nerves

Neurons consist of a cell body and several extensions which convey the nerve impulses to and from the cell body. A resting membrane potential is present across the membrane of the cell body and across the whole length of the processes – nerve fibres – the longest of which is usually called the axon.

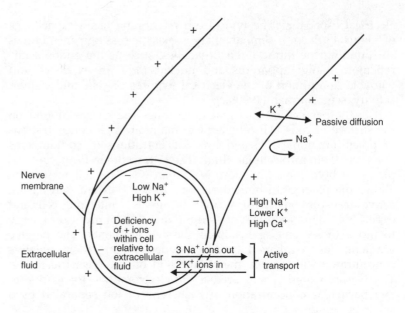

Fig. 1.3 Membrane potential.

As already stated, the resting membrane potential is ultimately due to the Na^+–K^+ pump and to the difference in permeability to Na^+ and K^+. These ideas are illustrated in Figure 1.3.

The situation is like that of a ship at sea in which the lower parts are below the water level but contain air able to pass freely in and out, like K^+. The seawater, like Na^+, is kept out by the hull and the small amount that does leak in is easily removed by the bilge pumps, an active transport mechanism. Thus different compounds – air and seawater – are separated by the ship's hull; due to the greater density of water a pressure difference is developed across the hull. If the hull is holed, water will rush in with great force because of the pressure difference, but if the hole is then quickly blocked the small quantity of additional water is ultimately removed by the bilge pumps to restore the situation.

In many tissues the individual cells are connected by gap junctions which allow some electrical conduction between cells. This does not occur in skeletal muscle or nerve tissue (Finean *et al.*, 1978). The concentration of Ca^{2+} outside the cell is maintained at a much higher level than inside by an important Ca^{2+} mechanism. Other ions, such as H^+ and Cl^-, are also moved by an active transport process.

The nerve impulse

The nerve impulse is a wave of electrochemical activity which passes along the nerve fibre using energy already stored as part of the membrane potential. It is a reversal of the membrane potential from -70 to $+30$ mV which occurs very briefly – taking about 1 ms – and spreads along the fibre without decrement. It is called the action potential.

The impulse is initiated by depolarization – altered charge – of the fibre membrane due to chemical disturbance at a synapse or receptor or to some other disturbance such as an electrical pulse. Depolarization means that the potential difference across the membrane is reduced from the $-70\,mV$ of the resting membrane. However, the impulse is only triggered when depolarized by about 10–15 mV (i.e. to about $-55\,mV$). Once this threshold is reached the impulse, or action potential, is generated automatically and spreads along the nerve fibre at a rate that is characteristic of that particular fibre. If the impulse is initiated normally it will pass only in one (orthodromic) direction, but if the middle of a nerve fibre is artificially stimulated two impulses will travel away from the point of stimulation, one in each direction, orthodromic and antidromic.

The effect of depolarization beyond the threshold level is to cause the membrane to become much more permeable to Na^+ by opening special channels or gates. Na^+ rushes through these channels into the fibre causing an abrupt and rapid local reversal of membrane polarity. After a delay, K^+ channels are also caused to open by the depolarization and the Na^+ channels close. Consequently the rush of Na^+ into the fibre is soon stemmed and there is a loss of K^+ from the fibre. In this way the membrane repolarizes again. Once the process is started, rapid depolarization followed by a relatively slow repolarization occurs automatically and takes several milliseconds. The voltage-gated sodium ion channels are believed to operate by an alteration of their protein configuration in response to varying local electrical potentials (Alberts *et al.*, 1983). Thus these Na^+ channels can be in at least three states:

- closed, but ready to open instantly
- open
- closed but unable to open instantly.

They go through these states in sequence in response to a voltage change beyond threshold, spending a very brief time open and a longer time – a millisecond or so – in a closed but inactivated state. These are absolute states for the channel which 'flips' almost instantaneously from one to the other: there is no half-open condition. The smooth rise and fall of the action potential – as in Figure 1.4(a) – is due to many Na^+ gates opening and closing to cause an average voltage curve (in reality, Na^+ channels are constantly opening and closing due to random local voltage fluctuations, but this is inconsequential until a large number of channels are affected simultaneously).

The nerve cell membrane is quite a large storage capacitor which is only trivially depleted by the passage of ions to provide the action potential. For example, it has been calculated that an outflow of only one hundred thousandth of the total K^+ in the cell can alter the membrane potential by 100 mV (Alberts *et al.*, 1983). Similarly small quantities of Na^+ ions enter the cell. Ultimately the situation is restored by the Na^+–K^+ pump. Even without the activity of the pump, the impulse can occur many hundreds of times before the

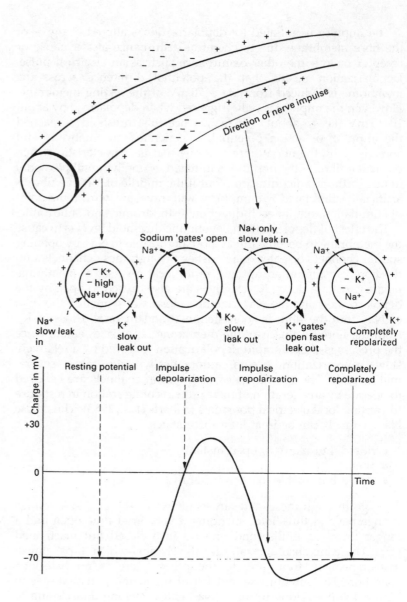

Fig. 1.4 (a) The passage of a nerve impulse.

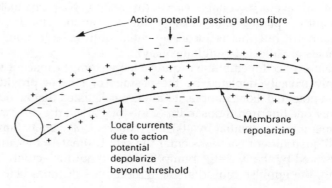

Fig. 1.4 (b) Depolarization and repolarization.

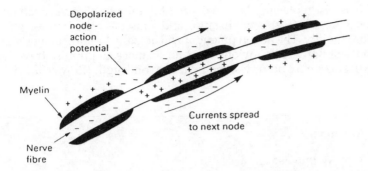

Depolarized
node -
action
potential

Myelin

Currents spread
to next node

Nerve
fibre

Fig. 1.5 Section through a myelinated nerve fibre.

membrane potential is significantly altered. The ship analogy used above is appropriate; many small rushes of water could be allowed to enter the hull before the ship is in danger of sinking, even if the bilge pumps are not working.

The impulse will travel along the length of the fibre because the depolarization spreads in all directions. Since the voltage-dependent sodium gates are opened once the threshold is reached the electrical charge spreading along the surface of the membrane causes the next area of the fibre to depolarize and so on. Once the impulse has passed, that particular part of the fibre membrane is refractory, i.e. it cannot be stimulated until it has repolarized (Fig. 1.4(b)).

The first part of the action potential (Na^+ ions rushing in) is analogous to a line of dominoes set up so that when the end domino is pushed over it falls against the next which falls against the next and so on. A wave of falling dominoes thus travels along the prearranged line. Such a system has the characteristics of the initial part of the nerve impulse in that energy is stored in the upright position of the domino, like the store of energy in the membrane potential. Also the domino has to be disturbed sufficiently to bring its centre of gravity outside its base – beyond the threshold – from which point it accelerates downwards, tipping over the next domino as it goes. The falling domino has the same positive feedback properties – rapid acceleration to the limit of the system – as the reversal of membrane polarity due to the inrush of sodium ions. Of course, the nerve membrane potential is automatically reset but the domino line needs the attention of a dextrous human hand to reconstruct it.

The speed of propagation of the nerve impulse along the nerve fibre varies in different nerves. Generally, the larger the nerve fibre diameter the lower its electrical resistance, hence larger currents and faster conduction. Further, many nerve fibres are surrounded by an electrically insulating sheath, the myelin sheath, interrupted at intervals by the nodes of Ranvier which are areas with much less insulation but many voltage-gated ion channels. The electrical potential of the nerve impulse travels along the membrane but only triggers the depolarization at the nodes of Ranvier because the intervening membrane has too much resistance (Fig. 1.5). Thus the nerve impulse can be described as skipping from node to node (saltatory conduction) using less energy and travelling much faster.

This is like replacing the usual size of dominoes with very tall ones that fall over a greater distance and thus pass the 'falling wave' more rapidly. The action potential will actually be spread over many nodes of Ranvier at any one time, for instance an impulse travelling at 100 m/s may occupy some 5 cm of axon length (Bray *et al.*, 1986).

Summary

A nerve impulse is:

- an 'all-or-none' event
- triggered by a disturbance of the nerve fibre membrane electrical potential beyond threshold potential
- an electrochemical disturbance – a depolarization – which travels along the length of the nerve fibre
- identical in magnitude and velocity for any given nerve fibre
- able to travel more rapidly in a myelinated nerve fibre.

The transfer of information in the nervous system and the regulation of muscle contraction are thus 'coded' by the number and frequency of nerve impulses.

Single nerve impulses can be recorded on the skin surface to investigate their conduction rates in peripheral nerve conduction studies.

'Signalling' between cells

Information is received by the outer cell membrane by means of chemical 'messengers', well known as either hormones (blood borne endocrine or local) or as neurotransmitters such as acetylcholine. These 'first messengers' often initiate the activity of intracellular 'second messenger' enzymic systems, such as cyclic AMP (adenosine monophosphate) or Ca^{2+}. These enzyme cascades provoke specific cellular activities such as change of shape or increased secretion. It is suggested that, since the cell is electrically complex, electrical and magnetic forces may act on the outer cell membrane as other first messengers. There are numerous ways in which electric and magnetic fields might exert an influence. The interaction of electric fields of enzyme and receptor molecules which guide the 'fit' at the cell surface is an example. It is also suggested that some cells might be sensitive to particular electromagnetic frequencies, so-called 'frequency windows'. For a full discussion of these matters and related theoretical possibilities see Charman (1990 and 1991b–h). These concepts are part of the theoretical basis, as yet incomplete, for the use of direct current (Chapter 2), ultrasound (Chapter 6), pulsed shortwave (Chapter 10), lasers (Chapter 14) and perhaps thermotherapy, in the acceleration of wound healing and repair.

Electric charges in tissues

Since some electrically excitable tissues, nerve and muscle, generate electrical pulses it is not surprising that these can be detected on the body surface. Thus the electroencephalogram is a record of the electrical signals generated by the brain, the electrocardiogram those generated by the heart and the electromyogram those from contracting muscle – the latter described in Chapter 4. Non-excitable tissues also show electrical potentials which are more or less static and include skin battery potentials, potentials related to tissue growth and healing as well as strain-generated potentials in connective tissue.

Electroencephalography

Patterns of electrical activity in the brain are recorded from electrodes fixed on the skin of the scalp. These signals may be up to 300 μV but generally around 50 μV and at various frequencies up to 50 Hz (Guyton, 1982).

There is a general positive correlation between the degree of cerebral activity and the frequency of the electroencephalogram record. The lowest frequencies of 0.5–2 Hz occur in deep sleep, infancy, coma or other serious organic brain disease. They are called delta waves. Somewhat higher frequencies, 4–7 Hz, are called theta waves and occur in light sleep and some emotional states. Alpha waves of 8–13 Hz occur in almost all adults during a relaxed resting but awake state with the eyes closed. Beta waves are found in active conscious states and have frequencies of 14–35 Hz or higher. These 'brain waves' are the summation of the underlying neuronal activity and are considered to be largely due to impulses originating in the thalamus, except that delta waves seem to be generated by the cerebral cortex itself. An abnormal increase in neuronal activity, such as occurs in epilepsy, is reflected in a high-voltage synchronous electroencephalogram recording.

Electrical charges generated by muscle cells

Like nerves, muscle fibres also produce an electrical disturbance which occurs when they contract. When many muscle fibres contract in unison the electrical signal produced is quite large and can be measured at the body surface. An example of this is the way in which information about the heart can be provided in the form of an electrocardiogram.

Skeletal muscles also give action potentials when they contract and these can be picked up, amplified by an electromyograph and displayed in a similar way. The action potentials recorded are those of one or more motor units. A motor unit consists of a single motor nerve together with the muscle fibres it supplies, which can be several hundred in a large muscle. There is, therefore, considerable variation in the recording of an electrical signal from a single motor

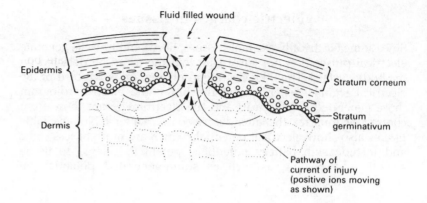

Fig. 1.6 The skin battery.

unit – a spike potential, as it is called. On average it lasts about 4 ms (Walsh, 1988). When the patient performs a voluntary muscle contraction both the number of motor units and the frequency of firing increase, leading to a more complex recording (see Chapter 4).

Skin battery

A transcutaneous voltage normally exists in human skin which is known as the skin battery. The stratum corneum is negatively charged with respect to the dermis, with an average potential difference of 23 mV (Foulds and Barker, 1983). Relatively hairless skin surfaces, such as the hands and feet, show a greater potential difference, but always negative to the dermis in all areas and with all subjects tested. Similar skin battery potentials occur in animals, and experiments on guinea pigs showed that these charges could drive currents across the edge of a cut in the skin (Barker *et al.*, 1982). It is believed that these potentials are generated in the actively metabolizing basal region of the epidermis and an incision through the skin leads to positively charged ions moving as shown in Figure 1.6 (a current of injury). This effect is thought to be due to sodium ion pump activity in epidermal cells. Similar injury currents have been found in humans as well as voltage changes over healing surgical incision sites. This, and other evidence, suggests that wound healing may be partly controlled by electrical signals and hence that electrical stimulation might influence wound healing.

Electrical charges generated by connective tissue cells

Strain generated potentials are found in bone and other connective tissues. These are charges resulting from, and proportional to, mechanical deformation of the tissue. The mechanism is not fully understood but is widely described as a piezoelectric effect (see

Chapter 6) but involves greater complexities (see Charman, 1990e). It is suggested that bone growth and remodelling are partly controlled by mechanical forces causing strain generated potentials, which in turn generate a direct current signal to stimulate bone growth or absorption. Similar mechanisms are believed to apply in the control of connective tissue remodelling in which the collagen fibres align themselves appropriately to withstand the applied mechanical stress.

Electrical gradients in embryonic development

In those animals and plants that have been extensively studied, embryonic development appears to be associated with current gradients. These are generated by cellular activity and seem to have a growth-regulating function. Experiments with some simple animals have shown that artificially reversing the electrical polarity can reverse the direction of head-to-tail development. All embryos seem to have electrical polarity which develops soon after fertilization.

Electrical gradients in limb regeneration

Most adult animals including humans are entirely unable to regenerate the complex masses of tissues involved in the regrowth of limbs. A few, however, notably the salamander, have the ability to regrow a new limb after surgical amputation. This appears to be achieved by blastoma formation near the amputation site whose undifferentiated cells develop to form the new limb tissues. Innervation and a large associated wound current seem to be essential components. A similar amphibian, such as a frog, that has no regenerative capacity shows a very much smaller wound current. There are claims of partial regeneration in non-regenerative animals produced by the application of artificial currents in various experiments; see Charman (1990d) for a review. The importance of wound currents in both healing (see Skin battery above) and regeneration is uncertain, particularly in determining what is cause and what is effect. The importance has been shown in humans in the amputation of part of the terminal phalanx of a child's finger. Such a wound has been shown to heal and the end of the finger regenerate if kept moist with associated increased skin battery currents (Illingworth and Barker, 1980).

Several other small tissue currents have been described, some in the nervous system but entirely separate from the impulses due to varying transmembrane potentials described above. For a review of this whole topic see Charman 1990 (a–f) and 1991 (a and b).

Summary

Electric charges are exhibited from:

1. Excitable tissues as: • electroencephalography
   - β waves   most ⎫
   - α waves   ⎬ brain activity
   - θ waves   ⎭
   - δ waves   least
   • electrocardiography
   • electromyography – see Chapter 4.

2. Non-excitable tissue as: • skin battery charges – associated with healing

   • connective tissue cell charges – piezoelectric
   • electric charges in embryonic development
   • electric charges in limb regeneration
   • various other charges and direct currents.

THE HEALING PROCESS

Throughout this book reference is made to the effects of various therapeutic modalities on the inflammatory, healing and repair processes, and pain symptoms of healing. It seems appropriate to give an outline of these changes at the beginning with some discussion of the mechanisms involved.

The tissue response to damage is often described in terms of mechanical injury to the skin and subsequent infection by bacteria. The series of changes that ensue are much the same whatever the tissue involved and however the injury is caused. Thus the visible changes of an accidental cut in the skin are very similar to the less visible changes due to a muscle or ligament tear. The reason is, of course, that the response to any kind of damage is similar in all vascular tissues; it is the response to some irritant. This could be the products of damaged cells or some introduced organism, say a bacterium, or a chemical or radiation irritant.

It is usual and convenient to describe these changes as a sequence of stages which decidedly overlap and occupy varying lengths of time. Thus the process can be characterized in the four stages of: initial injury, inflammation, proliferation and remodelling.

Initial injury

This results in damage to cells and small blood vessels. Cells die as a consequence of direct damage, oxygen deficiency due to the damaged blood vessels, or chemicals released from other damaged cells. The extracellular structure of the tissues may also be damaged with tearing of fibres and disruption of the ground substance. If the damage is at the surface, bleeding is visible, otherwise the extravasated blood is trapped in the damaged tissue. Within a few minutes the released blood starts to clot, which serves to plug the leaking blood vessels, helps to immobilize the area and traps bacteria. Clotting is precipitated by the aggregation of platelets and the activation of a 'cascade' system of enzymes. These convert prothrombin to thrombin which causes the soluble plasma protein, fibrinogen, to become the insoluble fibrin. This complex process of blood clotting, which involves an extrinsic and intrinsic system, is an important trigger to the inflammation that follows. It causes, among many other important reactions, the production of brady-kinin and initiation of the complement cascade, which is a system of interacting proteins in plasma associated with the activity of antibodies, especially in the presence of contaminants. Clots are dissolved after about 5 days by fibrinolysin.

Inflammation

This word, derived from a Latin word meaning to burn, is especially apt since, when the skin is involved, it becomes hot, red, swollen and painful. These are the four cardinal signs of inflammation. To these it is appropriate to add a fifth – loss of function. Inflammation is basically the result of the microcirculation of the tissues reacting to injury.

Vascular changes

First there is a very brief vasoconstriction of the non-injured vessels in response to irritation, followed by prolonged dilation. This dilation includes arterioles, venules and lymphatics in both active and dormant channels. The total blood flow to the region is, therefore, increased although the rate of flow in individual channels may be diminished. This leads to both redness and increased temperature of the skin. White blood cells – polymorphonuclear leucocytes – tend to move to the edge of the blood stream, lining up along the endothelial vessel wall, in a process called margination. They subsequently pass through the vessel wall into the adjacent tissue fluid. The endothelial cells forming the vessel walls tend to separate at their junctions, leading to increased vascular permeability. This is due to direct damage which loosens the inter-cellular junctions in both capillaries and venules. The endothelial cells of venules are also able to contract – pulling away from one another – when affected by chemical mediators such as histamine. This has tremendously important consequences, because it allows much more plasma protein (albumin, globulin and fibrinogen) to leave the blood vessel and enter the tissue fluid. Because of this, the osmotic pressure between the blood and tissue fluid is altered so that fluid leaves the vessels and enters the tissue spaces. This is further encouraged by the increased capillary hydrostatic pressure due to arteriole dilation. The resulting increase of fluid in the tissues is called oedema and the fluid itself is called an exudate. This, then, is the cause of the swelling associated with inflammation. It seems to be beneficial in the presence of infection since it dilutes bacterial toxins and allows the passage of immunoglobulins (antibodies circulating in plasma) and complement (a system of plasma enzymes) which will promote the destruction of bacteria. By the same mechanism that leads to coagulation of blood, fibrinogen in the exudate is converted to a fibrin network. This both limits the spread of bacteria and makes them more susceptible to phagocytosis by white blood cells, as discussed later. Where no infection is present, the value of the laying down of fibrin is less evident, as it can lead to restriction of movement in the tissues and hence later functional impairment, which is sometimes permanent.

Activation and control

While the vasodilation and exudation are a standard universal response, the causative agents are complex and multiple. Initially, histamine, formed from the amino acid histidine, is released by many kinds of injury, much of it being released from degranulated mast cells; these are wandering cells found in large numbers in connective tissue. Also at this stage, serotonin (5-hydroxy-tryptamine), probably from platelets, contributes, together with local inactivation of adrenalin. Collectively, these allow early vasodilation to occur, which is maintained by the activation of kinins by enzymes triggered by some of the processes of blood clotting. (Kinins are a group of polypeptides, which includes bradykinin.) There are many other groups of substances which provoke features of the inflammatory reaction, particularly a group of fatty acids formed from arachidonic acid in or on the cell surface. These form a group called prostaglandins and another group called leukotrienes. It seems that prostaglandins are affected by non-steroidal anti-inflammatory drugs and both groups by corticosteroids, which may account for the anti-inflammatory action of these drugs. Additionally, steroids may inhibit macrophage levels. Further mediators include enzymes from the complement pathway. These are also involved in histamine release and chemotaxis, which is the attraction of neutrophils to the area. Amongst many other mediators are platelet activating factor, plasmin and cytokines. The complex sequential appearance of so many different substances to promote vasodilation seems complicated but these are systems that control not only the initiation and completion of inflammatory change but also its nature and intensity.

Pain

The pressure applied to sensory nerve endings by exudate accounts for some of the pain associated with inflammation. This becomes very obvious if expansion of the tissues is restricted, leading to higher pressure. Pain is also provoked by all the chemical mediators that cause vasodilation, notably the kinins. Histamine may only provoke itching and the prostaglandins may act by potentiating the effect of other pain-provoking substances. Other chemicals liberated by cell injury may also cause pain.

Cellular response

Almost immediately after formation of the fluid exudate, poly-morphonuclear leucocytes (neutrophils) start to pass through the vessel wall by inserting pseudopodia in the gaps between cells and 'flowing' through, a process called diapedesis and a continuation of the margination noted above. A little later, these neutrophilic granulocytes are joined by monocytes which, once in the damaged area, develop into macrophages. Both types are attracted to the area by chemotaxis due to many of the mediator factors noted above. The principal function of the polymorphonuclear leucocytes is phagocytosis of pathogenic bacteria. This process of engulfing and destroying bacteria and other unwanted particles invariably leads to the death of neutrophils. If very large numbers are involved due to the extent and virulence of the invading bacteria then pus is formed, which is usually extruded from the surface. Macrophage cells are not only phagocytic and much longer lived than neutrophils, they also release chemical factors needed for the proliferative and remodelling phases. Phagocytosis appears more effective when particles and bacteria are trapped in the fibrin mesh. Lysosomes release digestive enzymes which break down dead cells and bacteria.

Influence of the nervous system

Although inflammation will proceed apparently normally in denervated tissues, the vascular responses, at least, are influenced by nerve impulses. At a very basic level the triple response occurs as a result of sensory and vasomotor nerve activity. At the site of the damage there is an initial red reaction which appears within a few seconds. This is caused by capillary dilation due to direct pressure. It is followed by local mild swelling – a wheal – because of the increased permeability of capillaries and venules, and a more diffuse redness – a flare – caused by arteriolar dilation. It is due to an axon reflex in which sensory nerve stimulation results in impulses being relayed antidromically via a branch (axon) of the peripheral nerve to the arterioles. Stimulation of polymodal pain receptors also leads to the release of neuropeptides from the C fibres which help to trigger inflammatory responses; substance P is probably the most important of these. The contribution of the higher levels of the nervous system can be seen from the fact that hypnosis can be used both to increase and decrease the vascular inflammatory response, although it does not directly affect cellular activity. Adrenalin, controlled by the sympathetic nervous system, can inhibit the vasodilation of inflammation. The effects of the higher centres of the nervous system on the perception of the pain of inflammation are well known and can both inhibit and exaggerate.

Summary

1. Initial injury:
   – damage to cells
   – damage to extracellular structures
   – bleeding into or outside tissues
   – blood clotting.

2. Inflammation – 'calor, rubor, tumour and dolor':
   – vasodilation
   – increased vessel permeability
       these → plasma protein leak into tissues
       which → oedema to dilute toxins and promote destruction
           of bacteria
   – local pain due to pressure of exudate and chemical mediators
   – cellular activity
   – polymorphs exhibit margination and diapedesis and
     phagocytosis
   – macrophages appear later and are longer lasting than
     polymorphs. Macrophages are not only phagocytic but also
     release important chemical agents controlling later phases
   – control of inflammation effected by complex sequential
     cascades of chemical activators including histamine, various
     kinins and prostaglandins
   – leucocytes attracted by chemotaxis
   – some influence from the nervous system.

Proliferation

This stage lasts about 3–4 weeks. It includes reconstructing the tissues, resurfacing if necessary and giving strength to the wound. It involves the activities of three kinds of cells: macrophages, fibroblasts and endothelial cells (to form new blood vessels, a process called angiogenesis). Acting in concert, these form new, highly vascular, wound-filling granulation tissue. It is called granulation tissue because of its grainy appearance when sectioned. Macrophages are considered essential for healing to occur. Not only do they digest and remove wound debris but they also migrate into the damaged area, releasing chemotactic agents which stimulate fibroblast activity and angiogenesis. These new blood vessels appear at first as buds of endothelial cells which grow into the damaged area, branching and eventually joining adjacent buds to form capillary loops when they canalize. As blood starts to flow through them, the oxygenation of the region increases and, at the same time, fibroblasts lay down new collagen fibres to provide a supporting framework. Thus new granulation tissue proceeds, growing in from the normal tissue edges, replacing the dead or dying injured tissues. The macrophages are notably able to tolerate low oxygen levels and thus tend to lead the process. Some of the fibroblasts become myofibroblasts which are able to contract; new collagen also tends to shorten, and both are thus able to effect wound contraction by

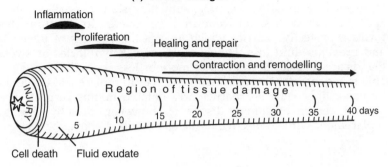

(a) Tissue changes

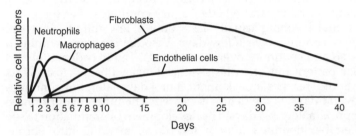

(b) Cellular changes

Fig. 1.7 Time scale of inflammation and healing.

pulling the edges together. This can, in certain circumstances, lead to contracture. Figure 1.7 illustrates the changing populations of the different cells during these phases.

Remodelling

The process continues until the whole damaged area is replaced. At the same time the granulation tissue becomes more fibrous and less vascular, to ultimately become dense fibrous tissue (i.e. scar tissue). At 3 weeks the strength of the wound is only approximately 15% of that of the original tissue. The process of remodelling may continue for months, the structure of the new tissue altering slowly. The number of blood vessels reduces to that appropriate to maintain viability of the tissues. Arterioles, venules and lymphatic channels redevelop, and there is regeneration of small nerve fibres. The fibroblasts not only lay down collagen, which tends to be of a different type at this later stage, but also the mucopolysaccharide matrix of typical connective tissue. Further, there is remodelling of the connective tissue with time. This phase can last for years. At first the fibres appear to be random but subsequently they become rearranged in a way that best controls the stresses to which the tissue is normally subjected. Importantly, this last mechanism depends on appropriate stresses being applied by activity.

If the skin surface has been damaged, the epithelial cells are able to regenerate to cover the area with new skin, a process called epithelialization. A small wound can be covered in 48 hours. This forms a protective barrier which lessens the chances of infection and prevents fluid loss. However, no new hair follicles or sweat glands are formed. Several other more or less specialized cells are able to regenerate (i.e. replicate themselves to replace lost tissue) in humans; liver cells are particularly notable in this respect. The general repair of human tissue is, however, broadly due to replacement with connective tissue as described above.

Timing of the processes

The processes just described overlap to a considerable extent and the length of each phase is very variable depending on the severity of the original injury and whether injury continues over time.

The initial bleeding usually lasts only a few minutes but cell death may continue over a few days. Vasodilation starts within an hour or so and continues over several days. Tissue oedema follows a similar pattern but often lasts rather longer. Phagocytosis starts within hours, reaches a peak about 3 or 4 days later, but continues over several days as the debris is cleared. The inflammatory phase lasts approximately 3–4 days. The development of granulation tissue can often be identified after a few days, merging into fibrous repair which may continue for weeks or months. This time scale is illustrated in Figure 1.7.

Summary

1. Proliferation, healing and repair:
   – involves activity of macrophages and fibroblasts as well as angiogenesis to form granulation tissue
   – wound contraction.

2. Remodelling:
   – more and more fibrous tissue formed – scar formation
   – regeneration of vessels, nerves and some tissue such as skin.

THE APPLICATION OF ENERGY TO THE BODY FOR THERAPY

Physical energy can be applied to the body in various forms (Table 1.2). The most obvious is mechanical energy, in the form of some appreciable mass, such as the hand, being pressed against the body surface. If this pressure varies at a suitable rate it is called a vibration

Table 1.2 Forms of energy applied to the body

	Mechanical	*Electrical*	*Radiation*
Continuous	Pressure	Constant current	
Low-frequency	Vibration	Low-frequency currents	
Medium-frequency	Sound	Medium-frequency currents	
High-frequency	Ultrasound	High-frequency currents	Radiowaves Microwaves
Still higher frequencies	Heat	Electron oscillation	Infrared Visible Ultraviolet X-rays γ-rays
Therapies	1. Pressure and vibration 2. Ultrasound 3. Conduction heating 4. Cold therapy	5. Direct current 6. Muscle-stimulating currents and trans-cutaneous nerve stimulation 7. Interferential therapy 8. Shortwave diathermy	9. Microwave 10. Infrared 11. Laser 12. Ultraviolet

(therapy 1, Table 1.2). If the frequency of vibration occurs between about 30 and 20 000 cycles per second, i.e. hertz, it is detected as sound when it strikes the tympanic membrane of the ear. At higher frequencies the sensory nerves cannot detect the vibration so we are unaware of it; it is then called ultrasound (therapy 2). This energy can be passed through the body tissues generating heat and causing other effects where it is absorbed.

If the atoms and molecules of the object placed against the skin are given more motion – that is, the object is made hotter – this heat energy can be transferred to the skin and tissues. The tissues are thus heated by conduction (therapy 3). If the molecules of the object in contact have less motion than those of the tissues then heat is conducted from the tissues to the object, thus cooling the tissues (therapy 4).

Where particles on or near the skin are given an electric charge this can cause ions in the tissues to move. The movement of charges is an electric current in the tissues (therapy 5). If these currents are varied, either in intensity or direction, at a suitable frequency, e.g. 50 Hz, it can disturb the ionic balance across nerve or muscle membranes, causing a nerve impulse or muscle contraction to occur (therapy 6). Increasing the frequency of current change to, say, 4000 Hz will allow the ions to pass easily through the tissues. However, if two such currents are passed through the tissues slightly out of phase they interfere to produce an amplitude-modulated current of low frequency which will stimulate nerve and muscle (therapy 7). Still higher frequencies, in the megahertz range, will allow large currents to pass through the tissues, producing significant heating spread throughout the tissues (therapy 8).

When the movement of electrons is made to occur at very high frequencies energy is given off in the form of electromagnetic radiations. These radiations can enter the tissues and cause effects when they are absorbed. Thus where the electron movement is at frequencies of thousands of millions of cycles per second (GHz) it produces radiations called microwaves (radar) which lead to heat when absorbed in the tissues (therapy 9). At higher frequencies they are called infrared and are absorbed at the skin surface but still cause heating (therapy 10). Still higher frequencies give radiations which stimulate the retina of the eye, i.e. they are visible. Where such radiations are of a single wavelength and in phase they are called 'laser' radiations (therapy 11). Those beyond the visible – ultraviolet (therapy 12) – cause marked biological changes when absorbed at the skin surface, i.e. sunburn.

Effects of applied electrical charges

The effects on the body of applied electrical charges depend on the amplitude and nature of the resulting current in the tissues. They can be rather simply summarized as having three basic effects, each of which may have various complex physiological and therapeutic consequences:

- Chemical changes occur in the tissues as a result of the application of unidirectional or direct current. Such effects are described in Chapter 2 and Electrolysis (Appendix). If the current is sufficiently great tissue destruction will occur.
- Excitable tissues, nerves and muscles, can be stimulated by currents that vary at a suitable rate. The change in current has to be quick enough to unbalance the ions around cell membranes, but not so quick that they do not allow time for the cell to respond. This may lead to many effects such as muscle contraction and altered pain perception. These currents are of various kinds and described in Chapters 3 and 4.
- Significant heating can be generated in the body tissues if high-frequency evenly alternating currents are applied because the rate of change is too high to allow time for excitable cells to respond and the polar or chemical effects are insignificant due to the even alternation, so that relatively high current intensities can be applied. High currents cause significant heating in the tissues because they dissipate much more energy than low current intensities. The heating will actually depend on the square of the current intensity (Joule's law: $H \propto I^2 Rt$, where $H =$ heat, $I =$ current, $R =$ resistance and $t =$ time). Such currents, described as 'diathermy', are discussed in Chapter 10.

In addition to these three major effects which may overlap, there are other less well-understood mechanisms. All are supported by some evidence and described more fully in the appropriate chapter:

- There are effects at a cellular level. Proliferation and increased migration of epithelial and connective tissue cells have been demonstrated due to the application of low-intensity d.c. DNA and protein synthesis may also be increased. This leads to accelerated wound healing, discussed in Chapter 2. Enhanced fracture healing has been demonstrated using small d.c. currents (an invasive hence non-physiotherapeutic procedure) as well as the use of pulsed currents both capacitatively and electromagnetically coupled. Such currents have also been applied successfully to treat connective tissue disorders.

There are also effects on the growth of neurons. Experimental work in animals on nerve both developmentally and after injury using both d.c. and pulsed electric fields have shown growth increases. It has been suggested that the mechanism may involve increased Ca^{2+} concentration in the growth region. Electrical pulses can also influence axonal transport and motor neuron plastic adaptation (Kidd *et al.*, 1988), discussed as trophic electrotherapy in Chapter 3.

In conditions of inflammation the cell membrane potential is reduced, which allows K^+ ions to escape into the extracellular fluid. This has the effect of attracting water by osmosis, which results in oedema which in turn can lead to pain. It is theorized that a pulsating magnetic field restores the negative charge to these cells, which re-establishes the K^+ and Na^+ balance and hence normal cell permeability (Hayne, 1984). Dyson (1985) states that ultrasonically induced membrane perturbation may increase calcium transport into mast cells, which activates them to release agents which initiate repair.

Acoustic streaming caused by ultrasound is known to change diffusion rates and membrane permeability which may alter rates of protein synthesis and hence repair (Dyson and Suckling, 1978). Laser therapy, which has been used successfully to accelerate wound healing (Dyson and Young, 1986), may work in the same way.

As noted above, the rapid oscillation of electric charges will lead to heating of tissues – diathermy. At the very low intensities produced by short pulses the additional energy is undetectable as heating but increases the heat energy. Suitably low levels applied for relatively long periods are considered to increase all cellular activity, thus increasing healing rates; see discussion in Chapter 10 regarding pulsed high-frequency electromagnetic energy.

It may be noticed that heat, ultrasound and laser have been considered with the effects of electric charges, but it must be realized that at the cellular level all therapies will produce a movement of ions, i.e. a movement of charges:

- The movement of ionized drugs through the skin can be effected by d.c., called iontophoresis and described in Chapter 2.
- It has been suggested that many claimed benefits of electrotherapy are due to a placebo effect. It would seem helpful to briefly discuss this often misunderstood concept. Placebo is latin for 'I shall please' and in medical usage has come to refer to treatments applied to please rather than benefit the patient.

More recently, a lack of physiological effect has become part of the meaning. Thus the word itself tends to have connotations of non-authenticity or fraud. (*Placebo domino* – I shall please the Lord – are the first words of Vespers for the dead and in medieval usage a placebo came to mean a sycophant, probably because of the use of professional mourners.)

The effect of undergoing any sort of treatment appears to help a proportion of patients. If this occurs when the treatment is known to be inactive – sugar pills, or electrotherapy not switched on, for example – then the effect is described as placebo. Many clinical trials have used such techniques often in a double blind format to reveal a surprisingly large number of patients (20–40%) responding to the apparently inactive therapies.

The explanation for these placebo responses are various, including the obvious power of suggestion. The reduction of stress and anxiety are considered to be a potent reason (Brown, 1998). It is known that under stressful conditions the hormonal and immune systems are activated. This could account for the effects of placebo treatments on a wide variety of symptoms.

It is well recognized that expectations of improvements have a powerful effect. This seems to be reinforced by the 'rigmarole' of treatment – a careful examination of the patient, an explanation of the intended treatment and association with complex machinery. (This latter is often cited as a major contributory factor to the placebo effect of electrotherapy.) Psychological factors appear to play a large part in producing the placebo effect; nevertheless many effects that are usually regarded as physiological often result. Consider also the discussion on biofeedback in Chapter 5 in this connection.

An ethical dilemma arises in that offering a treatment to a patient which the therapist believes to be ineffectual is clearly dishonest and improper, but the patient may well benefit from the treatment. A reasonable and full explanation to the patient would seem to be best, trying to avoid the implied stigma associated with the word placebo. See Brown (1998), French (1997) and Harrington (1997) for extensive consideration of the placebo effect.

Summary

Mechanisms underlying the therapeutic effects:

- direct current causing chemical changes
- low-frequency currents stimulating excitable tissues
- high-frequency currents causing heating
- continuous low-intensity d.c. and various pulsed currents leading to various changes at cellular level expressed as increased growth or repair
- direct current causing iontophoresis
- placebo effect.

Electroconvulsive therapy (ECT) refers to the application of current in a series of pulses to the brain via scalp electrodes for the treatment of severe depression and some other psychiatric disorders. The electrical charge causes extensive disturbance in the cerebral cortex – a seizure – which, in some ill-understood way, alleviates the depression. There may also be some mild memory loss. This treatment is not the province of the physiotherapist and is, therefore, not considered in this text.

BASIC GUIDELINES FOR THE APPLICATION OF ELECTROTHERAPY

Before applying any modality of electrotherapy to a patient the following questions should be considered:

- What effect is intended and can this treatment achieve this effect? In many instances it cannot be known if treatment is effective until it is tried. Sometimes effectiveness can be seen at once, e.g. relief of pain due to transcutaneous electric nerve stimulation or ice; in other cases it cannot be recognized for days or weeks.
- Is it safe, i.e. will the desired effect be achieved without undesirable effects? There is no effective treatment that does not carry some risks but for most electrotherapy treatment the risks are negligible provided reasonable and proper precautions are taken. Each modality has its own potential dangers and contraindications and no treatment should be considered without a thorough knowledge of these.
- Is it the best method of treatment to achieve this effect? Is it the most economical in terms of patient and/or therapist time, or other costs?

Physiotherapists should confine themselves to the use of electrophysical modalities in which they are competent. Usually electrotherapy is part of an overall treatment plan which is selected and modified on the basis of repeated examination and assessment. However, there are some basic guidelines which can provide the framework for sound practice:

- *Preparation of patient*

  - *Explanation*. An explanation of the treatment is an essential precursor of application. This not only reassures the patient but ensures informed consent. The type of sensation to be experienced is explained, and the patient is warned of any effects that should be reported.
  - *Examination and testing*. This refers to specific examination of the part to be treated for possible dangers and contraindications plus any relevant tests, e.g. for normal thermal sensitivity. A check should be made to ascertain if the patient might suffer an allergic reaction to any substance being applied to the skin.

Patients receiving radiation therapy require special consideration (Brooks, 1998). All forms of electrotherapy to the irradiated skin are widely considered contraindicated for a period of months after irradiation, as is the application of any substance to the irradiated skin during radiation therapy. Previously irradiated skin may be hypaesthetic, so electrotherapy modalities must be used with caution. Electrodes must not be placed in areas of skin erosion or hypaesthetic areas. The results should be recorded.

- *Assembly of apparatus*. All the apparatus and equipment needed should be assembled and suitably positioned. Visual checks are made of electrodes, leads, cables, plugs, power outlets, switches, controls, dials and indicator lights.
- *Preparation and testing of apparatus*. This includes setting up the apparatus and any necessary testing of it prior to application. When this has been done satisfactorily treatment can begin. The operator should minimize their own exposure to the effects of the modality being used.
- *Preparation of the part to be treated*. This involves any preparatory procedure, e.g. washing the area and positioning the patient, and in particular the part to be treated, comfortably and appropriately, so that he or she is relaxed and unnecessary movement is avoided.
- *Setting up*. The apparatus is set up to ensure optimum therapeutic effect and safety.
- *Instructions and warnings*. Before the treatment commences it is mandatory to instruct the patient in what he or she must and must not do, e.g. keep still and not touch the apparatus, and to give essential warnings, e.g. 'If this becomes more than a comfortable warmth it can burn'. The warning given should be noted on the patient's record card.
- *Application*. The patient must be observed throughout to ensure that treatment is progressing satisfactorily and without adverse effects. Accurate timing is essential.
- *Termination of treatment*. At the termination of treatment the part treated should be examined to ensure that the desired effects have occurred if visible, e.g. superficial vasodilation, and that there are no unwanted effects. If appropriate, an explanation of what to expect is given as well as instructions of when to come again and what must be done between treatments.
- *Recording*. An accurate record of all the parameters of treatment including region treated, technique, dosage, and the resultant effect must be made. This is for both assessment purposes and for legal requirements.

Reference may also be made to the Chartered Society of Physiotherapy's *Standards for the Use of Electrophysical Modalities*, and their guidelines for the safe use of various modalities.

REFERENCES

Alberts B., Bray D., Lewis J., Ra H. M., Roberts K., Watson J. D. (1983). *Molecular Biology of the Cell*. New York: Garland Publishing Inc.

Barker A. T., Jaffe L. F., Vanable J. W. (1982). The glabrous epidermis of cavies contains a powerful battery. *Am. J. Physiol.*, **242**, 358–65.

Bray J. J., Cragg P. A., MacKnight A. D. C. *et al.* (1986). *Lecture Notes on Human Physiology.* London: Blackwell Scientific Publications.

Brooks C. (1998). Radiation therapy. Guidelines for physiotherapists. *Physiotherapy,* **84**, 387–95.

Brown W. A. (1998). The placebo effect. *Sci. Am.*, Jan., 68–73.

Charman R. A. (1990a). Bioelectricity and electrotherapy – towards a new paradigm? Introduction. *Physiotherapy,* **76** (9) 502–3.

Charman R. A. (1990b). Bioelectricity and electrotherapy – towards a new paradigm? Part 1: The electric cell. *Physiotherapy,* **76** (9) 503–8.

Charman R. A. (1990c). Bioelectricity and electrotherapy – towards a new paradigm? Part 2: Cellular reception and emission of electromagnetic signals. *Physiotherapy,* **76** (9) 509–16.

Charman R. A. (1990d). Bioelectricity and electrotherapy – towards a new paradigm? Part 3: Bioelectric potentials and tissue currents. *Physiotherapy,* **76** (10) 643–54.

Charman R. A. (1990e). Bioelectricity and electrotherapy – towards a new paradigm? Part 4: Strain generated potentials in bone and connective tissue physiotherapy. *Physiotherapy,* **76** (11) 725–30.

Charman R. A. (1990f). Bioelectricity and electrotherapy – towards a new paradigm? Part 5: Exogenous currents and fields – experimental and clinical application. *Physiotherapy,* **76** (12) 743–50.

Charman R. A. (1991a). Bioelectricity and electrotherapy – towards a new paradigm? Part 6: Environmental current and fields – the natural background. *Physiotherapy,* **77** (1) 8–14.

Charman R. A. (1991b). Bioelectricity and electrotherapy – towards a new paradigm? Part 7: Environmental current and fields – man-made. *Physiotherapy,* **77** (2) 129–40.

Dyson M. (1985). Therapeutic applications of ultrasound. In *Biological Effects of Ultrasound: Clinics in Diagnostic Ultrasound* (Nyborg W. L., Ziskin M. C., eds) Edinburgh: Churchill Livingstone, 121–33.

Dyson M., Suckling J. (1978). Stimulation of tissue repair by ultrasound: a survey of the mechanisms involved. *Physiotherapy,* **64**, 105–8.

Dyson M., Young S. (1986). Effect of laser therapy on wound contraction and cellularity in mice. *Lasers Sci.*, **1**, 125–30.

Finean J. B., Coleman R., Michell R. H. (1978). *Membranes and their Cellular Functions* 2nd edn. London: Blackwell Scientific Publications.

Foulds I., Barker A. (1983). Human skin battery potentials and their possible role in wound healing. *Br. J. Dermatol.*, **109**, 515–22.

French S. (1997). *The Powerful Placebo in Physiotherapy: A Psychosocial Approach.* Oxford: Butterworth-Heinemann.

Guyton A. C. (1982). *Human Physiology and Mechanism of Disease* 3rd edn. Philadelphia: W. B. Saunders.

Harrington A. (ed.) (1997). *The Placebo Effect.* Cambridge, Mass.: Harvard University Press.

Hayne C. R. (1984). Pulsed high frequency energy – its place in physiotherapy. *Physiotherapy,* **70**, 459–66.

Illingworth C. M. and Barker A. T. (1980). Measurement of electrical currents emerging during the regeneration of amputated fingertips in children. *Clin. Phys. Physiol. Measur.* **1**, 87–9.

Kidd G. L., Oldham J. A., Stanley J. K. (1988). Eutrophic electrotherapy and atrophied muscle: a pilot clinical trial. *Clinic. Rehab.*, **2**, 219–30.

Miles F. A. (1969). *Excitable Cells.* London: Heinemann Medical Books.

Rees J. R., Sternberg M. J. E. (1984). *From Cells to Atoms. An Illustrated Introduction to Molecular Biology.* Oxford: Blackwell Scientific Publications.

Walsh J. C. (1988). Electrophysiology. In *Electrophysical Agents in Physiotherapy: Therapeutic and Diagnostic Use* (Wadsworth H., Chanmugan A. P. P., eds) Marrickville, NSW Australia: Science Press.

2 Therapeutic direct current

The very simplicity of a constant direct current ensured that it was used at an early stage for therapy. This encouraged rather exaggerated and fanciful claims for its use which have, perhaps, served to cloud the more reasonable applications – a victim of its history.

The nature, uses and production of therapeutic d.c. are described first. Discussion of the mechanisms of iontophoresis and those of d.c.-enhanced wound healing follows. Drugs used for iontophoresis, with some description of their effects, are noted. The principles of d.c. application are described, with comment on dosages, and in conclusion the possible dangers are listed.

HISTORY

The discovery of electricity came piecemeal, from the production of static charges on glass bulbs in the early 18th century, through the various means of producing a steady current – such as the voltaic pile – to more and more sophisticated means of varying and reversing the current. At each stage medical use was recommended, tried and much benefit was usually claimed. In 1786 Luigi Galvani stimulated the nerves and muscle of frogs with electric charges. When his work was published in 1791 it gave an enormous impetus to scientific experimentation in this realm. As a consequence Humboldt called the steady current 'galvanism' to distinguish it from frictionally generated static charges. Galvanic currents – continuous direct currents – came to be widely used therapeutically and even more extensively to introduce medication into the body tissues. As early as 1833 Fabre-Palaprat exploited this idea – nowadays called iontophoresis – and many subsequent claims were made for its effective use, often under strange-sounding names such as 'cataphoric medication' or 'endosmosis'. Stephane Le Duc in France popularized iontophoresis in the early years of the 20th century and is sometimes described as its originator; for a detailed description of the history of iontophoresis see Licht (1983).

NATURE (see Appendix)

Direct current refers to a current passing continuously in the same direction (see Fig. 3.1). For the purposes of definition, therapeutic direct current (d.c.) has been considered to pass for more than 1 s (Alon, 1987), and is sometimes called constant current or galvanism. It may be noted that all monophasic currents, whatever their pulse lengths, have the same d.c. effects (see Fig. 3.1). Thus a medium frequency 'd.c. type' current consisting of pulses of 125 μs duration, separated by intervals of 5 μs, hence giving a duty cycle of 96%, is effectively d.c. Very low intensity d.c. is often described as 'microamperage d.c.' or 'microamperage stimulation'.

TRANSMISSION

Current is passed to the body tissues by means of wet pads, sponges or a bath of suitable solution. Thus the conduction current generated in the apparatus is changed to a convection current in the wet pads and tissues. At the junction of the electrode (a conductor) with the electrolyte of the pad chemical changes will occur – the changes of electrolysis. The nature of these changes depends on the constituents of the electrolyte and the metal of the electrodes (see Appendix). The general result is the formation of acids at the positive electrode (anode) and bases at the negative electrode (cathode). Although these reactions occur at the junction of the electrode with the electrolyte, i.e. where the electrode touches the conducting gel or wetted pad in treatment situations, their effects can spread to the skin causing chemical damage. Such a chemical burn is far more likely to occur close to the negative terminal (cathode) as a result of the alkalis formed there.

The magnitude of these changes depends on the current density, that is the current intensity per unit area (mA/cm^2); also, because of the spread of chemicals through the wetted pad, the changes will depend directly on the total time that the current is flowing.

The current in any circuit is directly proportional to the voltage and inversely to the resistance (Ohm's law: see Appendix). The major resistance in a d.c. system applied to the body is the epidermis; thus the area of contact with the epidermis will determine the total resistance: the larger the cross-sectional area, the smaller the resistance. The value of this resistance will determine the current for any given voltage. Therefore what matters from a therapeutic point of view is the current per unit area, that is the current density.

IONTOPHORESIS

Iontophoresis involves the movement of ions across biological membranes by means of an electric current for therapeutic purposes. It is also called ion transfer.

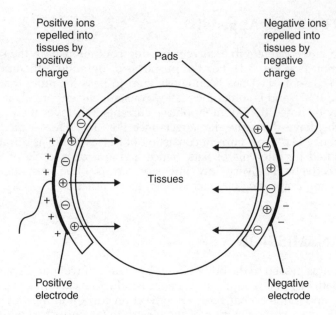

Positive ions repelled into tissues by positive charge

Pads

Negative ions repelled into tissues by negative charge

Tissues

Positive electrode

Negative electrode

Fig. 2.1 Movement of ions during iontophoresis.

Mechanism of iontophoresis

If a voltage is applied to an electrolyte a convection current will flow. This consists of positively charged ions moving towards the negative pole and negatively charged ions moving to the positive pole.

If a drug is in an ionic form, i.e. it has a charge, it can be made to travel in either direction depending on the polarity applied. Atoms and molecules in an electrolyte are constantly gaining or losing electrons to become ions and then reverting to their non-ionized form. There is also considerable random movement of particles. When an electric charge is applied it results in a steady drift of appropriately charged ions in each direction. If the electrolyte is divided by membranes – as in the therapeutic situation – then many more ions are driven through the membranes than would pass through due to random particle (Brownian) motion.

This is the situation that occurs when applying iontophoresis. The tissues are effectively a continuous electrolyte with the solution of the wet pad or sponge which contains the ionized drug (Fig. 2.1). Thus positively charged ions can be made to drift away from the positively charged pole towards the negative pole (from left to right in Fig. 2.1) and will pass through the skin and into the tissues, and vice versa for negatively charged ions. Some will lose their charge in the tissues and become chemically active. Hence some of the drug has been locally introduced into the tissues. An additional mechanism involves the passage of a solvent which can carry dissolved substances through the skin due to d.c. This form of electrosmosis has been called 'iontohydrokinesis' and is strongly dependent on the pH of the skin (Gangarosa *et al.*, 1980). The actual passage of current, hence of ions, occurs mainly via the sweat gland

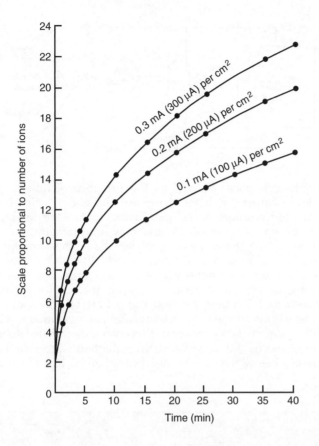

Fig. 2.2 Illustration of the number of ions driven into the tissues in a given time.

The number of ions introduced into the tissues is proportional to the cube root of the product of time and current density, e.g. for $100\,\mu A$ the current passing for $5\,min = 500$; cube root for $500 = 7.94$. Other points are found in a similar way.

ducts and to a lesser extent via the hair follicles and sebaceous glands.

The effects of any drug introduced by iontophoresis are likely to be either local in the skin under the active electrode or systemic because when the drug enters the tissue fluid it is disseminated throughout the body tissues. This has been demonstrated by the iontophoresis of radioactive material (O'Malley and Oester, 1955).

The number of ions entering the tissues from any given area of active electrolyte is proportional to both the current density and the time of application. In fact the number of ions transferred has been shown to be proportional to the cube root of the product of current density and time of application (Trubatch and Van Harreveld, 1972; Fig. 2.2). For practical purposes the current density is limited by the skin tolerance, which usually allows between 0.1 and $0.3\,mA/cm^2$. Dosage can thus be reasonably expressed for a given treatment area in terms of total current in mA multiplied by the time in minutes.

The concentration of ions in the solution used will obviously have an effect on the number of ions available; it has been shown, however, that concentrations of about 1 or 2% are as satisfactory as higher concentrations.

It must be understood that tissue penetration by ions used therapeutically is not a simple matter. Specific conductivity and pH

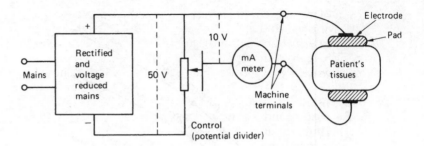

Fig. 2.3 Production of d.c. for patients.

of the solutions used, as well as the presence of non-drug ions which will compete with the drug, are all factors which have an influence. Furthermore some ions, such as zinc or silver, form precipitates which are insoluble and may limit penetration.

In spite of the generalization made above that iontophoresis would only lead to skin or systemic effects, there have been many suggestions and some evidence (Costello and Jeske, 1995) that drugs act on deeply placed structures beneath the site of application (Wadsworth and Chanmugan, 1980; Kahn, 1994; Demirtaş and Ömer, 1998). There is also some evidence from animal experiments (Glass *et al.*, 1980) in which higher concentrations of a radiolabelled substance than would occur due to systemic introduction were found in the deep tissues below the sites where iontophoresis had taken place.

Summary

Therapeutic d.c.:

- is the continuous unidirectional flow of charged particles in the tissues
- passes in the tissues as a convection current
- causes chemical changes at the junction of the conduction with the convection current
- will have a current density determined by the applied voltage and the size of the area to which it is applied for any given skin resistance
- can effect the passage of drug ions into the tissues for therapeutic purposes.

PRODUCTION

All that is needed to provide therapeutic d.c. is a steady unidirectional voltage, a means of regulating the voltage applied to the tissues via terminals marked positive and negative and a means of measuring the current flow.

The mains voltage is rectified and reduced and a potential divider is placed in parallel with the patient (Fig. 2.3). This divider can be altered by moving the control. With the potential divider at zero no voltage is applied so that no current will flow. The milliammeter in series with the patient will indicate zero current flow. Suppose 50 V is applied across the resistance and the control is turned to make contact one-fifth of the way along the resistance, as shown in Figure 2.3: then 10 V is applied to the tissues. If the total resistance of the patient and the meter were 5000 Ω then 2 mA would pass through the tissues and be shown on the meter (10/5000 = 0.02; Ohm's law). Similarly, if the connection is moved to halfway and 25 V is applied then 5 mA will flow. Thus the current to the patient can be regulated from zero.

Many pieces of apparatus have a switch to connect a different circuit, giving a different range of current, e.g. 0–10 mA or 0–100 mA. Note that the current in the patient depends not only on the voltage but also on the patient's resistance, so if skin resistance falls current will rise.

PHYSIOLOGICAL EFFECTS AND THERAPEUTIC USES

Low-density currents have been used for the effects they cause in the skin and for iontophoresis, usually for periods of 10–30 min. The current density is kept to a level that does not cause tissue damage or patient discomfort. Traditionally this is said to be below about 0.33 mA/cm^2 (2 mA/in^2) but Cummings (1987) uses between 0.1 and 0.5 mA/cm^2.

Direct current

Sensory stimulation

During the passage of such currents the patient is aware of a mild tingling or prickling sensation, which may merge into a mild irritation or itching. If sufficient current has passed for long enough an erythema of the skin will be evident under both electrodes, and is more marked under the negative (cathode). In the past this irritating effect was used for relief of pain. This erythema is confined to the area of the applied electrode.

Hyperaemia

Since this erythema is confined it indicates a capillary hyperaemia, unlike that due to heat in which arteriolar dilatation occurs. The initial erythema lasts for about 20 min or so but may be made to recur over a period of several hours, even a day later, by another stimulus such as heat (Kovacs, 1949). The mechanism of this erythema has not been fully elucidated. It differs from the erythemas produced by chemical stimuli such as an inflammatory or ultraviolet radiation-provoked erythema. The evident erythema has in the past led to the idea that vasomotor stimulation and increased circulation may promote improved nutrition of the area and speed up the resolution of inflammatory products (Kovacs, 1949); there seems to be no significant evidence to support this.

Electrotonus

Subthreshold nerve stimuli do not cause an action potential but they do affect the membrane potential. The cathode produces a local depolarizing potential that rises rapidly but falls exponentially with time. The anode causes the reverse – hyperpolarization. These are electronic potentials (Ganong, 1991) that occur because altering the charge across the nerve membrane alters the threshold, as explained in Chapters 1 and 3. Making the outer nerve membrane surface less positive lowers the threshold, which increases the nerve's excitability (catelectrotonus), while making it more positive (anelectrotonus), has the reverse effect.

Relief of pain

The relief of pain has long been claimed as a result of d.c. treatments. Sensory stimulation of cutaneous nerve endings (due to electro-chemical changes) inhibiting pain by means of the 'pain gate' theory could reasonably account for this phenomenon (see Chapter 3). It is suggested that the marked hyperaemia occurring under the cathode with strong d.c. may help to remove pain-inducing factors.

Acceleration of healing

Various forms of electrical stimulation have been shown to enhance healing. Over the past 25 years or so, many controlled research studies, both on humans and animals, have produced evidence that low density electric currents lead to augmented and accelerated healing. Increased rates of new bone formation have been shown to occur when small direct currents have been applied to fractures by implanted electrodes (Becker *et al.*, 1977). This has been used successfully in the treatment of non-union (Brighton *et al.*, 1981).

The healing rates of soft tissue wounds, particularly superficial open wounds, have also benefited from electrical stimulation. Although supported by some good experimental evidence and clinical research, the therapeutic application of electric currents for healing does not seem to have been widely embraced. This is perhaps surprising in view of the economic and social benefits accruing from even a small reduction in the time taken for healing of the enormous number of open wounds that need to be treated each year. It may be that uncertainties concerning the optimum dosages and the lack of a convincing mechanism to explain why healing should be stimulated by the application of electric charges has inhibited the advance of these therapies. A number of different current types have been utilized for this purpose but as, in the main, they have a direct current component and polarity appears to have particular consequences, they are considered in this chapter, although some currents, such as high-voltage pulsed galvanic stimulation (HVPGS) are further described in Chapter 3.

Electrical properties of normal and injured tissue.   All tissues have varying electrical potentials between different parts and there appears to be a constancy about some sites. Mechanically stressed bone, for example, generates an electrical potential (a piezoelectric effect), and areas of active bone growth or repair are negatively charged compared with other areas. These observations have led to the use of external electric currents to induce osteogenesis. This effect and an account of the skin battery and transcutaneous voltage are noted in Chapter 1.

Several studies of the effects of direct current on wound healing have been carried out, notably on rabbits and pigs. Some of these, but not all, have shown increased rates of healing and/or increased tensile strength of the healed tissue. The majority of these studies applied the negative electrode to the wound site, but at least one showed greater skin collagen production and faster epithelialization with the positive electrode applied.

Clinical studies of electrically enhanced healing.   Many clinical investigations in humans over the past 25 years have found that electrical stimulation led to enhanced wound healing. Ischaemic dermal ulcers have been treated in a similar manner by several investigators over the years with good results (Wolcott *et al.*, 1969; Gault and Gatens, 1976; Carley and Wainapel, 1985; Kloth and Feedar, 1988; Feedar *et al.*, 1991). All these studies compared treated with control groups and the most recent one was multicentred and double blind. In all cases the healing rate was approximately doubled in the electrically treated patients. Although the first three studies used low intensity d.c. and the latter two used high-voltage pulsed electrical stimulation, they all applied the negative electrode to the wound for the first 3 days of treatment and subsequently reversed the polarity.

A review of numerous investigations into the effects of electrical stimulation of skin (Reich and Tarjan, 1990) concluded that altering the polarity during the course of treatment was more successful than maintaining the same polarity throughout. They also attempted to elucidate the optimum electrical parameters appropriate for accelerating healing and repair but were hampered by the lack of detail reported, particularly the area of the application electrode, which made it impossible to know the current density. The importance of describing the current density, as opposed to the total current, when recording dosage is emphasized in this text. Reich and Tarjan concluded that quite a low total charge transfer – a few microamps over a few hours – worked well, but considered there was insufficient evidence to suggest timing of treatments over days and weeks. Many successful treatments used electrical stimulation for half an hour daily or 5 times per week. The use of the negative electrode during the first few days is supported by a study on rabbits (Brown *et al.*, 1988) which found that the positive pole delayed healing during the first 4 days but increased it during days 5–7.

Several other studies have shown similar healing improvement (Weiss *et al.*, 1990; Reich and Tarjan, 1990). Mulder (1991), on similar

---

Case study

Griffin *et al.* (1991) treated pressure ulcers in patients with spinal cord injury with high-voltage pulsed currents for an hour a day for 20 days. A negative polarity aluminium foil electrode was placed over the ulcer with a dispersive on the thigh. They reported a significant increase in healing rate.

---

lines to that of Feedar *et al.* (1991), included surgical wounds and found a significantly greater healing rate in the treated wounds compared with those receiving sham treatment. Myers (1991), analysing five studies that used high-voltage pulsed galvanic stimulation (HVPGS) to treat chronic wounds, found a highly significant difference between experimental and control groups and concluded that this treatment is effective. In contradiction, two studies on wound healing in animals (Byl *et al.*, 1994; Lettmann *et al.*, 1994) found no acceleration of healing due to microamperage stimulation.

Most studies reporting a successful outcome used a much greater current density than these.

Current sources. It should be noted that several different electrical sources have been used in these studies with differing electrical characteristics, including microamperage devices and relatively low-amperage battery-powered sources. These devices may be provided with a circuit to limit the maximum applied current so that changes in circuit resistance do not alter the output. The form of the output is illustrated in Figure 3.1(a),(b). Others have used similar devices with a pulsed output (see Fig. 3.1(c)). More widely used has been a high-voltage pulsed current, such as HVPGS, referred to in Chapter 3. Such stimulators produce twin high-voltage phases with a short duration. Although up to 500 volts may be applied, the very short pulse length means that the total current is about 1 or 2 mA (see bottom uniphasic graph of Fig. 3.4).

There seems to be little evidence to determine whether any one of these is the most effective. It may not be possible to know without clearly stated dosages as discussed by Reich and Tarjan (1990). Some writers favour pulsed currents on the grounds of safety (although no significant adverse effects seem to have been reported), and because pulsing is believed to increase local vascularity. It has also been suggested that HVPGS is more cost effective than continuous current because good results have been achieved with shorter periods of treatment. The use of some particular source is not necessarily a prerequisite for these treatments. Any source that produces constant d.c. that can be controlled may be appropriate.

Mechanisms of enhanced healing. The way in which electrical stimulation acts to encourage more rapid or more effective healing of superficial wounds is unclear. There is, however, evidence that proliferation and migration of epithelial and connective tissue cells involved in wound repair can be increased by an electric field (Alvarez *et al.*, 1983; Erickson and Nuccitelli, 1984). HVPGS has been reported to induce human fibroblasts in culture to increase their rates of DNA and protein synthesis (Bourguignon and Bourguignon, 1987). While these observations may indicate a way in which normal healing processes could be accelerated, it remains unclear how or why varying electric fields influence these cellular activities.

The skin battery referred to in Chapter 1 leads to the passage of small currents through a wound in the epidermis (see Fig. 1.6). Such currents can only flow if the wound is kept moist and it has been shown that a moist wound environment is also needed for optimum healing of epithelial wounds. Similar but larger currents of injury have been measured in injured animals and seem to be associated not only with repair but also with regeneration in salamanders, which are capable of limb regrowth.

If applied electric charges are able to enhance cell activity, it may be asked if reversing the electric field will inhibit growth. While it does not seem to be that simple, there is some evidence that applying the positive electrode can cause regression in some mouse tumours (Humphrey and Seal, 1959), reduce the growth of hypertrophic and keloid scars (Weiss *et al.*, 1989) and delay healing (Brown *et al.*, 1988). For an extensive review of this important topic see Watson (1996).

There are several other theoretical suggestions to account for the observed effects, but the whole subject is not well understood, and it is anticipated that future research will illuminate the underlying mechanisms enabling more rational treatments to be applied.

Other methods. Two other methods involving small electric currents have been applied to promote healing. First, the use of iontophoresis which is described later, and, secondly, TENS type currents (see Chapter 3) have been applied to promote healing (Kloth and Feedar, 1990).

Application. The size of any wound or ulcer to be treated should first be ascertained to enable the current density to be calculated and to monitor the rate of healing. The ulcer may be packed with gauze soaked in sterile saline to allow adequate conduction of the current. The negative electrode (cathode) is usually applied for the first few treatments, partly for its bacteriocidal effect (Kloth and Feedar, 1990) and for reasons considered above. A malleable electrode wrapped in saline-soaked gauze is applied over the wound and secured with a strap or bandage, ensuring even pressure overall. The electrode should be equal to, or somewhat smaller than, the size of the wound so that it is in contact, via the wet gauze, with the whole open area. The positive electrode (anode) should be of a similar or larger size but placed on normal washed and wetted skin on some convenient, usually more proximal, site. The current applied might be in the region of 10–$50\,\mu A/cm^2$ (i.e. something under $1\,mA$ for a $20\,cm^2$ ulcer). At this intensity the current would be undetectable to the patient. Such currents might be applied each day for 2–4 hours. After 3 or 4 days, and when any infection is cleared, the polarity should be changed. Any subsequent slowing of healing, a plateau, is a signal for a further change of polarity for a day or two.

If HVPGS is to be used the procedure is exactly the same, using the cathode at first and subsequently altering polarity. The current intensity should be less than that which will cause muscle contraction, and frequencies of around $100\,Hz$ are used, although some recommend lower frequencies around $30\,Hz$. It is suggested that treatment should be for 30–45 min daily or 3 times per week (see Newton, 1987; Chapter 3).

Contraindications to the use of electrical stimulation for wound healing. There seem to be no reports of serious or significant damage as a result of these treatments. Sometimes skin irritation has occurred under the dispersive pad as a consequence of using a current too large for the area of the pad or not cleaning the skin properly.

These currents should not be applied to tissues that contain neoplastic cells, since it is possible, but not supported by any evidence, that the currents may enhance the activity of such abnormal cells, leading to increased cancerous growth or metastases.

If the wound has been treated with topical applications containing free metal or other ions, these should be thoroughly washed out of the wound before treatment. This is because positively charged ions would be driven into the wound tissue by the anode and negatively charged ions by the cathode (i.e. iontophoresis, see below). This may cause irritation of the wound.

Further consideration is given to the general dangers of therapeutic electric currents at the end of this chapter and in Chapter 3.

The use of physiotherapeutic agents and methods to accelerate or promote wound healing is also considered in connection with ultrasound, laser, thermal and ultraviolet therapies. For an overview and background see Kloth and Feedar (1990).

Tissue destruction

At higher current densities d.c. will cause tissue damage. Coagulation of protein occurs under the positive pole and liquefaction under the negative. These effects will occur if the current density is high, such as would happen if a bare wire or needle electrode were placed on or in the skin (Kovacs, 1949). This effect has been used in the deliberate destruction of unwanted tissue such as warts. It is best known for its use in the removal of unwanted hair; with a large positive dispersive electrode applied in a convenient place, the fine-needle negative electrode is introduced into the hair follicle and a current applied to liquefy and destroy the hair-bearing epithelium.

Summary

Physiological effects and therapeutic uses of d.c.:

- sensory stimulation – tingling or pricking
- hyperaemia – cutaneous erythema
- electrotonus – alteration of nerve excitability
- tissue damage or destruction
- pain relief
- acceleration of tissue healing
- iontophoresis.

Iontophoresis

The physiological and therapeutic effects of iontophoresis depend on the nature of the drugs introduced into the tissues. A very large number of substances have been used for a vast range of therapeutic purposes over the years, most of them with little success. This has, perhaps, tended to diminish recognition of the fewer effective applications.

Costello and Jeske (1995) consider that there has been a recent resurgence in its use, particularly for the delivery of anti-inflammatory medication. They predict that miniaturized unit-dose systems may become available and also further increase its use. In a literature review Van Herp (1997) suggests it offers the promise of therapeutic efficacy and cost effectiveness.

Local anaesthesia

Local cutaneous anaesthesia can be achieved by the iontophoresis of a suitable agent such as lignocaine or procaine. The time of anaesthesia can be increased considerably by the addition of adrenaline. A study which compared iontophoresis with sub-cutaneous infiltration and topical application (Russo *et al.*, 1980; quoted by Boone, 1981) found that infiltration produced the longest-lasting anaesthesia – an average of 22.2 min – while iontophoresis caused anaesthesia of the same depth but lasting 14.5 min on average; topical application caused only a short 2.1-min effect. This has been used therapeutically in the treatment of herpes zoster and trigeminal neuralgia, but how successfully is not clear. Although little used in physiotherapy departments, this technique could be valuable for patients who have a strong aversion to hypodermic needles for inducing local anaesthesia. It is used sometimes for minor ear or eye surgery in which hypodermic injection is especially painful. The application of this form of treatment needs particular care in technique because skin anaesthesia is induced during the passage of the current (see below).

Relief of idiopathic hyperhidrosis

Perhaps the most successful use of iontophoresis is in the treatment of idiopathic hyperhidrosis. This distressing condition usually affects the palms and soles and sometimes the axillae. It can be sufficiently severe to interfere with the patient's work. Topical application of various antiperspirants may be ineffective so that surgical treatment – sympathectomy for hands and feet or skin removal for axillary hyperhidrosis – remains the only other option.

Glycopyrronium bromide iontophoresis has been shown to be a simple, safe and effective treatment (Abell and Morgan, 1974), particularly for the hands and feet. Exocrine sweat glands in the palms and soles are innervated by the sympathetic system but stimulated by acetylcholine so that the introduction of an anticholinergic agent (glycopyrronium bromide) into the skin will suppress sweating immediately. This effect lasts a variable length of time; Abell and Morgan (1974) found a mean of 33.7 days for the palm in 16 patients and 47.2 days for the soles in 4 patients. Later it was suggested that few patients need treatment repeated more often than every 4 to 6 weeks (Morgan, 1980).

Case study

A patient whose passionate hobby was snooker found his hyperhidrosis not only left embarrassing damp handprints on the green baize but hampered his cueing action. Glycopyrronium bromide iontophoresis given on request, approximately monthly, kept his hands satisfactorily dry for his work and hobby over a long period. Unfortunately no record was kept to correlate improved snooker score with the reduction of hyperhidrosis!

The length of post-treatment anhidrosis varies not only between patients but in successive treatments of the same patient. One of us (JL) treating two patients with a standard technique found mean periods of dryness to be 30 and 38 days, with a range of 17–62 days.

Treatment of the axillae has been less successful in the sense that dryness persisted for only a short period, 7.3 days (Abell and Morgan, 1974). This, and the fact that women and children seem on average to have shorter periods of anhidrosis, suggests that the drug may be held in the epidermis and released slowly, so that more is held by the thicker epidermis (Abell and Morgan, 1974).

Other drugs have been used with the same effect, e.g. poldine methylsulphate (Grice *et al.*, 1972). Using tap water iontophoresis –

that is, simply d.c. – has been described as successfully producing anhidrosis (Grice *et al.*, 1972; Midtgaard, 1986). The anode is used as the active electrode. Older texts refer to a drying effect of the anode but this is based on the observed effect when the metal electrode is implanted in the tissues. The sweat-reducing effect is likely to be due to obstruction of the sweat duct by the deposition of keratin (Abell and Morgan, 1974). Unfortunately, anhidrosis due to tap water iontophoresis seems to last only a few days so that repeated treatments are needed (Grice *et al.*, 1972; Abell and Morgan, 1974; Morgan, 1980). However, Midtgaard (1986) and Akins *et al.* (1987) claimed periods of 4 weeks' freedom from sweating. Akins *et al.* (1987) in testing the Drionic unit found that it took on average 14 days of treatment before sweating was inhibited and there were significant side-effects.

Application of antibiotics

The application of antibiotics to avascular areas by iontophoresis has been studied. Ear chondritis following burn injury has been successfully treated. Another method of dealing with chronic infection is metallic silver iontophoresis (Becker and Spadaro, 1978). Chronic non-healing ulcers have been treated with xanthinol nicotinate, a capillary dilator, and histamine diphosphate, which presumably acted similarly; both are quoted by Boone (1981).

Case study

La Forrest and Confrancesco (1978) describe three cases of ear chondritis. In one, a 33-year-old man had suffered second-degree burns to his face and hands and developed an infective chondritis of the left ear. (Cartilage, being avascular, is unresponsive to systemic antibiotics when it becomes infected due to loss of the overlying tissue.) The ear was treated by iontophoresis of gentamicin sulphate in sterile water 12 times over a 7-day period, by which time the ear was greatly improved and no infection was evident. No recurrence occurred.

Application of anti-inflammatory drugs

Anti-inflammatory drugs used to treat tendinitis and bursitis when delivered by iontophoresis were described as successful by several workers (quoted in Cummings, 1987). The advantages of this method of delivery over conventional injection are the painlessness and sterility of the treatment: absolute sterility is clearly very important for the introduction of anti-inflammatory agents. The disadvantages are that there is even less certainty of their efficacy and it is a time-consuming, hence expensive, method. The major doubt is whether these drugs reach the inflamed tissues, particularly if they are relatively deeply placed structures such as ligaments. However, a study of rhesus monkeys has shown that therapeutic dosages can be delivered to deeply placed joint structures (Glass *et al.*, 1980).

Various non-steroidal anti-inflammatory drugs are used for the treatment of musculoskeletal pain. For example, Demirtaş and Ömer (1998) reported the successful treatment of epicondylitis with iontophoresis of sodium salicylate and sodium diclofenac; they found the latter more efficacious. Concentrations of such NSAIDs in the tissues have been found to be greatly increased by iontophoresis compared with their percutaneous absorption (Pratzel *et al.*, 1986).

Case study

Dexamethasone iontophoresis was applied to first one and subsequently both knees of a patient with rheumatoid arthritis in a single case study by Hasson *et al.* (1991). This was combined with exercise and assessment. The dexamethasone lidocaine iontophoresis appeared to lead to improved muscle strength, swelling and range of motion in the treated knee compared with the control which had received only lidocaine iontophoresis during the first phase of treatment.

Neurogenic pain

Iontophoresis of vinca alkaloids (vincristine and vinblastine) has been used and recommended for the treatment of intractable, chronic pain syndromes, notably for patients suffering from post-herpetic and other neuralgias, and chronic pain in terminal cancer.

The vinca alkaloids are cytotoxic drugs which are microtubule inhibitors and have been used in the treatment of malignancy. Their application to sensory nerve endings in the skin by iontophoresis allows them to act in an unusual way on these nerve endings to interfere with axoplasmic transport – see Knyihár-Csillik *et al.* (1982). Clinical trials have reportedly been quite successful in reducing neurogenic pain (Csillik *et al.*, 1982; but see also Layman *et al.*, 1986).

Other uses

Numerous other drugs have been reported to show specific therapeutic effects when given by iontophoresis.

Case study

A boy was treated for myositis ossificans in the quadriceps muscle, with a 2% acetic acid solution administered via iontophoresis using the cathode at a dose of 4 mA for 20 min. This was followed by 8 min of $1.5\,W/cm^2$ of pulsed ultrasound at a 50% duty cycle. Radiographic findings showed a 98.9% decrease in the size of the ossified mass (Wieder, 1992).

Hyaluronidase has been used for the reduction of local oedema, but there remains considerable doubt about its stability and usefulness (Boone, 1981). Zinc iontophoresis in the treatment of ischaemic ulcers and for allergic rhinitis has been recommended and used in the past. The use of zinc as a wound dressing and its importance as a trace element in wound healing has now been recognized, so that its successful use on chronic ulcers is perhaps not so surprising (Cornwall, 1981). The dramatic skin erythema and weal produced by ethylmorphine hydrochloride (Renotin) or histamine iontophoresis was at one time widely used in the treatment of a large number of conditions (Kovacs, 1949; Taylor, 1949), but there seems to be no objective evidence of its effectiveness, with the result that this treatment is rarely used at present. Iodine and chlorine have been used to increase the extensibility of scar tissue in association with passive stretching (Tannenbaum, 1980; Cummings, 1987). Copper iontophoresis has been used for the treatment of fungal skin infections (tinea pedis) and salicylate for the relief of pain in rheumatic diseases, with no apparent evidence of any advantage over other simpler forms of treatment.

The therapeutic effectiveness of iontophoretically administered drugs has been purely a matter of opinion in the last 70 years or so when the fashion for it was at a peak. This has led to many unsupported claims of therapeutic efficacy and a subsequent backlash of scepticism. There is now though good evidence for some treatments, notably for hyperhidrosis, and the advantages of iontophoresis over local injection – it is non-invasive, there is no damage to tissues and it is sterile – may be important in the future.

Summary

Iontophoresis of appropriate drugs may be used for:

- local anaesthetic action
- the relief of hyperhidrosis
- an antibacterial action
- an anti-inflammatory action
- the relief of neurogenic pain
- other purposes including
  - oedema reduction
  - chronic wound healing
  - increase the extensibility of scars
  - fungal skin infections
  - relief of pain.

PRINCIPLES OF APPLICATION

Preparation of patient – explanation, examination and testing. First it is necessary to explain the nature of the treatment

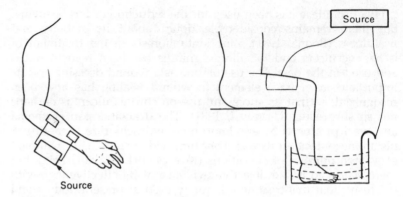

Fig. 2.4 A complete circuit for the application of d.c.

to the patient as well as the sensation (a mild prickling leading to a gentle warmth) that will be felt. It is very important to warn the patient to report any local increase in sensation or any painful sensation at once since there is a risk that a chemical burn may occur. Any increase of local current density may cause this chemical damage very rapidly; it may occur if there is an area of low skin resistance such as a cut, abrasion or papule. It can also occur if the skin resistance is uneven because some parts are covered with grease or due to uneven pressure from creases in the pad. It is therefore essential to examine the area for cuts and abrasions, establish by pinprick that the patient has normal pain sensation in the whole area of skin being treated and that he or she fully understands the need to report abnormal sensations.

Preparation of part to be treated. As the outer horny layer of the epidermis provides the main ohmic resistance to the current flow it is helpful to reduce this resistance by wetting and warming the skin prior to treatment by means of a warm soak or wash which also serves to remove excess surface oil or grease. Much of the current probably passes through the epidermis via the sweat glands.

Setting up. The principles of applying d.c. are the same whether it is the effect of the current alone that is intended or the iontophoresis of specific ions. The aim is to produce a uniform current density throughout the skin area to be treated. It is necessary to provide a complete circuit: current must enter and leave the tissues at separate sites (Fig. 2.4). For most treatments, only one site is of therapeutic interest, called the active electrode, while the other, designated the dispersive or indifferent electrode, is usually made to cover a much larger area – $2\frac{1}{2}$ times the area of the active electrode (Wadsworth and Chanmugan, 1980). This is done by applying the current through a container of water (or solution) or by using pads of suitable absorbent material to hold the water or solution. This material can be lint, gauze, sponge or suitable towelling. The pad must be thick enough to contain sufficient water; it should be at least 1 cm thick when lightly compressed. Such a thickness will usually ensure that it maintains good contact with the irregular skin surface and provides enough electrolyte to dilute harmful chemicals formed at the electrolyte–electrode junction.

The current is applied to the pad by some form of malleable carbon rubber electrode, aluminium foil or other metal sheet, which is made slightly smaller – 1 cm all round – than the pad. This is to reduce the likelihood of the bare electrode touching the skin. The wire should be connected to the electrode. The connection should make as little irregularity on the pad side of the electrode as possible so that the current spreads evenly over the whole area of the electrode. For the same reason the electrode should be flat and have rounded corners.

The pad and electrode are secured in position to ensure an even pressure over the whole area of the pad and hence uniform current density.

It is possible to treat the extremities by immersing the part to be treated in a container of water. The current is led in by an electrode clipped to the side of the container; the size of this electrode does not matter but it should be situated well away from the immersed body part (Fig. 2.4).

If a water bath is used for one electrode or two baths are used, one for each electrode (monopolar baths), it is important additionally to warn the patient not to remove a limb from the bath during treatment since this will break the circuit, interrupting the current and causing a marked sensory shock and perhaps muscle twitch. While not usually dangerous this may alarm the patient. It will also be noted that the current density is higher in the skin close to the surface of the water, hence there will be more sensation in this area. This is due to the fact that current can pass both in the tissues and through the water in the bath but where the limb emerges at the surface all the current must pass through the tissues, thus the path of lowest resistance is through the skin near the surface of the water.

Application. When applying the current it is essential to increase the intensity slowly and never to switch on or off with the intensity control above zero, as this can cause abrupt sensory and motor stimulation – a shock. The passage of the current is reputed to reduce the skin resistance during the first few minutes of treatment (Wadsworth and Chanmugan, 1980) so that the reading on the meter may increase a little without the control being moved.

The technique for the application of iontophoresis involves ensuring that the drug to be driven into the skin is placed beneath the correct electrode. Positively charged ions must obviously be placed under the positive electrode and negative ions under the negative. All the ions mentioned above that are used therapeutically are positively charged, hence they should be placed under the positive electrode – except for acetate, chloride, iodide and salicylate, which are all negatively charged. Sometimes the solution used is quite expensive – glycopyrronium bromide, for example – so that it is economical to use small quantities of the drug. When the hands and feet are being treated for hyperhidrosis a suitably sized pad and electrode can be enclosed with the hand or foot in a small plastic bag rather than using a shallow bowl or tray of solution.

Practical point
In order to prevent the bandage being wetted, thus transmitting current to the adjacent tissues, it is best to separate the bandage from the wet pad by a suitably sized piece of waterproof material such as polythene.

Practical point
This effect can be reduced by applying an irregular thin coat of petroleum jelly to the skin, just below the surface of the water.

Practical point
If the meter should indicate a sudden increase in current it is important to turn the control down slowly and inspect the area since this indication of lowered resistance may signal the beginning of a chemical burn.

DOSAGE

The introduction of ions into the tissues by iontophoresis depends on both current density and time, already noted and described (see Fig. 2.2). Many texts simply suggest total currents rather than current densities, and approximate times (Wadsworth and Chanmugan, 1980; Forster and Palastanga, 1985). As can be seen from Figure 2.2, increasing the time of treatment for any given current density makes proportionally smaller increases in ionic transfer. Thus it seems that the rather approximate dosage recommendations are quite reasonable for iontophoresis, since current densities that are detectable and yet are comfortably tolerable will be in the region of $0.1–0.2 \, mA/cm^2$ and even if the extremes of these current densities are used the number of ions transferred less than doubles between 10 and 40 min.

Using glycopyrrolate for hyperhidrosis it has been suggested that 12 mA for 12 min is appropriate for one adult hand; that is, a current density of $0.08–0.1 \, mA/cm^2$ (Morgan, 1980) or 15–20 mA for 15 min (Wadsworth and Chanmugan, 1980). Since the current is limited by the patient's tolerance this should always be at a comfortable level and the dosage made up by compensating with the time of treatment. Thus the dosage can be expressed in 'mA min', i.e. total current multiplied by the treatment time. Personal experience (JL) suggests that dosages of between 100 and 200 mA min are appropriate for each hand or foot and this conforms with the dosage suggested by Morgan (1980) and others. It must be remembered that systemic as well as local effects occur and these are unwanted and unpleasant side-effects (see below). The dosage must be kept below the level at which these effects occur, which varies from patient to patient. It is sensible to give a low dose (less than 100 mA min) for the initial treatment and assess the effects. With children the initial dose should be even less – 50–70 mA min. Most adults seem able to have both hands or both feet treated at one session without serious side-effects.

Treatments that produce an immediately detectable effect – such as anhidrosis due to glycopyrrolate or anaesthesia due to lignocaine will indicate their own effective dose at the end of treatment. If the effect of treatment is inadequate then it may be continued for a longer time.

For other iontophoretic treatments the dosage is similar to that for hyperhidrosis but often longer times are suggested – 5 mA for a $100 \, cm^2$ pad, i.e. $0.05 \, mA/cm^2$, for 20–30 min has been suggested for iodine (Tannenbaum, 1980) and acetate (Wadsworth and Chanmugan, 1980). Many writers give only the total current, not current density, but since most treatments are given over areas of $50–200 \, cm^2$ the 5–20 mA current usually suggested represents currents of about $0.1 \, mA/cm^2$. The times suggested vary from 10 to 30 min.

When direct current is used for pain relief and not for iontophoresis the recommended dosage varies depending on polarity. If the cathode (negative pole) is being used to achieve a pain-relieving effect then relatively high current densities of $0.5–0.8 \, mA/cm^2$ for 10–20 min have been suggested. If the positive pole is to be used then lower current densities of $0.15–0.25 \, mA/cm^2$ for 15–30 min have been suggested (Wadsworth and Chanmugan, 1980).

DANGERS

- Chemical damage to the tissues, a chemical burn, can occur as a result of the current density becoming too high. This can arise in a multitude of ways. Low skin resistance due to cuts or abrasions, uneven pressure or thickness of pads have already been mentioned. There is also danger of a burn if a bare piece of the metal lead or electrode inadvertently touches the skin.
- A shock can occur if the circuit is broken so that the current is interrupted, such as would happen if the current is switched off without being turned down slowly. This may happen in a number of ways – such as a lead breaking during treatment or the patient removing a hand from the bath – but with the relatively low currents employed there is no damage, except that the patient will suffer an alarming shock.
- Some patients experience a skin irritation caused by hyper-sensitivity to the chemicals produced by the current. It can usually be prevented by washing the treated part after treatment.
- Systemic effects can occur, especially if large areas are treated by iontophoresis. With anticholinergic drugs these can take the form of headaches, abdominal pains or mild dryness of the mouth. Patients should be warned to avoid vigorous exercise immediately after treatment, and if the symptoms are severe the area of treatment should be reduced. Pregnancy is a contraindication. Balogun *et al.* (1991) investigated the cardio-vascular responses during histamine iontophoresis therapy and found it did not appreciably alter the blood pressure or heart rate responses of normal subjects. However, they recommended that physiotherapists should question patients about any previous history of skin reaction following histamine injection, dizziness, fainting, chronic headache or hypotension, since it is expected that patients with these precipitating conditions will produce exaggerated responses. They also recommended that the cardiovascular responses and skin reactions of such patients should be closely monitored before, during and after histamine iontophoresis.

Summary

Possible dangers using d.c.:

- chemical burn
- unexpected shock
- skin irritation
- specific dangers due to iontophoresis of drugs
  - reduced skin sensitivity (anaesthetizing drugs)
  - systemic effects (anticholinergic drugs; histamine-like drugs).

REFERENCES

Abell E., Morgan K. (1974). The treatment of idiopathic hyperhidrosis by glycopyrronium bromide and tap water iontophoresis. *Br. J. Dermatol.*, **91**, 45–60.

Akins D. L., Meisenheimer J. L., Dobson R. L. (1987). Efficacy of the Drionic unit in the treatment of hyperhidrosis. *J. Am. Acad. Dermatol.*, **16**, 828–33.

Alon G. (1987). Principles of electrical stimulation. In *Clinical Electrotherapy* (Nelson R. M., Currier D. P., eds) Norwalk, Connecticut, USA: Appleton Lange, pp. 29–80.

Alvarez O. M., Mertz P. M., Smerbock R. V. *et al.* (1983). The healing of superficial skin wounds is stimulated by external electric current. *J. Invest. Dermatol.*, **81**, 144–8.

Balogun J. A., Adeniyi E. A., Akala E. O. (1991). Cardiovascular responses during histamine iontophoresis therapy. *Aust. J. Physiother.*, **37**, 105–10.

Becker R. O., Spadaro J. A. (1978). Treatment of orthopaedic infections with electrically generated silver ions. *J. Bone Joint Surg.*, **60A**, 871–81.

Becker R. O., Spadaro J. A., Marino A. A. (1977). Clinical experience with low intensity direct current stimulation of bone growth. *Clin. Orthop.*, **124**, 75–83.

Boone C. (1981). Applications of iontophoresis. In *Electrotherapy* (Wolfe S. L., ed.) New York: Churchill Livingstone, pp. 99–121.

Bourguignon G. J., Bourguignon L. Y. W. (1987). Electric stimulation of protein and DNA synthesis in human fibroblasts. *Fed. Am. Soc. Exp. Biol. J.*, **1**, 398–408.

Brighton C. T., Black J., Friedenberg Z. B. *et al.* (1981). Multicentre study of treatment of non-union with constant direct current. *J. Bone Joint Surg.*, **63A**, 2–13.

Brown M., McDonnell M. K., Menton D. M. (1988). Electrical stimulation effects on cutaneous wound healing in rabbits. *Phys. Ther.*, **68**, 955–9.

Byl N. N., McKenzie A. L., West J. M., Whitney J. D., Hunt T. K., Hopf H. W., Scheuenstuhl H. (1994). Pulsed microamperage stimulation: a controlled study of healing of surgically induced wounds in Yucatan pigs. *Phys. Ther.*, **74**, 201–19.

Carley P. J., Wainapel S. F. (1985). Electrotherapy for acceleration of wound healing: low intensity direct current. *Arch. Phys. Med. Rehabil.*, **66**, 443–6.

Cornwall M. W. (1981). Zinc iontophoresis to treat ischaemic skin ulcers. *Phys. Ther.*, **61**, 359–60.

Costello C. T., Jeske A. H. (1995). Iontophoresis: Applications in transdermal medication delivery. *Phys. Ther.*, **75**, 554–63.

Csillik B., Knyihár-Csillik E., Szücs A. (1982). Treatment of chronic pain syndromes with iontophoresis of vinca alkaloids to the skin of patients. *Neurosci. Lett.*, **31**, 87–90.

Cummings J. (1987). Iontophoresis. In *Clinical Electrotherapy* (Nelson R. M., Currier D. P., eds) Norwalk, USA: Appleton & Lange, pp. 231–41.

Demirtaş R. N., Ömer C. (1998). The treatment of lateral epicondylitis by iontophoresis of sodium salicylate and sodium diclofenac. *Clin. Rehab.*, **12**, 23–9.

Erickson C. A., Nuccitelli R. (1984). Embryonic fibroblast motility and orientation can be influenced by physiological electric fields. *J Cell Biol.*, **98**, 296–307.

Feedar J. A., Kloth L. C., Gentzkow G. D. (1991). Chronic dermal ulcer healing enhanced with monophasic pulsed electrical stimulation. *Phys. Ther.*, **71**, 639–49.

Forster A., Palastanga N. (1985). *Clayton's Electrotherapy: Theory and Practice*, 9th edn. London: Baillière Tindall.

Gangarosa L. P., Park N. H., Wiggins C. A., Hill J. M. (1980). Increased penetration of non-electrolytes into mouse skin during iontophoretic water transport (iontohydrokinesis). *J. Pharm. Exp. Ther.*, **212**, 377–81.

Ganong W. F. (1991). *Review of Medical Physiology*, 15th edn. Connecticut: Appleton Lange.

Gault W. R., Gatens P. F. (1976). Use of low intensity direct current in management of ischaemic skin ulcers. *Phys. Ther.*, **56**, 265–8.

Glass J. M., Stephan B. L., Jacobsen S. C. (1980). The quantity and distribution of radiolabelled dexamethasone delivered to tissues by iontophoresis. *Int. J. Dermatol.*, **19**, 519–25.

Grice K., Sattar H., Baker H. (1972). Treatment of idiopathic hyperhidrosis with iontophoresis of tap water and poldine methosulphate. *Br J. Dermatol.*, **86**, 72.

Griffin J. W., Tooms R. E., Mendius R. A. *et al.* (1991). Efficacy of high voltage pulsed currents for healing of pressure ulcers in patients with spinal cord injury. *Phys. Ther.*, **71**, 433–42.

Hasson S. H., Henderson G. H., Daniels J. C., Schieb D. A. (1991). Exercise training and dexamethasone iontophoresis in rheumatoid arthritis. *Physiother. Can.*, **43**, 11–14.

Humphrey C. E., Seal E. H. (1959). Biological approach toward tumour regression in mice. *Science*, **130**, 388–89.

Kahn J. (1994). *Principles and Practice of Electrotherapy*, 3rd edn. Edinburgh: Churchill Livingstone.

Kloth L. C., Feedar J. A. (1988). Acceleration of wound healing with high voltage, monophasic, pulsed current. *Phys. Ther.*, **68**, 503–8.

Kloth L. C., Feedar J. A. (1990). Electrical stimulation in tissue repair. In *Wound Healing: Alternatives in Management* (Kloth L. C., McCulloch J. M., Feedar J. A., eds) Philadelphia: Davis, 221–56.

Knyihár-Csillik E., Szücs A., Csillik B. (1982). Iontophoretically applied microtubule inhibitors induce transganglionic degenerative atrophy of primary central nociceptive terminals and abolish chronic autochthonus pain. *Acta Neurol. Scand.*, **66**, 401–12.

Kovacs R. (1949). *Electrotherapy and Light Therapy*, 6th edn. London: Henry Kimpton.

La Forrest N. T., Cofrancesco C. (1978). Antibiotic iontophoresis in the treatment of ear chondritis. *Phys. Ther.*, **58**, 32–4.

Layman P. R., Argyras E., Glynn C. J. (1986). Iontophoresis of vincristine versus saline in post-herpetic neuralgia. A controlled trial. *Pain*, **25**, 165–70.

Lettman D. J., Arnall D. A., Holmgren P. R., Cornwall M. W. (1994) Effect of microamperage stimulation on the rate of wound healing in rats: a histological study. *Phys. Ther.*, **74**, 195–200.

Licht S. (1983). History of electrotherapy. In *Therapeutic Electricity and Ultraviolet Radiations* 3rd edn (Stillwell G. K., ed.) Baltimore: Williams & Wilkins, pp. 1–64.

Midtgaard K. (1986). A new device for the treatment of hyperhidrosis by iontophoresis. *Br. J. Dermatol.*, **114**, 485–8.

Morgan K. (1980). The technique of treating hyperhidrosis by iontophoresis. *Physiotherapy*, **66**, 45.

Mulder G. D. (1991). Treatment of open-skin wounds with electric stimulation. *Arch. Phys. Med. Rehabil.*, **72**, 375–7.

Myers R. S. (1991). High voltage pulsed current enhancement of chronic dermal wound and ulcer healing: a meta-analysis. *WCPT 11th International Congress Proceedings, Book II*, London: World Confederation for Physical Therapy, 798–800.

Newton R. (1987). High voltage pulsed galvanic stimulation: theoretical bases and clinical applications. In *Clinical Electrotherapy* (Nelson R. M., Currier D. P., eds) Norwalk, CT: Appleton Lange, pp. 165–82.

O'Malley E. P., Oester Y. T. (1955). Influences of some physical chemical factors on iontophoresis using radio-isotopes. *Arch. Phys. Med. Rehabil.*, **36**, 310.

Pratzel H., Dittrich P., Kukovetz W. (1986) Spontaneous and forced cutaneous absorption of indomethacin in pigs and humans. *J. Rheumatol.*, **13**, 1122–5.

Reich J. D., Tarjan P. P. (1990). Electrical stimulation of skin. *Int. J Dermatol.*, **29**, 395–400.

Russo J., Lipman A. G., Comstock T. J. *et al.* (1980). Lidocaine anaesthesia: comparison of iontophoresis, injection and swabbing. *Am. J. Hosp. Pharmacol.*, **37**, 843–7.

Tannenbaum M. (1980). Iodine iontophoresis in reducing scar tissue. *Phys. Ther.*, **60**, 792.

Taylor G. A. (1949). A new drug for iontophoresis. *Physiotherapy*, **49**.

Trubatch J., Van Harreveld A. (1972). Spread of iontophoretically injected ions in a tissue. *J. Theor. Biol.*, **36**, 355–66.

Van Herp G. (1997). Iontophoresis: a review of the literature. *N. Z. J. Physiother.*, Aug, 16–17.

Wadsworth H., Chanmugan A. P. P. (1980). *Electrophysical Agents in Physiotherapy*. Marrickville, Australia: Science Press.

Watson T. (1996). Electrical stimulation for wound healing. In *Clayton's Electrotherapy*, 10th edn (Kitchen S., Bazin S., eds) Philadelphia: W. B. Saunders, pp. 323–48.

Weiss D. S., Eaglestein W. H., Falanga V. (1989). Exogenous electric current can reduce the formation of hypertrophic scars. *J. Dermatol. Surg. Oncol.*, **15**, 1272–5.

Weiss D. S., Kirsner R., Eaglestein W. H. (1990). Electrical stimulation and wound healing. *Archives of Dermatology*, **126**, 222–5.

Wieder D. L. (1992). Treatment of traumatic myositis ossificans with acetic acid iontophoresis. *Phys. Ther.*, **72**, 133–7.

Wolcott L. E., Wheeler P. C., Hardwicke H. M. (1969). Accelerated healing of skin ulcers by electrotherapy: preliminary clinical results. *South. Med. J.*, **62**, 795–801.

3 Electrical stimulation of nerve and muscle

From the twitch of a frog's leg, described by Galvani, to the tingling of a transcutaneous nerve stimulator the word 'electrotherapy' commonly conjures up the concept of currents stimulating the body. Hence this chapter may be considered central to the subject.

It begins with the principles, definitions and descriptions of the different types of therapeutic currents. If the chapter were thought to have a mission it would be to emphasize the need for accurate descriptions of currents and their modulation. (The whole of electrotherapy seems to have been bedevilled by inadequate descriptions of the modalities used – study after study has been done in which the results cannot be compared with one another due to insufficient measurement of the modality.) There is therefore no apology offered for taking time and space to try to elucidate the plethora of names, both historical and modern, generated by fads, fashions and commercialism. Others have made similar pleas (e.g. Alon, 1987; Singer *et al.*, 1987).

The production of electrical pulses is briefly outlined. This is followed by an important section explaining the way in which electrical stimulation acts on the peripheral nerves, including the effect of varying rates of current rise and pulse frequency.

The physiological and therapeutic effects are next considered, in particular the stimulation of innervated muscle, including the effects on strength and fatigue and the effect on pain. At this point the nature of peripheral pain is briefly discussed as well as the mechanisms whereby it may be relieved.

This is followed by consideration of the general principles of application of currents to the tissues including a discussion of current flow in the tissues and descriptions of the placement of electrodes. Then there are descriptions of the application and uses of many different current types. These include TENS, HVPGS, interferential currents, diadynamic currents, low-frequency muscle stimulating currents, and several others.

Finally, safety considerations are explained and discussed.

PRINCIPLES

It is important first to understand the effects of electric charges on the body tissues in general terms. These effects depend on the *rate of change* of the applied electric pulse:

- If there is no change, or only a very slow change, of current amplitude and no change of current direction (polarity) the resulting steady flow of ions into the tissues will cause chemical changes at the electrode–tissue junction, as described in Chapter 2.
- If there is a faster rate of change, the ionic balance across excitable cell membranes is disturbed stimulating nerves and muscles. If this current is unidirectional it will cause chemical changes, as above, but if it is evenly alternating no such changes can occur because any change in one direction is cancelled when the current reverses.
- If there is a very rapid and even change in amplitude and direction then there is insufficient time for transmembrane excitation to occur, nor can there be chemical changes. Thus larger currents can be used, which are able to cause tissue heating, the basis of diathermy (see Chapter 10). Of course, heating will occur due to any current passing through the tissues if it is of sufficient intensity, but the chemical and excitable tissue stimulation will occur at low intensities with the appropriate current form.

This chapter then, is concerned with those current forms that change at a rate sufficient to stimulate nerve and muscle tissue. Apart from the overall term – neuromuscular electrical stimulation (NMES) – they are given a whole multitude of names.

All stimulators of nerve tissue (except implanted stimulators) are in fact transcutaneous electrical nerve stimulators (TENS), but this term is usually applied only to low-intensity, usually battery-operated, sensory nerve stimulators used for pain control. Such names as faradic, galvanic or diadynamic, historically applied to specify certain therapeutic currents, often overlap and are used inconsistently.

It is convenient to describe the unit of stimulating current as a 'pulse' of current; when this is unidirectional it can be called a current 'phase'. This will cause one (or two) nerve impulses. The simple graphs given in Figure 3.1 and subsequent figures illustrate the relationship of time with amplitude and hence the rate of change of current described as the waveform. Thus in Figure 3.1(a) a slow rise, steady, unidirectional current, and a slow fall, illustrate the therapeutic direct current described in Chapter 2.

If the rise is made rapid – i.e. there is a high rate of change – then nerve stimulation occurs leading to a nerve impulse, shown in Figure 3.1(b) (see Chapter 1). This will happen both when the current rises and when it falls. If the time for which the current flows is made shorter, say 1 ms, as in Figure 3.1(c), then there is no time for the nerve membrane to recover and only a single nerve impulse results. The consequence of (b) and (c) would be to stimulate sensory nerves giving a series of single nerve impulses recognized consciously as a series of little shocks. Similarly, if the current amplitude was a little larger, motor nerves would be stimulated leading to a series of single muscle twitches. If these stimuli are repeated every 10 ms they will cause a steady tingling sensation as

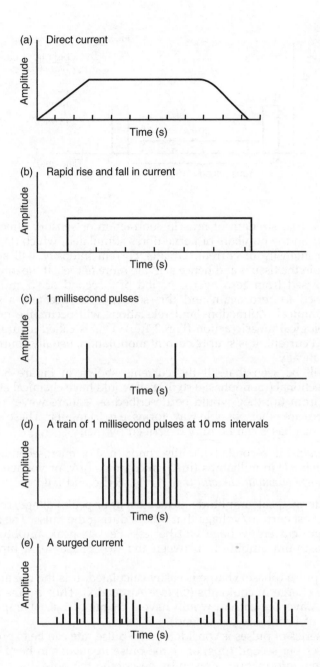

(a) Direct current

Amplitude

Time (s)

(b) Rapid rise and fall in current

Amplitude

Time (s)

(c) 1 millisecond pulses

Amplitude

Time (s)

(d) A train of 1 millisecond pulses at 10 ms intervals

Amplitude

Time (s)

(e) A surged current

Amplitude

Time (s)

Fig. 3.1 The relationship of time and current.

they stimulate sensory nerves and a tetanic muscle contraction as they stimulate the motor nerves; this is shown in Figure 3.1(d) (see also Chapter 1). Such currents at low intensities produced by small battery-operated electronic stimulators are used for pain control in TENS stimulators. At higher intensities they are used for muscle stimulation.

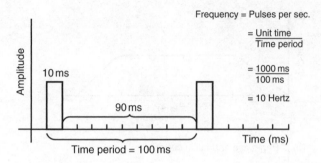

Fig. 3.2 Relationship of frequency (f) to time period.

The actual strength of muscle contraction or sensory effect will depend on the numbers of nerve fibres stimulated, which depends on the intensity of current. Greater current intensity will spread further in the tissues and hence activate more nerves. If the intensity is increased from zero over a period of a second or so and then decreased to zero again and this sequence is repeated, a series of rhythmical contractions and relaxations will occur like normal physiological muscle action (Fig. 3.1(e)). This is called a surged or ramped current. It is simply current modulation, usually controlled automatically.

It will be seen that all the currents shown in Figure 3.1 are unidirectional (monophasic) so that all would have chemical effects. Apart from (a), they would be described as 'square wave' pulses but there are other possible waveforms, e.g. triangular. These single pulses or phases can be fully described by their:

- *duration* in seconds (s), milliseconds (ms) or microseconds (µs);
- *amplitude* in milliamps (mA), microamps (µA) or voltage (V);
- *change of amplitude with time* – rate of rise and fall.

The terms peak amplitude, peak current or peak voltage, refer to the highest current/voltage that occurs during the pulse. The mean (average) current/voltage will be less. Peak-to-peak amplitude is the maximum amplitude between the two phases of a biphasic current.

The pulse (phase) charge is easily calculated. It is the quantity of electric charge in coulombs (C) (see Appendix). Thus a 1 ms pulse of 1 mA average current would have a charge of 1 µC (1 ampere is a flow of 1 coulomb per second).

If a series of pulses is considered, the pulse rate can be expressed in pulses per second (pps) or as the pulse frequency in hertz (Hz). The same information is given by describing the pulse interval, or interpulse interval, expressed in s, ms or µs. Thus a series of 10 ms pulses separated by 90 ms pulse intervals will have a frequency of 10 Hz (Fig. 3.2).

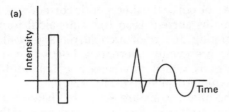

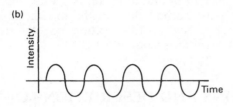

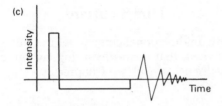

Fig. 3.3 Different forms of biphasic current. (a) Discrete pulses; (b) continuous pulses; (c) asymmetrical pulses.

Summary of terms describing electrotherapeutic currents:

- pulse – an isolated electrical event separated by a finite time from the next event described by its
  - amplitude in mA, μA, or V
  - duration in ms or μs
  - rise time and decay time in ms or μs
- phase – current in one direction for a finite time. Synonymous with a unidirectional, hence monophasic, pulse
- waveform – shape of the visual representation of a pulse on an amplitude–time plot
- interpulse intervals – time between successive pulses
- frequency – number of pulses per unit time; pulses per second in Hz.

So far consideration has only been given to unidirectional pulses. Many pulses used therapeutically are biphasic. Current passes first in one then in the opposite direction (Fig. 3.3(a)). Such individual pulses may be separated by various pulse intervals like monophasic phases or they can be continuous (Fig. 3.3(b)). When such continuous pulses follow a sine curve the therapeutic current is called sinusoidal current. The mains current is in this sinusoidal form. Due to the constantly changing direction, such currents are called alternating currents. These are evenly alternating but it is common to have uneven alternations, which may be of unequal amplitude, unequal duration or asymmetrical shape (Fig. 3.3(c)).

Clearly if the alternations are equal in charge there will be no total current flow and hence no chemical changes. If the alternations are such that current in one direction is greater than in the other there will be a net current flow in the former direction. For an authoritative approach to this section see the report by the Electrotherapy Standards Committee (1990).

DEFINITIONS AND DESCRIPTIONS OF TYPES OF CURRENT USED THERAPEUTICALLY

Direct current

This refers to any unidirectional current but it is often used to mean *constant direct current*, that is an unvarying current also known as *galvanism* or a *galvanic current* (see Chapter 2).

Low-frequency stimulation

Each pulse of current depolarizes the nerve fibre. The pulse repetition rate can be up to 1000 pps (1 KHz). The pulses may be all in one direction – uniphasic – or in both directions – biphasic.

Each pulse can also be either constant current or constant voltage. These are both consequences of the way in which resistances in the internal circuit of the machine are arranged; they diminish changes of the electrical pulse due to alterations of external resistance, such as that due to the pads or gel drying out. Where the electrodes are fixed or stationary, constant current is usually used, but if 1 electrode is moved during treatment – a dynamic application – constant voltage is preferable. This prevents the current density from becoming uncomfortably high if the area of the pad in contact with the tissues is reduced.

Pulsed currents

If the continuous unidirectional current is interrupted it gives a series of pulses or phases of unidirectional current which can be of any duration or shape, repeated at any frequency. Certain durations, shapes and frequencies have acquired particular names so that although any unidirectional pulse is an interrupted direct current (i.d.c.), the term is customarily used to describe only the longer-duration pulses.

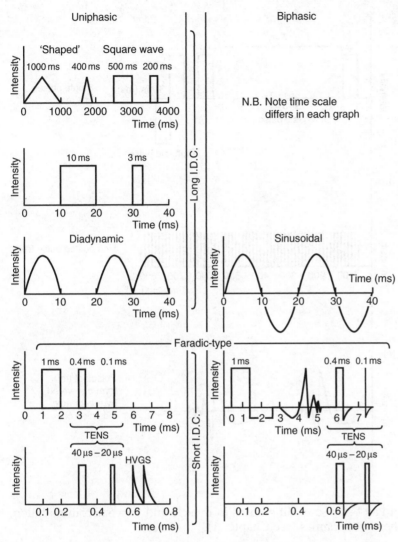

Fig. 3.4 Comparison of low-frequency currents: pulses, shapes and durations. Note that the time scale differs in each graph.

Long duration (of 1 ms or more)

Rectangular wave pulses. These are pulses of any duration between 1 and 600 ms separated by pulse intervals of anything from 1 ms to several seconds (Fig. 3.2 and Fig. 3.4). Such pulses can stimulate motor and sensory nerves and can be used to stimulate denervated muscle.

Accommodation pulses. Triangular, trapezoidal, sawtooth, serrate, slow-rising, shaped, selective and accommodation pulses are all synonymous terms. Again, these are relatively long-duration pulses, usually 300–1000 ms, separated by pulse intervals of one-half to several seconds (Fig. 3.4). These pulses are used to stimulate muscle (as opposed to nerve) tissue selectively and they are able to

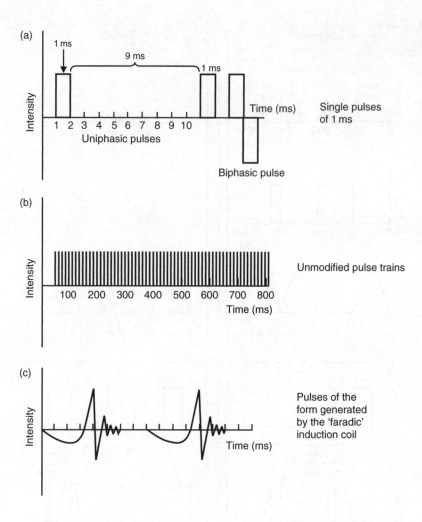

Fig. 3.5 Short-duration muscle stimulating pulses.

do so because of differences in muscle and nerve accommodation,
hence the names (see Chapter 1).

Short duration (of 1 ms or less)

Faradic-type pulses. Pulses used for the stimulation of muscle
via the motor nerve employ pulses of 0.1–1 ms at frequencies
between 30 and 100 Hz and may be called faradic-type pulses. Such
pulses were originally generated by an induction coil and interrupter
which, because it was an electromagnetic device, was called a faradic
coil (Fig. 3.5(c)). They may be uniphasic or biphasic. Stimuli used
in trophic electrotherapy are often 80 μs but can be as short as 50 μs.

TENS. It has already been pointed out that all nerve-stimulating
pulses are TENS, but the term is usually restricted to pulses of
relatively low intensity used to control pain. Almost all such
generators are battery-operated. A variety of pulse forms are
available. A few are monophasic, i.e. short pulse i.d.c., but the

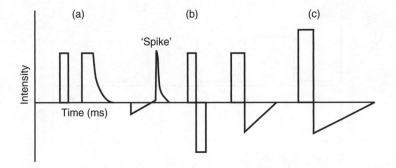

Fig. 3.6 Types of TENS pulses: (a) mono-phasic; (b) biphasic; (c) increasing intensity of biphasic pulse needs a balancing increase of pulse duration of the second phase.

majority are symmetrically or asymmetrically biphasic (Fig. 3.6 and Fig. 3.4). Pulse durations, often fixed for a given source, can be any length from 10 μs to 400 μs. The frequency is usually variable and ranges from 2 to 200 Hz. Voltage, and thus the applied current, can be varied but is limited to low amplitudes; the maximum peak current is between 50 and 100 mA. The safest of these pulses will be biphasic with no nett d.c. component. Various waveforms are illustrated in Figure 3.6. To maintain an even charge in biphasic pulses when the amplitude is increased it is necessary to alter the pulse shape. The increased amplitude is compensated by an increased duration of the alternate phase, also illustrated in Figure 3.6.

In describing these pulses, the simple square wave form has been assumed and illustrated, but when the pulse is applied through the skin the shape of the phase is influenced by the tissue capacitance. Thus for a constant current pulse the voltage would rise rapidly at first and then more slowly as the tissue capacitance charges. The reverse occurs as the current falls. For a constant voltage pulse there will be a large initial current flow which falls in the manner illustrated in Figure 3.7 (Patterson, 1983).

H-wave.   This is a form of TENS consisting of a series of biphasic exponentially decaying pulses of around 11 ms. Each phase has a rapid rise (about 12 μs) followed by an exponential fall lasting some 5.3 ms (see Fig. 3.8). The amplitude is variable up to a peak-to-peak voltage of around 60–65 V. The frequency can also be altered up to about 60 Hz – hence 120 phases per sec.

The waveform is intended to be similar to the electromyographic output from the H reflex, described in Chapter 4, hence the name.

While this form of current is like other TENS pulses (indeed with its evenly biphasic form and sharp voltage spike at mid-frequencies it bears a remarkable similarity to the mechanically generated faradism of yesteryear), it may be noted that the second phase follows during the partial refractory period of many neurons. The significance of this special feature is not known.

Electroacupuncture.   Various current forms are in use. It can be a pulse consisting of a few seconds of d.c. or a form of low-frequency, high-intensity TENS.

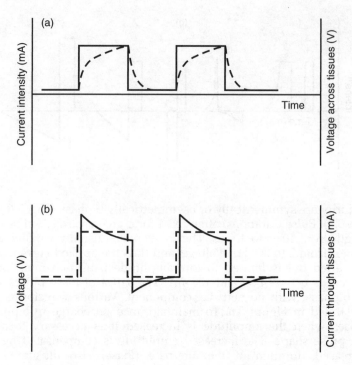

Fig. 3.7 Tissue voltage and current resulting from applied pulses: (a) constant current pulse (continuous line) and resultant voltage across the tissues (broken line); (b) constant voltage pulse (broken line) and resulting current in tissues (continuous line).

High-voltage galvanic stimulation (HVGS) or high-voltage pulsed galvanic stimulation (HVPGS). This form of current was originally developed in the USA and given this name (see Fig. 3.4).

The twin pulse waveform has almost instantaneous rises with exponential falls. The pair of pulses lasts for only 0.1 ms and each peak lasts for only a few microseconds; the shape and duration are normally fixed. The frequency of the double pulse can be varied, usually from 2 to 100 Hz. With such short peaks very high voltages are needed (hence the name) to provide high enough currents to stimulate nerve fibres (see Fig. 3.13). Peak currents of 2–2.5 A (Alon, 1987) may be generated during the few microseconds of peak voltage but, of course, the total average current is very low, at around 1.2–1.5 mA.

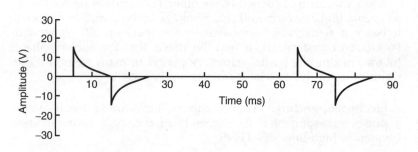

Fig. 3.8 H-wave – evenly biphasic pulses; in this example, illustrated at approximately 16 Hz and 32 V peak to peak.

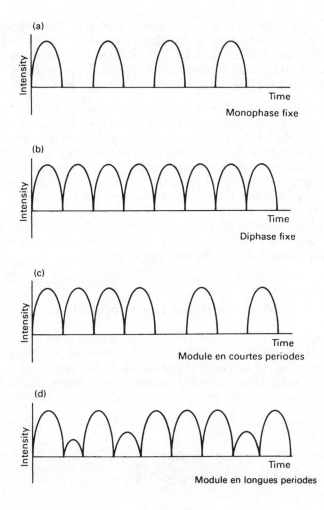

Fig. 3.9 Diadynamic pulse modes.

Alternating

Sinusoidal currents

Sinusoidal currents are evenly alternating sine wave currents of 50 Hz, the form of the UK mains current (see Fig. 3.4). This gives 100 phases in each second of 10 ms each, 50 in one direction and 50 in the other. It can be produced from the mains by reducing the voltage to 60 or 80 V with a step-down transformer.

Diadynamic currents

Diadynamic currents were introduced by Pierre Bernard nearly 70 years ago. They are monophasic sinusoidal currents, being rectified mains-type current. Diadynamic currents have two basic forms:

1 Half-wave rectified sinusoidal current known as MF (*monophase fixe*). This consists of a series of 10 ms half sine wave-shaped pulses with 10 ms pulse intervals.

2 Full-wave rectified sinusoidal current known as DF (*diphase fixe*). This is a continuous series of 10 ms sinusoidal pulses resulting in a frequency of 100 Hz (Fig. 3.9). (Note that the above refers to rectified 50 Hz mains current. If 60 Hz mains, as in the USA, is used then the pulse lengths and intervals will be 8.333 ms.)

If these two current forms – MF and DF – are applied alternately for 1 s each the resulting current is called CP module (*module en courtes périodes*). If two MF currents are applied so that one series of pulses occupies the pulse intervals of the other and one is of constant intensity while the other is surged, the result is called LP module (*module en longues périodes*). The length of each surge and surge interval varies with different sources but is usually 5 or 6 s (Fig. 3.9).

The physiological effects of such currents will cause sensory and motor nerve stimulation and thus muscle contraction, as well as chemical changes due to the unidirectional current.

Medium frequency stimulation

Medium frequency currents have pulse repetition rates greater than 1 kHz. At this frequency, each phase of current cannot stimulate a nerve impulse, as succeeding pulses fall in the refractory period. The usual methods of allowing for the repolarization of the nerve membrane are either by amplitude modulation (IFT) or interruption (Russian).

Medium frequency direct current

This is referred to in Chapter 2 (p. 31).

Rebox-type current

The Rebox is a device that was developed in Czechoslovakia in the 1970s. There is a hand-held dispersive and current is delivered by a point-type electrode. The point electrode is made the negative pole. The current consists of unipolar rectangular pulses of between 50 µs and 250 µs at 3000 Hz; thus it is a medium-frequency current. The circuit also contains a microammeter and an earphone and can be linked to a small computer and printer to display a graph of current and other parameters.

'Russian' currents

This consists of a 2500 Hz evenly alternating medium frequency current applied as a series of separate bursts. There are thus 50 periods of 20 ms duration consisting of a 10 ms burst and a 10 ms interval. Each 10 ms burst contains 25 cycles of alternating current, i.e. 50 phases of 0.2 ms duration.

Interferential currents

The principle of interferential therapy is to cause two medium-frequency currents of slightly differing frequencies to interfere with one another. Where they do so, a new resultant current is set up. The resultant amplitude at any given point is the sum of the two individual current amplitudes, so that where two peaks or two troughs coincide, they will augment each other, but where a peak and trough coincide they cancel each other out (see Fig. 3.10(a)).

Providing the amplitudes of the two individual currents are the same, the resultant current frequency will be the mean of the two. For example, if current A is 4000 Hz and current B is 4100 Hz, the resultant current frequency will be 4050 Hz.

This resultant current varies in amplitude. The frequency with which it varies is called the amplitude modulation frequency, or beat frequency, and is equal to the difference in frequency between the two individual currents (in the above instance, 100 Hz). When the amplitude of this modulated pulse reaches the nerve threshold it triggers an impulse.

Again, if the amplitude of the two individual, medium-frequency currents is equal, the beating will be 100%, as in Figure 3.10(a). This is unlikely when two currents are passing in the tissues because they will inevitably have paths of different resistance. In this case there is partial beating (see Fig. 3.10(b)) and the 'modulation depth' will not be 100%.

High-frequency currents

High-frequency currents of millions of hertz are used therapeutically but they cannot stimulate nerve or muscle, because they change too rapidly. They can be safely applied at a high current intensity to produce tissue heating (see Chapter 10).

Summary of the types of therapeutic electrical pulses

- pulses lasting 1 ms or more (long duration)
  - rectangular/square-wave pulses
  - accommodation pulses
- pulses of less than 1 ms (short duration)
  - muscle-stimulating
  - TENS
  - H-Wave
  - HVPGS
- sinusoidal waveforms of low frequency – 50–60 Hz
  - evenly alternating – sinusoidal current
  - uniphasic – diadynamic currents
- sinusoidal waveforms of medium frequency – more than 1 kHz (in which nerve stimulation is due to modulation of the pulse train).
  - interferential currents
  - 'Russian' current
- uniphasic rectangular pulses of medium frequency
  - Rebox-type current.

The waveforms of these are largely summarized in Figure 3.4.

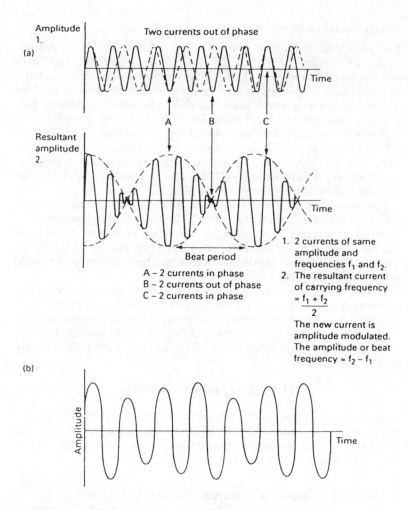

Fig. 3.10 (a) Interference of two medium-frequency currents. (b) Partial beating.

PRODUCTION OF ELECTRICAL PULSES

Commercially available electrotherapeutic equipment continues to be advertised as 'new' and innovative and considerable efforts are made to connect the trade name of the equipment to the treatment.

Most modern electrotherapeutic stimulators are able to provide a range of pulse widths, frequencies and intensities which can not only be separately controlled but can also be programmed (i.e. pre-set) to give a repeatable treatment.

Any report, study or account of electrotherapeutic applications should always include a description of the electrical pulses utilized, in terms of the parameters (duration, amplitude, shape, polarity and frequency, as described earlier), as well as the current density employed.

Modern pulse generators are based on integrated circuits of transistors, resistors and capacitors.

The pulse felt at the wrist is simply a wave of fluid, i.e. blood pressure, which is generated by the action of the heart. An electrical pulse – using the word in another context but similar sense – is produced by the same basic mechanism. As the heart contracts (ventricular systole) the pressure in the arteries rises and causes the blood to flow at a higher pressure for a time while the aortic valve is open. When it closes the pressure in the arteries falls (ventricular diastole). This cycle is repeated at a rate determined by the sinoatrial node. Thus a system exerting a pressure (voltage) causes a flow (current) which is turned on and off by a valve (switch). The time for which the pressure is exerted, i.e. heart muscle contraction, is controlled by the rhythmicity of the sinoatrial node acting as a timing device. In a modern pulse generator the mains current is applied via a transformer to provide a suitably reduced voltage; it is rectified and smoothed. The switch is a transistor which can turn the current on or off very rapidly, and the timing device is a capacitance–resistance circuit.

With these circuits it is possible to time pulses of voltage to last a few microseconds or for several seconds. Not only can the voltage pulse be timed but the period when it is off can be similarly controlled, so that a train of pulses can be generated with identical pulse lengths and pulse intervals. Further, the train of pulses itself can be timed to occur in bursts or surges of pulses separated by timed rest periods.

General structure of electrical pulse generators

Pulse generators may be considered to have four functional parts:

1 A power source; this may be from the mains supply or a battery.
2 An oscillating circuit to provide a train of pulses.
3 A modulating circuit to alter the train of pulses, perhaps splitting it up into short bursts or surging it.
4 An amplifying circuit to increase the output voltage appropriately.

When power is drawn from the mains it will need to be modified. The voltage will have to be reduced to an appropriate level for the subsequent circuits and output. This is done with a transformer and rectified by means of a diode (semiconductor diodes are usually used). With a suitable controlling circuit these could be applied as diadynamic current to a patient. If the voltage-reduced rectified mains current is applied to a 'smoothing' circuit (a capacitor in parallel and a series inductance) it becomes an unvarying direct current and, if regulated with a potential divider, could be applied to a patient (see Chapter 2).

Modern pulse generators go through the above steps to produce a smooth unidirectional current that can be applied to an oscillator to generate any type of current. For low-intensity TENS currents (used for patient-controlled pain modulation) the smooth d.c. can be supplied by a small battery. There is nearly always a light provided to indicate that the power circuit is on.

The oscillator to generate a train of pulses works, in principle, as a multivibrator. Such circuits are usually manufactured all in one piece as an integrated circuit which can be fitted to appropriate

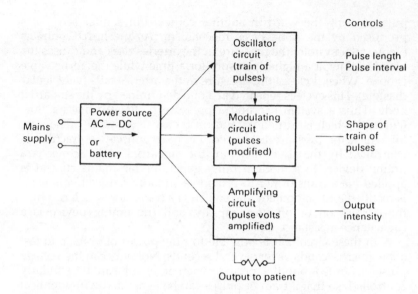

Controls

Pulse length
Pulse interval

Shape of
train of
pulses

Output
intensity

Output to patient

Fig. 3.11 Block diagram to illustrate electrical pulse generators.

resistors to give the desired pulse lengths and intervals. Where these are to be varied a switch on the panel of the machine connects the necessary resistance to give the pulse length required.

The train of pulses may then be modified, surged for example, by another integrated circuit which may also be controlled by a switch on the machine. A circuit may also make the d.c. pulses biphasic. Finally the output is amplified and applied to a potential divider to regulate the output to the patient. This is illustrated in Figure 3.11.

EFFECTS OF LOW-FREQUENCY ELECTRICAL PULSES ON THE TISSUES

When currents are passed through the tissues two groups of effects can be considered:

- There are clear and well documented effects on excitable tissue, that is nerve and muscle, which lead to numerous indirect effects. For example, modifying pain perception in the central nervous system or causing muscle contraction is secondary to the stimulation of the nerve fibre. There is also evidence of direct effects on these tissues affecting their growth and metabolism (trophic electrotherapy is considered in this chapter).

  Peripheral nerves are composed of many fibres – nerve cell processes – both sensory (afferent) and motor (efferent). The motor fibres are the axons of cells in the anterior (ventral) horn of the spinal cord, hence called anterior horn cells, while the cell bodies of the sensory nerves are found in the posterior (dorsal) root ganglia. The motor nerves to skeletal muscles and the sensory nerves conveying touch and proprioception are all fast-conducting, of large diameter and myelinated (Table 3.1).

Table 3.1 Classification of peripheral nerve fibres

Type of sheath	Fibre diameter (μ)	Conduction speed (m/s)	Classification by letter — Efferent motor	Classification by letter — Efferent autonomic	Classification by letter — Afferent sensory	Classification by number — Afferent sensory
Myelinated	22 → 2	120 —60— 30→4	Aα: Extrafusal muscle fibres		Aα: Cutaneous, joint and muscle receptors; large interoceptors	Ia: Primary sensory fibres of muscle spindles
						Ib: Sensory fibres from Golgi tendon organs
			Aβ: Intrafusal muscle fibres		Aβ: Low-threshold mechanoreceptors for light pressure rubbing vibration	II: Secondary sensory fibres of muscle spindles
			Aγ: Intrafusal muscle fibres		Aδ: Fast pain nociceptors; high-threshold mechanoreceptors for strong pressure, pinch; thermoreceptors above 45°C	III: Nociceptors pressure-pain
				B: Preganglionic		
Non-Myelinated	0.1	0.5		C: Postganglionic	C: Slow pain polymodal nociceptors; thermoreceptors; interoceptors	IV: Nociceptors

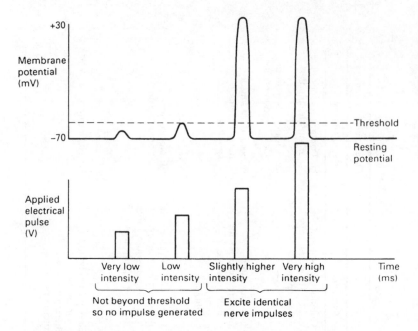

+30

Membrane
potential
(mV)

-70

Threshold

Resting
potential

Applied
electrical
pulse
(V)

Very low   Low   Slightly higher Very high   Time
intensity   intensity intensity   intensity   (ms)

Not beyond threshold   Excite identical
so no impulse generated   nerve impulses

Fig. 3.12 The all-or-none response.

The majority of fibres making up a typical peripheral nerve are of small diameter, are slow-conducting and non-myelinated; a high proportion are nociceptor C fibres, while the others are autonomic.

- Effects on non-excitable tissue at a cellular level are much less well recognized or understood. There is evidence that direct pulsed currents may accelerate healing in skin and other tissue, as noted in Chapter 2. It has also been suggested that pulsatile currents may affect cell metabolism leading to arterial, venous and lymphatic exchange at a microcirculatory level, but there is no substantial supporting evidence (Alon, 1987).

Nerve stimulation by electrical pulses

Nerve fibres in a resting state have a potential difference of some 70 mV across the fibre membrane, the inside being negative and the outside positive. The nerve impulse is an electrochemical change that spreads along the fibre, as described in Chapter 1. The impulse can be set off by depolarizing the potential difference across the membrane with an electric pulse. The nerve impulse will travel in both directions but will only cause an effect in one direction (the orthodromic direction) because it is blocked by a synapse in the other direction; but see discussion on trophic electrotherapy below.

This occurs because the electrical pulse causes a movement of ions through the tissues and hence across the membrane. However it must be a sufficient disturbance – beyond the threshold value of about 10 mV – to fire the nerve impulse. Once the potential across the nerve membrane is altered beyond its threshold value the full

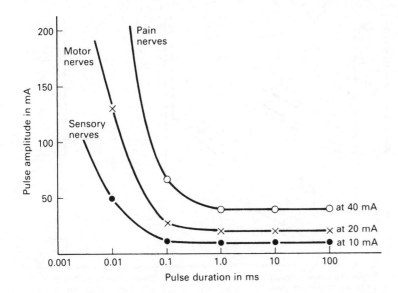

Fig. 3.13 Strength–duration curves.

nerve impulse occurs, thus it is an all-or-none response (Fig. 3.12). What the electrical pulse does is to trigger the nerve impulse but it needs a certain minimal amount of electrical charge to do so. This can be given by a small current for a relatively long duration or by a larger current for a short period. There is, however, a certain minimum current needed to fire a nerve impulse at long durations; it is called the *rheobase*. This idea is demonstrated in the strength–duration curve shown in Figure 3.13 – shorter pulse durations need larger currents to provoke a nerve impulse.

It will be seen that as the curves are exponential an enormous current would be needed at very short pulse lengths so no practical nerve or muscle stimulation occurs. It must also be understood that pulses of greater current than is needed to trigger the nerve impulse have no further effect on that nerve fibre. No matter what the current amplitude the same nerve impulse is triggered. As explained earlier, increased sensory effects or stronger muscle contractions are due to a larger *number* of fibres being stimulated. Similarly if the electrical pulse has a longer duration no further effect occurs, as illustrated in the strength–duration curve in Figure 3.13, in which the same current triggers impulses at 1, 10 and 30 ms etc. It is the initial half-ms or so of the rheobase current which has sufficient charge to disturb the nerve fibre membrane beyond its threshold. Rather longer pulses of, say, 300 ms will provoke two nerve impulses, one when the current rises and the other when it falls. The reason for this is explained later.

Rate of rise of pulse

What has been described so far is true provided the rate of rise of the electrical pulse is very rapid, i.e. it is a square wave pulse. If the rate of rise of the current is very slow it will not provoke a nerve impulse because the ionic balance across the nerve fibre

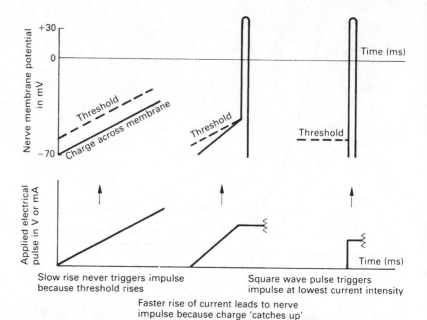

Fig. 3.14 Nerve accommodation for three applied electrical pulses of different rates of rise.

membrane is able to adjust itself so that the threshold potential rises in response to the applied electric charge. This process is called accommodation. The rate at which accommodation can occur is limited so that the threshold may eventually be reached by the slow rising pulses of higher currents (Fig. 3.14). This ability to accommodate is much more marked in nerve than in muscle tissue. This fact is used to discriminate between innervated and denervated muscle, as explained in Chapter 4. This also explains why d.c., given for iontophoresis for example, does not cause nerve stimulation when turned up slowly, as described in Chapter 2. From what has been noted above it is evident that the electrical pulse with the least charge that will stimulate a nerve impulse is one that rises rapidly – square wave – and which is of less than 1 ms duration. Note that in Figure 3.14 the pulses are cut off because their fall would stimulate another nerve impulse.

Summary

A single electrical pulse will excite a nerve impulse, provided it has sufficient energy to disturb the nerve membrane potential beyond threshold. This requires:

- Sufficient electric charge either at:
  - rheobase current for pulses of long duration
  - at currents above the rheobase for pulses of short duration
- Sufficiently rapid rate of pulse rise to avoid nerve accommodation.

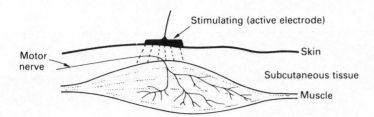

Fig. 3.15 The motor point.

Application of electric pulses to the tissues

To apply electrical pulses to the tissues a complete circuit is needed so two electrodes with suitable conducting material are fixed to the skin. The effects will be evident where the current density is highest, i.e. in the superficial tissues under the smaller (active) electrode. Consequently the cutaneous sensory nerves are affected first and with greater current densities the more deeply placed motor nerves are stimulated. However, the sensory and motor fibres are large-diameter, myelinated, fast-conducting fibres and thus more readily stimulated than the small-diameter pain fibres.

If a low current density is applied to the skin the sensory nerves in the skin, which normally transmit touch, temperature and pressure, are the first to be stimulated. This causes a mild tapping sensation which may be due principally to rapidly repeated stimulation of touch receptors. Higher current densities will cause the current to affect more nerves leading to more intense tingling and will eventually spread to motor nerves causing muscle contraction. As still higher currents are applied more motor units will be affected resulting in both stronger and more widespread muscle contractions. Further increases of current will cause pain nerve fibres to be stimulated resulting in perceived pain. These three types of nerve fibres are affected in the same order with any form of stimulating pulse (see below).

Clearly the positioning of the electrodes will determine the site of greatest current density and hence which nerves are affected; for example, in order to stimulate a normally innervated muscle effectively but painlessly the active electrode is applied to the motor point. This is a point on the skin surface at which maximum muscle contraction can be achieved because it is close to the point where the motor nerve trunk enters the muscle. Current applied at this point – often at the junction of the proximal third with the distal two-thirds of the muscle belly – will influence a large number of nerve fibres close together. Thus less current density will be needed than if the muscle belly were stimulated at some other place (Fig. 3.15). Notice that the phrase used above – 'to stimulate a muscle' – is a convenience. The current is stimulating the motor nerve which conveys nerve impulses to stimulate the muscle fibres.

Summary

A series of electrical pulses applied to the skin will stimulate:

- cutaneous sensory nerves causing a tingling sensation at low current amplitude
- motor nerves causing a muscle contraction at somewhat higher current amplitude
- nociceptors causing perceived pain at even higher current amplitude.

Stimulating different nerves

Strength duration curves have been produced for sensory and motor nerves and pain responses (Fig. 3.13). It will be seen that greater currents are needed for pain fibres, less for motor nerves and less still for sensory nerves. The amplitude of current needed to stimulate a nerve fibre is inversely proportional to its diameter. Thus the small C fibres carrying pain impulses need the greatest current. It is not a difference in threshold but simply that the larger fibres have a lower electrical resistance (due to large cross-section and differing membrane characteristics), allowing a larger current for any given voltage (Ohm's law; see Appendix). The difference in sensitivity between motor and sensory fibres is due to their different depths; sensory nerves in the skin receive a higher current density, as explained earlier.

It can also be seen from the strength–duration curves that this separation is greatest at short pulse widths. It is therefore easier selectively to excite motor or sensory nerves without eliciting pain by short-duration pulses, say around 0.05 ms.

Refractory periods

The foregoing relates to single electrical pulses causing single nerve impulses. It will be recalled from Chapter 1 that once the nerve impulse has occurred, charging the membrane potential to $+30$ V, it returns to its resting value in about 0.4–1 ms for A fibres and 2 ms for C fibres. During this time, which is called the absolute refractory period, no stimulus, however large, will cause another nerve impulse. During the next 10–15 ms the nerve impulse can be triggered again but only by a larger stimulus than is normally needed. This is called the relative refractory period. After this the nerve is in its normal resting state (Fig. 3.16).

These facts have important implications for the frequency of electrical pulses used to stimulate nerves. If a series of electrical pulses is applied to a motor nerve at one pulse per second (1 Hz), a corresponding series of muscle twitches will occur. Similarly, stimulation of a sensory nerve will lead to a series of separately

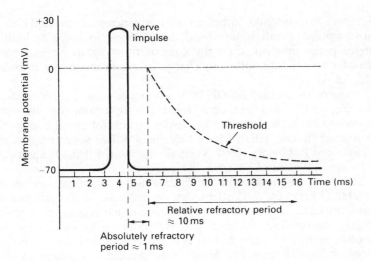

Fig. 3.16 The absolute and relative refractory periods.

recognized mild shocks. If the frequency is increased to, say, 10 Hz there is a corresponding tremor of the muscle, but if the frequency is increased to, say, 30 Hz the muscle contracts continuously – a tetanic contraction. Although the peak current remains the same the strength of the tetanic contraction increases with rising frequency up to about 100 Hz but not beyond. This is illustrated in Figure 3.17. The increase in muscle force occurs because the tension developed during one twitch has no time to relax before the next occurs, so that successive twitches are cumulative. Beyond 100 Hz the muscle contraction and sensory tingling do not increase with increased pulse frequency; in fact they may diminish unless the current intensity is increased. The reasons for this are obvious from what has been described already. Pulses of 1 ms at 100 Hz will have pulse intervals of 9 ms and at higher frequencies the interval would be shorter still; this means that each pulse is applied during the relative refractory period. In order to excite a nerve impulse during this time a greater current is needed. Thus higher peak currents are

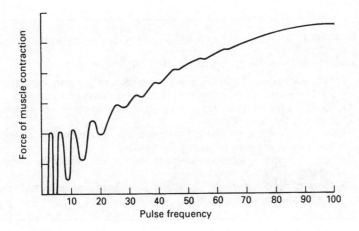

Fig. 3.17 Strength of tetanic contraction increasing with rising frequency up to 100 Hz.

necessary to generate impulses at frequencies above 100 Hz. If shorter pulse durations are used, say 0.05 ms, to leave a slightly longer pulse interval, then the current must again be increased in order to provide sufficient charge to excite the nerve impulse (Fig. 3.13).

Frequencies around 30–40 Hz cause smooth muscle contraction (see Fig. 3.17) and are considered the optimum for therapy, increasing frequency leading to greater muscle fatigue if therapy is prolonged (Baker, 1981). Many therapists utilize such frequencies (Delitto and Robinson, 1989). Normally generated firing frequencies of motor nerves rarely exceed 40 Hz (Scott, 1996).

At higher frequencies above 500 Hz for 1 ms pulses, or about 1000 Hz (1 kHz) for 0.05 ms pulses, no increase in the number of nerve impulses can occur no matter how much current is applied, because succeeding electrical pulses would be given during the absolute refractory period. This is sometimes called the maximum depolarization frequency. Above this stimulation frequency the nerve depolarizes at its own frequency. Single pulses of 0.125 ms separated by intervals long enough to allow the nerve to fire and repolarize will cause nerve stimulation. However, if the pulses are applied at 4000 Hz (i.e. medium frequency) they are modulated in some way to cause nerve stimulation. They can be interrupted, like Russian current, by 50 bursts per second, where the first phase of each burst depolarizes the nerve, or modulated by interference providing amplitude modulation at the beat frequency.

Thus it can be seen that electrical pulses of 0.1–1 ms at 30–100 Hz would stimulate medium and large myelinated nerve fibres with the least possible current. It is notable that these parameters partly encompass both TENS (sensory) and faradic (motor) stimulation. However, the current density in the deeper tissues must also be considered.

Fast twitch muscle fibres, which are phasic and are recruited for added muscle strength and fast movement, respond best to frequencies in the range 50–150 Hz. Slow twitch fibres, which are postural and the first to become active, have a tetanic frequency of 20–30 Hz.

Summary

The effects of pulse frequency at frequencies around:

- 1 Hz – a series of muscle twitches and sensory shocks result
- 10 Hz – a tremor of muscle and tapping sensation results
- 30 Hz – muscle twitches merge to a tetanic contraction and sensory tingling occurs
- 50–100 Hz – tetanic muscle contraction increases with rising frequency, sensory 'buzzing' or tingling
- 500 Hz – the maximum depolarization frequency for 1 ms pulses
- 1000 Hz and beyond – usually amplitude modulated or interrupted to affect nerves.

Penetration of electrical pulses through the tissues

The impedance of the skin is very large for both direct current and the longer pulses – much greater than the rest of the tissues – but it is very much less for shorter pulses. Thus the skin may have an impedance of about $1000\,\Omega$ for a 10 ms pulse but only $50\,\Omega$ for a 0.1 ms pulse. This happens because the skin acts as a capacitor which offers much less impedance to short pulse lengths in the same way that it does for high-frequency currents.

The distribution of current through the tissues with shorter pulses is therefore more even, so that effectively the current penetrates further. Consequently the deeper nerves, e.g. motor nerves, are more easily stimulated with the shorter pulses. With longer pulses most of the current is 'used' in the skin, stimulating cutaneous nerves, as discussed later.

Electrical pulses for nerve stimulation

It can be seen that some of the currents used for stimulation and described earlier are more appropriate to excite a nerve impulse than others. Thus for stimulating motor and sensory nerves, i.e. large-diameter fast-conducting nerves, the pulses should be square wave and of short duration (0.5–0.1 ms). To achieve discrimination from pain nerves and greater depth even shorter pulses (0.05–0.02 ms) are appropriate. Symmetrical biphasic pulses have the advantage of avoiding any risk of chemical damage. They are sometimes referred to as depolarized pulses. The most appropriate frequencies for muscle stimulation depend on the predominant fibre type and are considered to be around 30 Hz for tonic muscle fibre and 80 Hz for phasic.

For other purposes, e.g. stimulating nociceptors, longer pulses would seem appropriate. Similarly if polar effects are needed to promote wound healing obviously direct current pulses are chosen.

PHYSIOLOGICAL EFFECTS AND THERAPEUTIC USES

The motor unit

The motor unit consists of an anterior horn cell, the alpha motor neuron emanating from it and all the individual muscle fibres it supplies (see Fig. 4.3). The number of muscle fibres supplied varies from a very few where precise control of movement is required up to one or two thousand for large postural muscles. All the muscle fibres of a particular motor unit are the same type.

Type I are slow twitch, red because they are highly vascular, and predominate in postural muscles. They are slow to contract and relax because the motor neuron supplying them is of small diameter and low conduction velocity and fires at a continuous, low frequency. They have many oxidative enzymes and fatigue slowly.

Type II are fast twitch, white, glycolytic fibres. They are less vascular. The motor neuron supplying them is of larger diameter and has a higher conduction rate. They are divided into two subgroups. Type IIA have fewer oxidative enzymes than type I, but are relatively fatigue resistant. They predominate in ordinary low force movement. Type IIB have the least oxidative enzymes and fatigue rapidly. They produce a large force for short periods and are only brought into play during strenuous movement.

An individual muscle is made up of many motor units of different types, giving the muscle its particular characteristics.

Voluntary contraction of muscle

During voluntary contraction of muscle there is an asynchronous firing of motor neurons resulting in a smooth contraction. The force of a contraction is graded, in general, by an increase in: (a) the number of motor units recruited (spatial summation) and (b) the frequency of nerve impulses (temporal summation); (a) occurs in the early stages and in low force muscle contractions and (b) occurs later and at greater muscle force. In other words, as more motor units become involved, further increase of muscle force is largely achieved by increased rates of nerve impulse firing (Milner-Brown and Stein, 1975).

Type I muscle fibres are recruited first and later type II. Prolonged muscle contraction leads to fatigue, rapidly in type IIB and most slowly in type I. The order of recruitment is largely fixed but can be influenced by cutaneous stimulation (Garnett and Stephens, 1981).

Electrical stimulation of innervated muscle

Electrical stimulation of muscle differs from voluntary contraction in several ways. First, there is synchronous firing of all motor neurons stimulated. Secondly, electrical stimulation will not stimulate motor units in the same recruitment order as voluntary contraction. In fact, it is largely reversed because: (a) larger diameter motor neurons (type II) are more easily stimulated, and (b) sensory nerves are inevitably stimulated. Additionally, the frequency of firing is fixed, unlike voluntary contraction. Therefore, in order to cause stronger muscle contractions the current density has to be increased to stimulate more motor units.

Electrical stimulation of muscle via its motor nerve has both immediate and long-term effects. Muscle contraction and vascular changes are examples of the former, while muscle strengthening and structural changes in muscle fibres may ultimately result from long-term, chronic stimulation. These are considered below.

The structure of living muscle is not fixed. There is, for example, a balance between the synthesis and breakdown of the constituent proteins. The rate of this can be as much as 10% of skeletal muscle protein per day, occurring at a higher rate in type I slow twitch fibres than in type II. More anabolic than catabolic activity will lead to muscle hypertrophy with more muscle and collagenous tissue produced, while the reverse will cause atrophy. Similarly, the form or structure of the constituent muscle fibres can alter in response to changes in long-term stimulation. This plastic adaptation of skeletal muscle tissue is considered to be under both hormonal (e.g. steroidal) and neuronal control. Thus the flow of impulses in the motor nerve serves both to provoke immediate muscle contraction and, in the long term, to promote muscle fibre growth and change, as described later.

Where voluntary active exercise is restricted, electrical stimulation may be substituted. It is usually applied by surging (or ramping) a series of short pulses at frequencies between 30 and 100 Hz. If the surge of pulses is made to last for, say, 2 s and the interval between surges for 4 s then a slow physiological muscle contraction and joint motion will be mimicked. Obviously the surge length, rate of rise and fall and interval can be varied (Fig. 3.1(e)). Electrical stimulation is used for a variety of therapeutic purposes which may be grouped as follows.

Muscle strengthening

Normal muscle.   The question of whether electrical stimulation of normal muscle can lead to an increase in muscle strength is not entirely resolved in spite of much research. The gist of this seems to be that electrical stimulation does increase muscle strength although not quite to the same extent as the equivalent voluntary exercise. In an extensive review Lloyd *et al.* (1986) concluded that in general electrical stimulation was not a satisfactory substitute for voluntary activity. However, a number of the studies showed that electrical stimulation (or electrical stimulation combined with voluntary activity) led to similar or in a few cases even greater strength gains than that due to voluntary exercise alone. Taking a number of such studies together, the average gain in strength due to electrical stimulation would seem to be around 20–25% over a month or so, varying from no increase in strength to 50%. This latter appears to be the maximum achievable in normal untrained muscle (see Balogun *et al.*, 1993; Callaghan and Oldham, 1997). Marked individual differences in response to electrical stimulation were noted. Uncertainty remains due to the variety of techniques and protocols adopted by the different studies.

In a well-controlled study by Hon Sun Lai *et al.* (1988) it was shown that electrical stimulation of muscles over a 3-week period produced significant gains in muscle strength, being greater in the group treated with high-intensity electrical stimulation than in the group treated with lower intensities. The force of isometric contraction showed greater gains than that of concentric contraction. Eccentric contraction (isotonic lengthening) showed no significant gains. Although the gain in strength declined when treatment stopped it was still significant for the high-intensity group 3 weeks later. There was also a clear increase in isometric strength demonstrated in the opposite untreated limb, a cross-transfer effect which did not show a marked difference between the high- and low-intensity groups. This cross-transfer effect was also found in the study by Balogun *et al.* (1993) in which a 24% strength increase occurred in the treated muscles and a 10% increase in the untreated, contralateral muscles after 6 weeks. This study compared groups treated with three different stimulation frequencies (20, 45 and 80 pulses/sec), and found no difference.

Almost all studies of electrical stimulation for muscle strengthening on healthy subjects have tested the relatively young. An important study involved healthy adults over 65 years (Pfeifer *et al.*, 1997). This found almost identical strength gains of about 25% in the triceps surae of those given electrical stimulation and those performing voluntary exercise. This occurred over a 6-week period and the electrical stimulation was found to be well tolerated by these subjects.

It is considered that the strength gain can be attributed to neural mechanisms, at least initially. This is suggested by several features: the speed with which the increase occurs – it can be demonstrated in about a week – and the speed with which it can decline, as well as the lack of evidence of any changes in muscle volume. Several neural mechanisms have been proposed. One is the increased activation of the spinal motor neuron pools, which regulate the force of muscle contraction due to stimulation of afferent neurons. This would account for the cross-transfer effect. Long-term potentiation has also been suggested. This involves increased sensitivity of synapses as a result of continuous stimulation of input fibres; the effect may last for some weeks. Synchronization of motor unit firing patterns is a further mechanism that has been proposed. The selective recruitment of large fast-twitch type II fibres over the slow-twitch type I fibres could also be implicated, although this does not conform to the finding that electrical stimulation leads to similar strength gains to those of voluntary muscle contractions. There is widespread agreement that tolerance to electrical stimulation increases markedly after a few applications in most subjects.

The force of voluntary muscle contraction is greater in most but not all subjects than the force that can be produced by electrical stimulation of the same musculature (De Domenico and Strauss, 1986; Strauss and De Domenico, 1986). This difference does not seem to be accounted for by the nature of the stimulating current since different stimulators did not produce significantly consistent differences in contraction force. Soo *et al.* (1988) have shown that stimulating the quadriceps at quite low intensities – 50% of maximum voluntary contraction applied as eight contractions of 15 s duration twice a week for 5 weeks – led to a statistically significant increase in quadriceps torque. Thus surprisingly little electrical stimulation, a total of only 2 min stimulation in each of 10 sessions, has shown significant effect.

Weakened muscle. In weakened or weakening muscles the value of electrical stimulation is much clearer and significant gains have been reported with improvement of muscle function. Electrical stimulation at 30 Hz applied to the quadriceps of immobilized knees and given in 2 s on and 9 s off cycles for 1 h each day for 6 weeks has been shown to reduce muscle atrophy (Gibson *et al.*, 1988). In this study, cross-sectional area of the quadriceps was found to diminish by 17% in the untreated group, but there was no significant loss in those patients that were treated. The effect was considered to be due to the maintenance of protein synthesis in muscles rather than preventing protein breakdown. Obajulwa (1991) found a significant increase in mean quadriceps muscle girth after using a surged faradic pulse train of 3 s at a maximum tetanic contraction level, but within the limits of tolerance. The surge was repeated 10 times, with a rest period of 10 s between each. This regimen was repeated 3 times a week for 10 weeks. Similarly, improvement in muscle force over a 4-week period of electrical stimulation of chronically weakened quadriceps was found (Singer, 1986). In this study, however, no significant increase in muscle cross-sectional area was found but electromyograph changes suggested increased neuromuscular efficiency to account for the increased muscle force.

A faradic-type current has been used successfully in the treatment of chondromalacia patellae (Johnson *et al.*, 1977). Fifty patients given 19 treatments over a 6-week period showed considerable improvement; at least half became symptom free. The quadriceps muscle was stimulated to produce 10 s isometric contractions with a 50 s rest period ten times every treatment. The current amplitude was the maximum the patient could tolerate; in fact the authors concluded that the efficacy of treatment varies directly with the current amplitude – highest currents give the best results. They also noted that the greater the initial atrophy the more effective the treatment and consequently felt that normal muscle would gain least from the technique. The body of evidence points to the need for maximum tolerable levels of contraction for strengthening. However, Snyder-Mackler and Robinson (1989) warn that, after the motor threshold is exceeded, very small increases in stimulation amplitude produce relatively large increases in the force of muscle contraction as recruitment increases rapidly, so care must be exercised.

The strengthening effect has been used to promote greater achievement in athletics but any advantage this might have over similar amounts of voluntary effort has not been unequivocally demonstrated. Its use for the prevention of disuse atrophy appears to be justified; for a full discussion see Currier (1987).

Interestingly, behavioural styles appear to affect how subjects characterize discomfort with electrical stimulation (Delitto *et al.*, 1992). They felt that electrically elicited muscle contractions themselves contributed to the discomfort.

Facilitation of muscle control

Stimulation is extensively used therapeutically to initiate and facilitate voluntary contraction of muscle, although it is not possible to distinguish this effect from the strengthening effect already considered. This idea may be applied in several circumstances:

- Where voluntary muscle contraction is inhibited by pain or injury. Stimulating the quadriceps, especially the vastus medialis, after knee surgery or knee injury, for example, is often utilized. Another example is stimulation of the calf and Achilles tendon in chronic and postsurgical cases of Achilles tendon injuries (Grisogono, 1989).
- In situations where muscle action is not readily under voluntary control without practice: stimulation of the pelvic floor muscle in the control of incontinence (see Mills *et al.*, 1990; Blowman *et al.*, 1991; Cawley and Hendriks, 1992); stimulation of the abductor hallucis for the management of early hallux valgus (see below for further discussion of both of these); and, in circumstances such as postural flatfoot or metatarsalgia, where voluntary lumbrical control is desirable.
- In circumstances in which a new muscle action has to be learned, for example where a muscle or a motor nerve has been transplanted.
- In the later stages of a recovering peripheral nerve lesion to encourage voluntary muscle contraction where reinnervation has only recently occurred.
- In situations in which it is necessary to demonstrate to the patient that a particular muscle action or movement can occur normally, where hysterical paralysis is present, for example.
- For children with cerebral palsy, where electrical stimulation may enhance muscle contraction and provide sensation so that a child can add a weak response with effective results (Carmick, 1993).

Maintenance or increase of range of joint motion

Motion may be limited by different tissues and from different causes. Electrical stimulation of muscle to stretch the shortened tissues has been used in:

- Contractures of fibrous tissue and scarring. Limitation of joint motion due to shortening of soft tissues on one side of the joint has been treated by cyclical electrical stimulation of the muscles that stretch the contracture. This has been successful in increasing the range of movement in hemiplegic patients (Baker and Parker, 1986), especially for the patient with shoulder pain and for the reduction of shoulder subluxation.
- Loss of motion due to spasticity of muscles in hemiplegia or other neurological conditions. To maintain the normal range of motion in such patients regular passive movements are recommended, often carried out at home by the patient's own family. Electrical stimulation has been applied as an alternative to manual passive movement to help prevent the loss of motion due to spasticity of the opposing muscles (Baker *et al.*, 1979).

Case study

Tekeodlu *et al.* (1998) found that brief intense TENS (0.2 ms, 100 Hz at bearable pain level) applied 30 min a day, 5 times a week for 8 weeks to the antagonists of spastic muscles improved the outcome of rehabilitation of patients with hemiplegia after stroke.

Case study

Pandyan *et al.* (1996) reported the results of electrical stimulation (10.3 ms pulses at 35 Hz) applied in 3 s bursts to the wrist and finger extensors of two hemiplegic patients. They were treated over several weeks and provided their own control. The active range of wrist movement was found to have increased and wrist posture and hand oedema to have improved. (See the original study for discussion.)

- Scoliosis. In the treatment of scoliosis the lateral trunk muscles on the convexity of the curve are stimulated electrically. Surface electrodes are attached to the patient's back and muscle contraction is provoked in short cycles at a level that allows the patient to sleep during the treatment (Eckerson and Axelgaard, 1984). In moderate scoliosis (20–45°) it has been shown that a progression of the curve can be halted in over 80% of patients (Axelgaard and Brown, 1983). A later overview of scoliosis treatment (Cassella and Hall, 1991) found over half the subjects treated with nightly electrical stimulation were not benefited.

Functional electrical stimulation

Functional electrical stimulation is the electrical stimulation of the intact lower motor neuron to initiate contraction of paralysed muscle to produce functional movement.

Electrical stimulation to replace splinting. This involves the use of faradic-type or similar electrical pulses applied to the skin to cause muscle contraction. These systems encompass both control and rehabilitation of the neuromuscular complex in that strengthening occurs when muscle is regularly and repeatedly stimulated as considered above. There may also be a beneficial effect on muscle spasm (see below). Electrical stimulation of the dorsiflexors in hemiplegic patients triggered by a switch in the shoe has been used. A controlled trial (Burridge *et al.*, 1997) of this technique found considerable improvements in walking speed and physiological cost index when the stimulator was being used, but no significant 'carry-over' effect. The subjects of this study had hemiplegia and had suffered a stroke at least 6 months previously.

Similarly stimulation of the deltoid has been used to prevent glenohumeral subluxation in hemiplegic patients (Baker, 1987).

Rather more complex systems are being devised to enable paraplegic patients to gain control of standing and walking (see Ferguson and Granat, 1992; Isakov and Mizrahi, 1993).

Electrical stimulation for the control of spasticity.   The effects of electrical muscle stimulation on spasticity are not clearly established and reported results are variable. This is partly due to the difficulty of measuring and defining spasticity. In general there have been three approaches:

- stimulation of antagonists to utilize the effect of reciprocal inhibition
- stimulation of the spastic muscles themselves
- alternately stimulating agonist and antagonist muscles.

This latter approach has been tried using low-frequency (3–35 Hz) 0.2 ms pulses, for some minutes daily over several weeks. The pulse frequencies are based on trophic stimulation as considered below and on the principle that afferent stimulation reinforces the pre-synaptic inhibition of motor neurons, thus reducing spasticity.

Another approach involves the use of a mesh glove to stimulate the whole hand with trains of 50 Hz, 0.3 ms pulses, electrodes on the forearm completing the circuit (Dimitriyević *et al.*, 1996). Stimulation both below and above the sensory threshold was applied to hemiplegic patients for periods of 30 min per day and was found to suppress spasticity, improve hemispatial neglect and enhance the remaining voluntary activity.

These and other studies (e.g. Shindo and Jones, 1987) have claimed the successful reduction of spasticity, but a single-blind trial by Livesley (1992) found only one short-lived subjective improvement.

A slightly different approach was used by Lagassé and Roy (1989), who studied the effects of a functional electrical stimulation training programme on the co-contraction level of spastic hemiplegic patients during a rapid forearm extension movement. The pattern of stimulation was adjusted individually from the EMG output of the non-affected limb. The treatment reduced the antagonist co-contraction level associated with spasticity.

While the results of electrical stimulation for the treatment of spasticity have been inconsistent, none has supported the opinion, sometimes advanced, that such stimulation exacerbates spasticity (Baker, 1987).

Changes in the structure and properties of muscle: long-term electrical stimulation

Animal studies.   The ability to modify the properties of mammalian skeletal muscle by means of long-term electrical stimulation was first demonstrated by Buller and colleagues in 1960. By reversing the nerve supply between a predominantly fast contracting muscle with that of a slow contracting one in the cat, it was shown that not only the contractile properties were exchanged but extensive sequential changes also occurred in the metabolic and histological properties. Thus fast twitch type II fibres were converted to slow twitch type I. Similar changes occurred when animal muscle was subjected to long-term, low-frequency stimulation (Salmons and Vbrova, 1969). Other animal studies have shown that the transformation process takes some 6–8 weeks and is sequential, starting with changes in the muscle membrane and capillary circulation and completed with an exchange of fast to slow type myosin isoenzymes (Pette and Vbrova, 1985). Although there is overwhelming evidence that variation from the usual neuronal activity is a key factor in provoking these changes, and that the nature of these variations differs between muscles, it is not known how best to effect and exploit this ability to alter muscle properties.

Human studies.   These effects have also been demonstrated in humans (Scott *et al.*, 1985). In this study, low-frequency (10 Hz) stimulation of the lateral popliteal nerve was given for 3 periods of an hour daily for 6 weeks, at sufficient intensity to give a visible contraction of the tibialis anterior and movement of the foot. This led to a significant increase in resistance to fatigue in the stimulated muscles when compared with the unstimulated controls, suggesting a change in the properties of the type II fibres.

Later work by Rutherford *et al.* (1988) on normal subjects compared the effect of long-term, low-frequency stimulation with a non-uniform pattern of stimulation incorporating a range from 5 Hz through to 40 Hz. This study showed similar changes in the fatigue characteristics in response to both patterns of stimulation. However, muscles stimulated with a low-frequency pattern lost muscle strength, whereas muscles stimulated using a mixed pattern of stimulation became stronger.

Similar techniques have been applied to the quadriceps muscles of 21 healthy subjects (Cramp *et al.*, 1995; Cramp, 1998). One of three selected patterns (a uniform 8 Hz pattern, a uniform mixed pattern of 160 ms at 40 Hz followed by 8 Hz and a non-uniform pattern of frequencies up to 50 Hz) was applied unilaterally for 3 hours every day, 5 days a week for 6 weeks. Stimulated muscle showed significant increases in strength and fatigue resistance, and indications were that a mixed or non-uniform pattern included greater changes than a uniform 8 Hz pattern. Individual responses to electrical stimulation varied and in most cases subjects who gained in strength did not show increased fatigue resistance. Comparative studies have also been undertaken to monitor these changes in patient groups with neuromuscular disease (for a review see St Pierre and Gardiner, 1987). Overall, it would appear that changes in contractile properties may often accompany loss of strength and alterations in neuronal activity.

Trophic stimulation.   The frequencies of the motor unit action potential have been recorded electromyographically and used to determine the frequency of electrical stimulation of the muscle (Kidd and Oldham, 1988a,b). This form of stimulation has been called *eutrophic or trophic electrotherapy* to indicate its growth promoting or nourishing effect. The application of trophic electrotherapy to the intrinsic hand muscles of patients with rheumatoid arthritis has been reported (Kidd *et al.*, 1989) in which the patterned stimulation was derived from a fatigued motor unit of the first dorsal interosseous muscle of a normal hand.

Trophic electrotherapy has been applied in cases of non-recovering Bell's palsy (Farragher *et al.*, 1987). The mean frequency of motor unit firing in particular facial muscles was used to dictate the frequency (5–8 Hz) of 0.08 ms rectangular pulses applied to the facial nerve, with 2 s on and 2 s off, for up to 8 h over several weeks. Very considerable objectively assessed improvement was noted. Stress incontinence has also been treated with trophic electrotherapy.

Summary. The motor nerve apparently sends two types of encoded information to muscle fibres. One type causes immediate muscle contraction, the other is trophic, causing adaptation over a long period of time and is non-uniform and patterned. By stimulating muscle appropriately with chronic, low-frequency electrical pulses, adaptation can occur with a resultant increase in strength and endurance. There is considerable uncertainty concerning the optimum patterns of stimulation and this may well be the key factor. There are, however, other features of this therapy, such as the effect of loading and normal use of the muscle during stimulation, as well as patient compliance and acceptability (Baker, 1987) which need to be resolved (see Ciba Foundation, 1988).

Effects on muscle metabolism and blood flow

Electrical stimulation will have the same effect as normal voluntary muscle contraction in causing a temporary increase in muscle metabolism. There will be the associated consequences of increased oxygen uptake and carbon dioxide, lactic acid and other metabolite production, as well as raised local temperature and greater local blood flow. Many studies have demonstrated an increased blood flow, for example Currier *et al.* (1986). Using 10 and 30% of maximum voluntary contraction these authors quantified a 20% blood flow increase which occurred about 1 min after electrical stimulation had started and continued for some 5 min after it had finished.

Not only is the intramuscular blood flow increased but as a consequence of regular muscle contraction and relaxation the flow in adjacent softwalled veins will be increased – the muscle pumping action. This effect is used therapeutically to help control limb oedema by raising the rate of flow in venous and lymphatic vessels.

It has been found that stimulating parts of the quadriceps with 0.4 ms pulses at 50 Hz in 4 s on/4 s off cycles leads to an 18.5% increase in blood flow in the femoral artery (Tracy *et al.*, 1988). This study used sufficient current to stimulate the muscle to 15% of its maximum voluntary contraction and measured the blood flow in the femoral artery with an ultrasonic Doppler device. The increased blood flow was noted within 5 min of the start of electrical stimulation and fell to normal levels within 1 min of cessation of stimulation.

Brown *et al.* (1998) studied the effects of percutaneous stimulation of triceps surae or tibialis anterior at 8 Hz for 28 days, 3 × 20 mins/

day on limb blood flow and microvascular filtration capacity. Their findings suggested adaptations occurring as a result of mild low-frequency stimulation at the level of the microvasculature which could include capillary growth and/or improved microvascular perfusion, contributing to the greater resistance to fatigue. Such adaptations would clearly benefit ischaemic human muscles and in 15 patients with intermittent claudication a similar regimen led to significant increases in maximum walking distance and resistance to fatigue during electrically-evoked contractions of calf muscles.

Summary

Therapeutic uses of electrical stimulation of innervated muscle:

- strengthening muscle in healthy subjects
- strengthening atrophied or potentially atrophied muscle due to disuse
- facilitation of motor control
- maintaining or increasing the range of joint motion
- functional electrical stimulation
  - to replace splinting and provoke motion
  - to control spasticity
- effect changes in muscle structure and properties with chronic electrical stimulation
- increase muscle metabolism and blood flow
- increase venous and lymphatic flow in adjacent tissues.

Fatigue of muscle

Muscle fatigue as a consequence of voluntary contraction is well known but it is a complex and not fully understood phenomenon. Initially it is due to depletion of muscle glycogen and available blood glucose with other biochemical limitations. Ultimately the rate of oxygen utilization is important. Fatigue at submaximal contractions is controlled by varying the particular motor units involved. Prolonged contraction shows increased recruitment of motor units to maintain the same muscle force as fatigue occurs (Berger, 1982). It would therefore be expected that electrical stimulation of muscle via the motor nerve would lead to relatively rapid muscle fatigue, since a fixed set of motor units are being stimulated with the fast twitch type II fibres preferentially selected. This has been shown to occur by Currier and Mann (1983) and Rankin and Stokes (1992). The former authors showed that muscle fatigue due to electrical stimulation was greater than that due to isometric, voluntary contraction of equal force. The degree and duration of fatigue appears to be directly related to the extent of the electrical stimulation. Rankin and Stokes found some evidence of fatigue persisting for surprisingly long periods after a therapeutic protocol of electrical stimulation applied to healthy subjects. Full recovery was delayed for up to 24 h and, in some cases, 48 h.

The use of functional electrical stimulation for paralysed muscles with intact lower motor neurons, as occurs in spinal cord injuries, has led to interest in the way muscles fatigue in response to electrical stimulation (e.g. Mizrahi, 1997). As would be expected in these paraplegic patients, electrical stimulation causes rapid muscle fatigue for the reasons noted. Additionally there is no sensory feedback to indicate local muscle fatigue. Fatigued muscle shows a better response to pulse trains of variable frequency (with brief pulse intervals at the start of the train) than to trains of electrical pulses of constant frequency (Binder-Macleod *et al.*, 1997). This conforms to the finding that the force a given stimulating frequency generates depends on the state of fatigue of the muscle so that there is no 'ideal' single frequency for electrical stimulation.

Fatigue after exercise, including electrically induced exercise, may be a necessary stimulus for muscle strengthening, but whether stimulation of already fatigued muscle could be harmful is not known. The possible risks due to functional electrical stimulation (see p. 83) have also been considered by Stokes and Cooper (1989) but there seems to be no evidence of any structural or functional damage due to electrical stimulation.

There appears to be an inverse relationship between endurance and force in motor units. Low levels of electrical stimulation – for up to 2 h a day – appear to maintain fatigue resistance in muscles without reducing force (Gordon, 1998).

Stimulation of denervated muscle

Denervated muscle is different in many respects from innervated muscle, including its response to electrical stimuli. Without a functional nerve supply muscle can only be caused to contract by direct stimulation of the muscle fibre. There are therefore differences between stimulating muscle via its nerve and direct denervated muscle stimulation:

- muscle tissue is less excitable than nerve so that a greater electric charge is needed (see Fig. 4.4)
- slow 'worm-like' contraction results because of the slow spread of contraction through the muscle and diminished rate of contraction compared with innervated muscle
- slow-rising electrical pulses can stimulate muscle because it has less ability to accommodate than nerve.

Muscle tissue may be stimulated by slow-rising pulses, also called selective, triangular or accommodation pulses. This occurs because, unlike nerve, the muscle stimulation threshold cannot rise fast enough (see Stephens, 1965). This provides a means of selectively stimulating different tissues. To stimulate nerve, as previously discussed, a square wave pulse is best. To stimulate muscle fibre but not nerve, a triangular pulse with a rise time of 50 ms (100 ms pulse length) is used. To stimulate denervated muscle fibre only, a rise time of longer than 100 ms is best; 300 or 500 ms triangular pulses are often selected.

Denervated muscle can be made to contract with square wave pulses of sufficient duration (30 ms or more) or triangular wave pulses of long duration (rise times of 100–500 ms). In both cases the current needs to be applied through the muscle tissue itself, because there is no motor point. The current is usually most successfully applied in the long axis of the muscle fibres, that is with the stimulating electrodes at each end of the muscle belly.

There has been confusion and controversy over the therapeutic use of electrical stimulation of denervated muscles for many years. The rationale for such treatment is to maintain the muscle in as healthy a state as possible by electrically induced artificial exercise while awaiting reinnervation. It seems reasonable that making muscles contract with electrical stimuli would substitute for the beneficial effects of normal muscle contraction. Newham (1991) points out that skeletal muscle has a great capacity for regeneration. The evidence, however, is somewhat contradictory and in particular clinical benefit has not been unequivocally demonstrated in humans (see Bélanger, 1991).

When muscle is denervated many structural and functional changes occur (see Sunderland, 1978). They are principally:

- loss of voluntary and reflex activity
- atrophy, degeneration and fibrosis
- fibrillation – spontaneous contraction of muscle fibres.

There is considerable literature concerning the effects of electrical stimulation on denervated muscle (Spielholz, 1987), including evidence that it will retard muscle atrophy and degeneration but not completely prevent it.

The type and amount of stimulation used to achieve this is very variable. The best results (Hnik, 1962) seem to have been achieved with vigorous isometric muscle contractions – to the point of fatigue – for two or three sessions each day separated by at least 10 min intervals. Davis (1983) concluded from a review of the literature that *all* the denervated muscle fibres must be activated, that isometric contractions are more effective than isotonic and that regular stimulation should commence as soon as possible after denervation. From a therapeutic point of view such regimens are difficult to apply except to a few superficial muscles at a time. This, then, tends to be limited to a small number of muscles and to those that patients can be taught to stimulate for themselves. Further, if this treatment is to be useful it will require considerable compliance and tolerance on the part of the patient to continue treatment over a long period of, perhaps, 1 or 2 years. Some clinical studies have been unable to demonstrate any benefits due to the application of electrical stimulation over long periods provided other appropriate care is given to the paralysed muscles. In summary, the value of electrical stimulation for denervated muscle is not proven and its application to gain what may be only a small benefit is probably not justified.

The contradictory experimental findings may be due to variations in the type of electrical stimulation – the parameters of frequency pulse duration, rise time, intensity and so forth – or the varying amounts of stimulation given or, perhaps, it is the trophic effects that are important. In view of this and the availability of conveniently small muscle stimulators that can be used by the patient, the benefit of denervated muscle stimulation may well be demonstrated in the future. Trophic electrotherapy is now the treatment of choice if some motor units are still available for stimulation.

Stimulation of afferent nerves

Electrical stimulation is extensively used for the control of pain. Although the idea had been proposed for many years the rationale was provided by the gate control theory of pain proposed in the mid 1960s by Melzack and Wall (1965). To account for the effects of electrical stimulation it is necessary to consider pain mechanisms first.

Pain

All sensations are modulated by the central nervous system before they reach conscious level. Pain is an abstract term referring to what is recognized by individuals. The International Association for the Study of Pain proposes the following definition: 'Pain is an unpleasant sensory and emotional experience associated with actual or potential tissue damage, or described in terms of such damage' (Merskey, 1990). The input from the periphery is modified in the nervous system at various levels and has sensory, cognitive, emotional and autonomic components.

Nociceptors

The A delta receptors respond to strong mechanical stimulation and to damaging heat, i.e. above 45°C. When these fibres are stimulated they cause a pricking or stinging sensation known as first or fast pain. A delta receptors are present as discrete sensitive spots in the skin all over the body surface (and small numbers in joints and muscles). Their impulses are carried by small myelinated fibres at speeds around 15 m/s (see Table 3.1).

Fast pain seems to be functionally concerned with helping the body avoid tissue damage since it provokes an immediate flexor withdrawal reflex and evokes rapid well-localized conscious awareness.

The C fibre receptors appear to be sensitive to many kinds of stimuli – mechanical, chemical and heat – hence they are called polymodal. Probably they are sensitive to the chemicals released from tissue damaged by any stimulus. This includes inflammatory changes leading to the release of hydrogen ions (protons), histamine, serotonin, acetylcholine, bradykinin, kallidin, prostaglandins E and F as well as several cellular metabolites such as ATP, ADP and lactic acid. All of these have been found to stimulate or sensitize the C nociceptors (Thompson, 1994). Such stimulation gives rise to a dull aching pain.

Slow pain is transmitted by unmyelinated C fibres at a speed of about 1 m/s (see Table 3.1). Their free nerve endings are found in all innervated body tissue except the central nervous system.

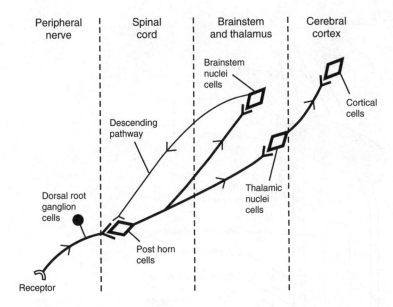

Fig. 3.18 General outline of the pain pathways.

Pain pathways

Nerve impulses giving rise to conscious pain travel in four regions of the nervous system, in each of which they can be modulated:

- peripheral nervous system
- spinal cord
- brainstem and thalamus
- cerebral cortex.

A simple overview of the general arrangements is shown in Figure 3.18.

The cell bodies of the A delta and C fibres are found in the dorsal root ganglion and their central connections enter the spinal cord via the dorsal root (except for some 30% of the C fibres which return to the peripheral nerve and enter the cord via the ventral root). Here they synapse with central nociceptive transmission cells. Nociceptive-specific cells are mainly in lamina I and respond only to nociceptors. Wide dynamic range cells are chiefly in lamina V and receive input from nociceptors and large-diameter A beta fibres.

From here, information is transmitted via the direct pathway – the spinothalamic tract – to the thalamus or indirectly via the spinoreticular-thalamic tract (Johnson, 1997). From the thalamus, information is transmitted to the somatosensory cerebral cortex and other regions of the brain (see Fig. 3.19).

The synaptic transmitter of the nociceptive system is probably substance P, but there are many other candidates (Thompson, 1994).

Types of pain

Acute pain. The initial few seconds of acute pain is described as *transient pain*. If tissue damage is negligible the transient pain ceases. Continuing acute pain is closely associated with tissue

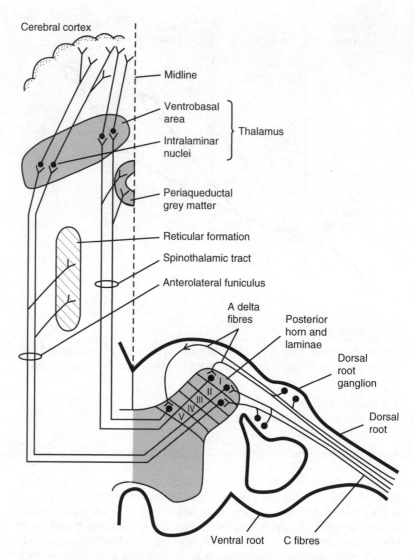

Fig. 3.19 The principal nociceptor connections and pathways.

damage. Figure 1.7 is relevant, in that inflammatory changes and exudation in the first hours can cause increasing pain. Clearly a further function of this acute pain is to limit movement or stress on the injured tissue and thus facilitate healing.

Chronic pain. Chronic pain is really only defined by its persistence. Pain that remains after apparent tissue healing, or is associated with degenerative disease, is termed chronic. Similarly, persistent pain without evident tissue damage is chronic. It may be due to a dysfunctional nociceptive system.

Somatogenic pain. Somatogenic pain may arise from both the body wall and from the viscera. Surface pain is usually well-localized; deep pain from tendons, muscles and joints tends to be more diffuse. Pain arising in the viscera themselves, associated with the autonomic system, is also not well localized although often severe (e.g. spasm of the ureter due to a kidney stone). Sensations originating in the parietal membrane – pleura, pericardium, peritoneum – are often sharp and better localized. These structures have more A delta innervation.

Pain originating in deep structures may be recognized in some other (superficial) site; this is called *referred pain*. This may occur when some visceral disorder provokes peripheral pain, such as pain in the left arm as a consequence of heart disease. It also occurs when a proximal part of a peripheral nerve is irritated, causing pain to be recognized in the sensory distribution of that nerve, as a result of pressure from an intervertebral disc or other structure in the spinal column. The mechanisms believed to account for the phenomenon of referred visceral pain are:

- nociceptors from both skin and viscera, carrying impulses to the same dorsal horn cell
- peripheral sensory nerves whose axons are bifurcated, one branch from skin and the other from some deeper structure (Bowsher, 1994).

The matter of referred pain is of considerable importance for physiotherapists, because visceral disorder may be interpreted by the patient as cutaneous or deeper pain arising in the same dermatome. An understanding of this mechanism is clearly important in identifying the correct source of pain. It may also help to explain how stimulation, electrical or other, can affect visceral pain (Hanegan, 1992).

Neurogenic pain. Another type, neurogenic pain, is entirely different in quality – often a burning sensation – and may be associated with autonomic disturbance. It is due to some form of neuronal damage; causalgia and post-herpetic neuralgia are examples.

Psychogenic pain. Pain is markedly influenced by psychological factors such that a separate category of psychogenic pain is sometimes used.

Summary of pain categories

- Somatogenic pain
  - acute pain, associated with tissue damage
  - chronic pain persisting after tissue healing.
- Referred pain, provoked in deep structures but recognized superficially.
- Neurogenic pain.
- Psychogenic pain, influenced from higher centres.

Alteration in pain

The nature of chronic pain is neither consistently defined nor completely understood. Some prolonged pain occurs unrelated to tissue damage and evident damage can occur with little or no pain.

Pain is also influenced by hormones, the duration of the pain, the personality, age, sex and cultural background of the individual.

It is important to understand that pain perception is not a fixed response to nociceptor stimulation. It can be both increased and decreased by other influences in the central nervous system (Johnson, 1997).

The mechanisms that can decrease pain perception – and the way in which electrotherapy might influence them – are discussed further in terms of suppression of the nociceptive system (see Fig. 3.19). There are other strong influences, such as the contributions of the higher centres and sympathetic nervous system in circumstances of severe stress when pain from quite serious injury is not recognized; also hypnosis.

The chemicals released due to tissue injury and inflammation, noted in Chapter 1, are able to activate and sensitize local nociceptors. This causes tenderness (allodynia) and an exaggerated response to painful stimuli not only at the site of injury but in surrounding tissues. Similarly, a release of neurotransmitters in the dorsal horn of the spinal cord provoked by nociceptor activity is able to make the nociceptive pathways hypersensitive. This and other mechanisms are thus able to amplify the central nervous system response to both noxious and other inputs (Johnson, 1997). These mechanisms to enhance the pain are plainly protective and disappear when healing occurs. It is suggested that in some instances of chronic pain it is this sensitization of the nervous system that persists.

Control of pain

The gate control theory of pain was suggested in 1965 by Melzack and Wall and has been expanded and modified since. The essence of it is that pain perception is regulated by a 'gate' which may be opened or closed by means of other inputs from peripheral nerves or from the central nervous system, thus increasing or decreasing the pain perceived. Some low-threshold mechanoreceptors from skin and elsewhere pass, without synapsing, up the posterior columns of the spinal cord. These A beta fibres give off collaterals, which impinge on nociceptor cells of the A delta and C pain fibres in laminae of the posterior horn. It is believed that the input of these mechanoreceptors effectively reduces the excitability of the nociceptor cells to pain-generated stimuli; it may be referred to as presynaptic or segmental inhibition.

Thus electrical pulses which stimulate these A beta mechano-receptor fibres are effective in reducing pain perception. As noted already, these relatively large-diameter nerves are capable of being stimulated at low current intensities (Fig. 3.13) and will convey impulses at quite high frequencies. Therefore low-intensity but perceptible high-frequency (100–200 Hz) TENS is appropriate and effective. Walsh (1997) notes that 'Despite the fact that the theory has since been disputed with regard to the precise location and mechanism involved in the "gate", it is still held as a concept that some form of inhibition can occur by stimulation of large-diameter afferents at a segmental level; hence the term "segmental inhibition".'

Morphine acts on the C fibre system and hence controls tissue-damage pain but not other types of pain. This occurs because morphine imitates naturally occurring groups of neurotransmitters, encephalin, β endorphin and dynorphin. In the substantia gelatinosa (lamina II) there are interneurons which can produce encephalin to inhibit the C system cells in this region. Collateral branches of A delta fibres in the posterior horn connect with these interneurons and stimulate them. Thus stimulation of the A delta fibre by electrical pulses will damp down C fibre system-type pain. This is reputed to be the mechanism by which acupuncture works, since these A delta nerve fibres are considered to be stimulated by pinprick. (Acupuncture points seem to be where bundles of these nerves pierce the deep fascia (Bowsher, 1994). The stimulation must be done in the same neural segment.) However, Levin and Hui-Chan (1993) were unable to demonstrate stimulation of A delta fibres in normal subjects and concluded that pain relief was due to stimulation of A alpha and beta fibres by both conventional and acupuncture-like TENS. They concede that patients afflicted with chronic pain may tolerate higher TENS intensities, possibly sufficient to stimulate A delta fibres. Stimulation of these fibres by high-intensity, low-frequency TENS, however, remains as a rational explanation of the inhibition of C fibre-type pain.

It is also recognized that activation of these A delta pain fibres may provoke impulses in the midbrain that then travel back down the spinal cord to inhibit nociceptor neurons at the original level: a descending pain suppression system (De Domenico, 1982; Bowsher, 1994; Walsh, 1997). The A delta nociceptors in the spinothalamic tract give off collateral branches to the periaqueductal grey matter (PAG) in the midbrain. Descending neurons from this region pass to various subregions of the rostral ventral medulla (not shown in Fig. 3.20(c)) and thence to the spinal dorsal horn generating encephalin in the substantia gelatinosa. These and other known descending pain-suppressing pathways use serotonin (5-hydroxytryptamine) and noradrenaline as neurotransmitters.

Summary

The mechanisms so far described are summarized in Figure 3.20 and below:

- The pain gate effect on both A delta (fast) and C (slow) pain fibres in the posterior horn due to stimulation of mechano-receptors (A beta) fibres by high-frequency, low-intensity electric pulses, sometimes called hi-TENS or traditional TENS.
- A morphine-type effect on the C fibre system occurs. This is due to encephalin produced by interneurons in the posterior horn, which have been stimulated by A delta pain receptor fibres. These A delta fibres are themselves stimulated by low-frequency, high-intensity electrical pulses, which are called lo-TENS or acupuncture TENS.
- Morphine-type (encephalin) effect on C fibre system as in point 2 above but via centres in the midbrain and involving serotonin as a neurotransmitter; also activated by A delta stimulation by low-frequency, high-intensity stimuli.

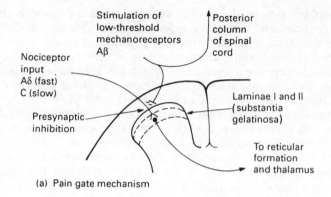

(a) Pain gate mechanism

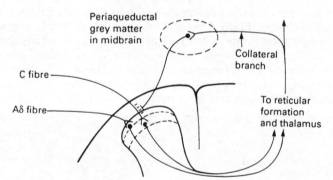

(b) Encephalin mechanism in the posterior horn

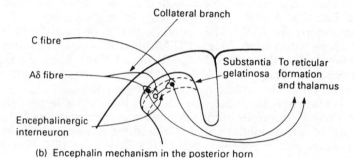

Fig. 3.20 Control of pain.

(c) Encephalin mechanism via descending pathway

Electrical stimulation at high frequencies may be able to produce a physiological block in both types of peripheral pain fibres. This effect is rather unclear and its clinical value is uncertain (De Domenico, 1982). However, a well-conducted study (Walsh *et al.*, 1993) has shown that different combinations of TENS frequencies and pulse lengths have differing influences on peripheral nerve conduction latency. It was shown that negative peak latency was markedly increased (i.e. conduction was slowed) in the superficial radial nerve of those who had received 0.2 ms pulses at 110 Hz for 15 min, and to a lesser extent with other stimulation parameters. It is presumed that the slowing of conduction reduces the volume of nociceptor traffic, hence reducing pain perception (Walsh, 1997). Thus it would seem that TENS may act directly on peripheral nerves, as well as at their connections in the spinal cord, as indicated above. Furthermore, the effect appears to depend on the stimulation parameters in an, as yet, unelucidated way. These facts may go some way to account for the inconsistency of results from clinical trials, as discussed below.

Electrical stimulation also reaches the cerebral cortex in the sense that the patient is aware of a prickling or tingling sensation. This may contribute to the placebo effect that occurs with all treatments.

As noted earlier, most of the treatments for pain relief are given by means of small battery-operated TENS stimulators which provide fairly short – around 0.05 ms – pulses of low intensity and variable frequency – often 50 or 100 Hz but may be up to 200 Hz. Similar effects are, of course, produced by similar electrical pulses. Many different sources of electrical stimulation, e.g. diadynamic, interferential and faradic-type currents, can lead to pain relief, which may be due to one or more of these mechanisms.

Therapeutic effectiveness

Clinical studies and experimental trials.   The effectiveness of TENS for pain relief has been well supported in quite a large number of clinical studies and trials (see Thorsteinsson, 1983; Fahrer, 1991). However, there are also a substantial number of studies that have shown no benefit from the application of TENS. Fahrer (1991) considered 25 trials reported between 1975 and 1990. He suggests that, as the number of trials interpreted as 'efficacious' (14 of 25) dominate slightly over the 'unproven' and 'not efficacious' studies, TENS should be regarded as an adjunctive analgesic aid. He notes that these studies evaluating TENS are not easy to compare because of large differences in trial design and other parameters. In fact, the average number of patients or subjects for each trial is somewhat lower in the 'efficacious' trials quoted, which rather diminishes their effect. In general, when treating acute and some neurogenic pain, the results appear to be better than those achieved in the treatment of chronic pain. Several studies, including one particularly large and thorough piece of work (Deyo *et al.*, 1990), have found no benefit beyond placebo for the use of TENS in chronic low back pain. Similarly, Herman *et al.* (1994), comparing active with placebo TENS coupled with a standardized exercise programme for acute low back pain, found that TENS did not lead to a better outcome. Successful treatment of neurogenic pain has been reported (Meyer and Fields, 1972). Perhaps not surprisingly, postoperative and obstetric pain have been quite successfully treated (Santiesteban, 1981), but some studies were unable to show benefit for the pain of labour. Sim (1991) also concluded that, following cholecystectomy through a right upper paramedian incisional approach, the limited benefits of TENS do not justify the additional cost or time. However, TENS has been shown to be as effective for postoperative analgesia as nitrous oxide and oxygen mixture (Entonox) inhalation (Jones and Hutchinson, 1991). Both provided short-term pain relief during postoperative physiotherapy, but TENS was preferred due to the lack of side-effects. TENS stimulation of an acupuncture point on the thumb has been shown to be effective in improving anti-emetic control following opioid analgesia in orthopaedic surgery in females (McMillan, 1994). TENS has been reported to give pain relief after coronary artery bypass surgery, but neither Forster *et al.* (1994) nor Domaille and Reeves (1997) found it to be better than placebo. In a double-blind trial the efficacy of TENS has been found to be much greater than would be accounted for by the placebo effect. Pain was relieved in 48% of instances due to TENS and in 32% of instances due to placebo treatment (Thorsteinsson *et al.*, 1977).

An important recent study on the effects of TENS on the inflamed joints of rats found that both high- and low-frequency TENS were effective in reducing hyperalgesia. The effect of low-frequency TENS lasted 12 h, while that of high-frequency TENS lasted more than twice as long. The writers (Sluka *et al.* 1998) conclude that TENS is effective in reducing referred or radiating pain, but does not affect the inflammatory response nor guarding of the limb. They also suggest that the effects of TENS may differ in the normal from those in the sensitized state.

Parameters of TENS.   Some efforts to determine the effective TENS parameters and mechanism have involved healthy volunteers. These studies have measured pain thresholds, ratings and tolerances to harmless but painful stimuli such as:

- ischaemic pain (e.g. Walsh *et al.*, 1995c)
- mechanical pain – pinch or pressure (e.g. Simmonds *et al.*, 1992)
- electrically induced pain (e.g. Barr *et al.*, 1986)
- cold-induced pain (e.g. Johnson *et al.*, 1989).

So far the results of such studies are inconsistent and have only moved a short way towards clarifying the mechanisms by which TENS might modify pain perception. Among the features to emerge are that:

- Pain thresholds appear to be raised by continuous (conventional) TENS to ice pain (Johnson *et al.*, 1989), to dull pressure – but not sharp mechanical pain (Simmonds *et al.*, 1992), to ischaemic pain (Roche *et al.*, 1984) and by high-intensity low-frequency TENS to acupuncture points (Noling *et al.*, 1988).
- Pain rating scores for ischaemic pain lowered due to the application of low-frequency (4 Hz) TENS (Walsh *et al.*, 1995c) or low-intensity trains and high-intensity continuous TENS (Roche *et al.*, 1984).
- Pain tolerance to electrically induced pain was increased by conventional low-intensity TENS, notably at a frequency of 60 Hz, but had no effect on pain threshold (Barr *et al.*, 1986). Others have not found this and question the usefulness of tests involving electrically induced pain (Rieb and Pomeranz, 1992).
- Ice pain thresholds are raised particularly at frequencies between 20 and 80 Hz (Johnson *et al.*, 1989).

- Considerable individual variations in response were noted (Johnson *et al.*, 1989).
- Males have higher pain thresholds and tolerances than females (Simmonds *et al.*, 1992).

Walsh *et al.* (1995a) demonstrated a significant increase in conduction latency in the superficial radial nerve following the application of TENS for three consecutive 5-minute periods. The observed neurophysiological effect was dependent upon the combinations of pulse frequency and pulse duration parameters. The 110 Hz, 0.2 ms TENS group showed a statistically significant increase in latency compared to the control group. A further study (Walsh, 1995b) showed that the increase in latency was evident for up to 15 min after the TENS unit was switched off.

A careful study (Marchand *et al.*, 1993) concluded that high-frequency, low-intensity TENS reduced both the intensity and unpleasantness of pain (which were separately measured) due to chronic backache. Much of the reduction of pain unpleasantness was considered a placebo effect, which, had it been combined with the effect on pain intensity, would have disguised the real effect. The authors conclude that TENS is a useful, short-term analgesic for low back pain. Failure to distinguish between the affective and other components of pain could well account for the confusion and uncertainty over the effects of TENS and similar treatments.

There is a definite difference in the mode of action of high-frequency, low-intensity TENS compared to that of the low-frequency, high-intensity type which acts by the release of morphine-like neurotransmitters. This is shown by the fact that the latter can be blocked by a morphine inhibitor (Sjölund and Eriksson, 1979). This difference does not seem to be reflected in any differences in clinical use; both types were reported to be successful in similar conditions. It has been suggested (Thorsteinsson, 1983) that high-intensity, low-frequency TENS gives somewhat better results but is less well tolerated.

Duration of pain relief.   The duration of pain relief due to TENS is very variable. One study (Thorsteinsson *et al.*, 1977) found a mean of 4–7 h, but it is not clear why pain should be relieved for such long periods due to any of the described mechanisms.

A later study (Johnson *et al.*, 1991a) found analgesia lasting less than 30 min in about half the patients and over 1 h in a further 30%. This particularly valuable study of a large number of long-term TENS users showed that nearly half (47%) had their pain reduced by more than half as a result of this treatment. Interestingly, some of the patients who had no pain relief continued to use TENS, apparently because it provided distraction from the pain, illustrating that TENS may do more than relieve the pain. A further study by the same authors (Johnson *et al.*, 1991b) found that patients consistently use particular pulse frequencies and patterns to control their pain. While these vary widely between individuals, there appears to be no relationship between these parameters and the cause or site of pain.

TENS has also been utilized in the successful treatment of patients suffering from persistent, abnormal skin sensations, such as formication or feelings of worms wriggling under the skin (dysaesthesia) (Bending, 1993). The mode of action would presumably be similar to that leading to pain relief, so that similar therapeutic parameters should be used.

Other types of current.   The effects of other types of current on pain have not been nearly so extensively researched. Although it is widely agreed that interferential currents have a pain-relieving effect, there seems to be a dearth of objective studies. It has been shown that a rise in the pain threshold may occur after interferential treatment (Pärtan *et al.*, 1953), but a more recent study on jaw pain (Taylor *et al.*, 1987) could find no significant difference between interferential and placebo treatments. A small pilot study investigating the effect of interferential therapy on induced ischaemic pain in healthy volunteers (Scott and Purves, 1991) found a pain relieving trend in the treatment group which was not statistically significant. Stephenson and Johnson (1995) found that interferential treatment raised the cold-induced pain threshold in healthy subjects. Quirk *et al.* (1985) found that the symptoms of osteoarthritis of the knee were significantly relieved by treatment using interferential therapy and exercises, shortwave diathermy and exercises, or exercises alone. Overall analysis revealed no significant difference between the three regimens except that the only patients to deteriorate during treatment were those in the exercise-only group. For a discussion of the way interferential currents may relieve pain see De Domenico (1982) and for an important critique on this topic see Johnson (1999).

There is, of course, good reason to suppose that many types of electrical currents which are not customarily regarded as TENS, such as various uniphasic and biphasic pulsed currents, HVPGS and diadynamic currents, could all relieve pain by the mechanisms described above. Microcurrent electrical stimulation has also been advocated. This consists of very low current (10–100 µA) usually biphasic, reversing polarity every 0.4 s. While such currents may be effective in tissue healing, their analgesic effects have not been strongly supported.

The pain-relieving effect of electrical stimulation has been found to decline during long-term use in some patients. The reasons for this are unknown; Johnson *et al.* (1991a) found that this had occurred in about a third of their patients.

Other effects

Effects on cutaneous blood flow

Cutaneous vasodilation occurs in the area of application of some electrical stimulation of sufficient intensity. This is considered to be due to stimulation of sensory nerves causing arteriolar vasodilation activating the axon reflex at first and the subsequent release of histamine-like substances (Wadsworth and Chanmugan, 1980). This effect, evidenced by a rise in skin temperature, has been noted in some studies as a result of strong TENS stimulation. It has been utilized in the treatment of peripheral vascular disease; it is thought to involve the sympathetic system. However, there is marked inconsistency in the results of investigations on normal subjects, some showing no effect, some skin cooling (for a discussion see Scudds *et al.*, 1995). With monophasic (unidirectional) currents the pH and other chemical changes seem to cause the vasodilation, as described in Chapter 2.

Reduction of oedema

There are claims that various therapeutic current applications will help to reduce tissue oedema. These are based on at least three distinct mechanisms:

- The muscle pumping action, noted above (p. 87), in which intermittent muscle contraction mechanically compresses adjacent soft-walled venous and lymphatic vessels to increase the centripetal flow of their contents. The consequent reduction of interstitial pressure is considered to be effective for all oedema, whatever the stage or cause.
- There is a hypothetical mechanism which suggests that the application of current displaces the negatively charged plasma proteins of the interstitial fluid of a traumatized region. The increased mobility of albumin in particular should accelerate the normal lymphatic capillary uptake, so increasing the fluid return in the lymphatic system and reducing oedema. While there is some evidence supporting this hypothesis and it is often asserted (e.g. Newton, 1987), careful experiments on animals have been unable to demonstrate this particular effect, although a symmetrically biphasic current appeared to hamper absorption (Mohr *et al.*, 1987; Cosgrove *et al.*, 1992). These studies applied cathodal high-voltage pulsed currents at 24-hour intervals after the initial trauma and were thus treating already resolving oedema. Other animal experiments, however, applied similar currents immediately after trauma (i.e. while the oedema was developing), and found the oedema formation clearly retarded (Bettany *et al.*, 1990; Taylor *et al.*, 1991).
- A third suggested mechanism (Mendel *et al.*, 1992; Reed, 1988) is that the current acts to decrease the permeability of capillaries in some way, thus diminishing fluid and plasma protein loss to the interstitial space. This suggests that the time at which the current is applied is important.

It must be understood that effects on animals, both supporting and refuting a mechanism, are not necessarily transferable to humans. However, these studies provide some important evidence, not previously demonstrated, which may eventually lead to more enlightened clinical applications.

Effects on the autonomic nervous system

It is to be expected that some autonomic nerves would be stimulated by electrical pulses of suitable intensities since somatic nerves of similar size are stimulated. Such effects are frequently postulated as an explanation for therapeutic benefit, particularly in connection with interferential currents. The evidence for these effects, such as it is, seems to be inconsistent.

Altering the ionic distribution around the cell

Altering the ionic balance around the cell – as electrical stimulation inevitably does – would be expected to lead to some effects, but clear evidence and clinical correlation are lacking at present. It has been indicated in Chapter 2 that monophasic currents can accelerate the healing of cutaneous wounds and bone. Remodelling of bone and fibrous tissue have also been proposed. Many other effects have been considered to occur, such as increases in cell metabolism and exchange across the cell membrane, both being associated with increased microcirculation (Alon, 1987); see also Chapter 1.

Hierarchy of effects

The effects of electrical stimulation have sometimes been described in a confusing and illogical manner with no distinction being made between the direct and indirect effects. A more rational approach has been proposed (Alon, 1987) in which the physiological responses to electrical stimulation are organized into cellular, tissue, segmental and systemic levels. Thus nerve excitation occurs at a cellular level and the muscle contraction it induces is an effect at the tissue level. Muscle group contraction and its effect on venous and lymphatic flow occur at a segmental level whilst the analgesic effects due to the release of endorphins and encephalins is an effect at the systemic level.

Summary of the effects of pulsed currents on:

- Sensory nerves → prickling sensation
  → pain relief via pain gate mechanism
  → cutaneous vasodilation via axon reflex
- Motor nerves → skeletal muscle contraction
  ↓

  - re-education of movement
  - increased strength and endurance
  - increased intramuscular blood flow
  - increased muscle metabolism
  - increased blood flow in adjacent tissues (pumping effect)
  - increased or maintained joint motion
  - control of joint motion (FES)
  - muscle fatigue

  → affect muscle fibre growth – trophic change

- nociceptors – Aδ and C fibres
  → pain sensation
  → modify pain perception
  (due to release of endogenous opioids and other mechanisms)
- muscle tissue → muscle contraction
- autonomic nerves → possible effects on blood flow
- capillaries → possible effects on tissue fluid exchange
- cells → growth and activity altered by monophasic pulses – tissue healing accelerated.

PRINCIPLES OF APPLICATION

Electrical energy for therapy must be applied to the body tissues with at least two electrodes to form a complete circuit. The transition of an electric current of conduction in the wires (electron movement) to a convection current in the tissues (ionic movement) is complex and very important in determining the resulting effects.

Electrode–tissue interface

The changes that occur between the conducting metal and conducting fluid on and within the tissues consist of complex dynamic electrochemical interactions. The simple consequences of these have been described in Chapter 2 and the Appendix. If the applied current is evenly alternating (biphasic) there are no significant chemical changes; also if the total current, although unidirectional, is very small (low-intensity and/or very short pulses) the chemical effects will be negligible.

A layer of ion-containing fluid is needed to pass current from the electrode to the tissues, normally skin. This is water or conducting gel. This serves to ensure a uniform conducting pathway between

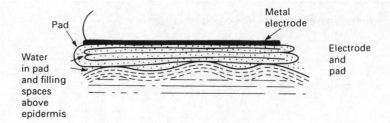

Fig. 3.21 Cross-section of electrode and pad.

the electrode and the epidermis and secondly to make the electrochemical changes occur outside the epidermis. Since the epidermal surface is very irregular a flat electrode pressed onto it would be in contact at only a few points, leading to a high current density at these points. Further, the epidermal surface has a high electrical resistance because it is largely dry keratin, and because of the presence of oily sebum. This resistance is lowered by wetting the skin surface.

Types of electrode

There are three basic electrode systems:

- A malleable metal electrode such as tinplate or aluminium coupled to the skin with water retained in a pad of lint, cotton gauze or some form of sponge material, e.g. Spontex (Fig. 3.21). The water provides the uniform ion-containing low-resistance pathway for the current while the absorbant material simply serves to keep the water in place. Ordinary tapwater is suitable in most instances but in some soft-water areas a little salt or bicarbonate of soda may need to be added. The whole assembly is fixed in place by a strap, bandage or by suction. The thickness of the pad needed, and hence the quantity of water, depends on the irregularity of the skin surface and on whether significant chemical changes will occur. If the latter is the case then about 1.25 cm is considered an appropriate thickness. Otherwise rather thinner (0.5–1 cm) wet thickness seems to be sufficient for most treatments.

  In a system in which current passes through the body the total current at each of the two electrodes must be equal but the important factor is the current density, i.e. current per unit area. Thus if two pads are of unequal size, most effect will occur close to the smaller one, which is called the active electrode. The other electrode is called the indifferent or dispersive electrode. In order to limit the effects to an area such as the motor point of a muscle, the active electrode can be a small metal disc covered with lint or other suitable material and attached to a handle. This is often called a button electrode.

- The second system involves electrodes that will conform to the body surface more easily than the metal electrodes described above. These are made of carbon-impregnated silicone rubber. They may be used with sponge pads or coupled to the skin by a thin layer of conducting gel and fixed in place either with a strap or adhesive tape. A somewhat similar system for more lengthy application of TENS involves karaya gum (obtained from a particular kind of tree in India) which when wetted is both conductive and adhesive. Some synthetically produced polymers act in the same way (Patterson, 1983).

In general, the carbon rubber and similar electrodes used with conducting gel are convenient for long-term use and repeated self-application by the patient, whereas the water pad conduction methods, whether with metal or carbon rubber electrodes, are more appropriate for treating larger areas with higher currents and are usually used in the physiotherapy department. Metal electrodes are somewhat more efficient in passing current to the tissues than carbon rubber and other similar types in that they have a lower impedance (Nelson *et al.*, 1980). However, carbon rubber appear, on the whole, to be better than many other commercially available polymer electrodes, some of which exhibit remarkably high impedance (Nolan, 1991). It should be noted that, where the electrode is coupled to the skin by a wet pad, current density is determined by the area of the pad, but, where the electrode is in direct contact with the skin, it is determined by the area of the electrode. Patterson (1983) noted that carbon rubber electrodes have significant resistance compared with the electrode-tissue junction, so that most current will take the shortest pathway. Thus, where it is directly coupled to the skin by gel, the current density is likely to be higher close to where the metal wire enters the electrode.

- The third system is by means of a water bath (or baths) in which the body part is immersed with an electrode. Current is passed from electrode to tissues through the water. This system is considered later.

Current flow in the tissues

The quantity of current that flows in the tissues and the path it follows will depend on the impedance of that pathway. The impedance includes the ohmic resistance, capacitive resistance (or reactance) and the inductive resistance. The latter is negligible in the tissues but the two former have an important influence on the effects of the electrical stimulation. Generally, watery tissue such as blood, muscle and nerve has low ohmic resistance; bone and fat has rather higher and epidermis has the highest of all. The ohmic resistance is determined therefore chiefly by the thickness and nature of the skin under the electrodes and, to a much lesser extent, by the inter-electrode distance. Where two low-resistance regions are separated by a high-resistance region, i.e. a near insulator, a capacitor is formed and capacitive effects occur. Thus where an electrode is separated from nerve and muscle by skin and fat there is a capacitor. The concept of these electrical pathways is illustrated in Figure 3.22.

For direct current (unidirectional current) and slowly changing pulses of current the skin resistance is high and thus most of the

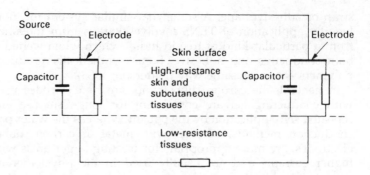

Fig. 3.22 Electrical pathways of current applied to the tissues.

electrical energy is released in the skin and subcutaneous tissues, hence cutaneous nerves are affected. As the current spreads through the low-resistance pathway of the deeper tissues it can have less effect. However, capacitive resistance diminishes for short pulses of current or alternating (biphasic) currents of higher frequencies, thus the current can pass through the skin more easily and relatively more energy is released in the deeper tissues. This explains why short pulse (phase) lengths are able to penetrate the skin more easily. The effect occurs with both single pulses and alternating pulses of appropriate frequency (i.e. a 4000 Hz medium-frequency current is a series of 0.125 ms phases (half cycles) and behaves in the same way as separate single pulses of this duration).

Taken together the effects described above suggest that some deeply placed low-threshold nerves, such as motor nerves, would be more efficiently stimulated by shorter pulses, say about 1/20th of a millisecond (0.05 ms) because of the skin capacitance. On the other hand to stimulate high-threshold unmyelinated pain fibres (C fibres) in the skin it would seem sensible to use longer pulses of a few milliseconds.

Arrangements of electrodes

It has been noted already that what matters for producing an effect in the tissues is the current density. Adding to the size of the electrodes will decrease the current density. Since the water in the pad has a very low ohmic resistance the effective area of application is that of the pad.

The position of the electrodes will obviously determine the path that the current will follow in the tissues. In many situations a small electrode is used to give a high, localized current density, such as to stimulate the motor point of a muscle or an acupuncture point. In these circumstances the dispersive (or indifferent) electrode can be placed on any convenient area of skin that is reasonably close. The further away it is placed the more current will be needed and less effective localization will occur. If the two electrodes are of similar size the current density under each will be similar and therefore effects such as sensory stimulation will occur under both. If the electrodes are placed close together the effects will be localized

Practical point
The area of the pad can be increased by using either a single, larger pad or with one or more additional parallel-connected electrodes.

to the region between them, e.g. placing electrodes at either end of the long axis of the belly of a muscle will cause local stimulation of that muscle, or stimulating sensory nerves in a local area of skin to give pain relief. If the electrodes are placed too close together current will be localized to the adjacent edges and to the intervening small area of skin rather than passing through the whole area of electrode and epidermis in contact.

Polarity

While current density is the most important factor in determining the effect of an applied current, polarity must also be considered. The polarity will only be significant with uniphasic, unevenly biphasic pulses, or if the pulse has an evenly biphasic charge but is unequal in amplitude (e.g. Fig. 3.3).

The negative electrode (cathode) will stimulate a nerve fibre with rising current more readily than the positive electrode because the outer surface of the nerve membrane is positively charged at rest and thus more easily driven beyond threshold by increasing negativity (see Chapter 1).

The positive electrode (anode) will also provoke a nerve impulse as the current rises, but will require a somewhat greater amplitude because it has to influence the surface of the nerve further from the electrode (a positive phase with the current falling can have the same effect as the rise of current in a negative phase).

Even when a pair of identically sized electrodes are used, the current density is unlikely to be exactly equal under each, due to variations in skin impedance and electrode/tissue junction resistance.

Water baths

The hand, forearm, foot and leg can conveniently be put into baths or bowls of water with electrodes to provide a means of passing current to the tissues. Such an arrangement can be used to provide a large area for an indifferent electrode, as described in Chapter 2. They can also be used as a method of applying muscle-stimulating currents. If two electrodes are placed in the same water bath with the part to be treated, current will pass both through the water and through the tissues – two pathways in parallel (Fig. 3.23). The current density in the tissues is critically dependent on the position of the two electrodes in the bath and on the relative resistance of the two paths. Such a system is often used to stimulate the intrinsic muscle of the foot for re-education when it is called a faradic foot bath.

Unipolar and bipolar

The system described above, with both electrodes in the same bath, is referred to as 'bipolar' whereas if one electrode is in the bath and the circuit is completed by a pad electrode or an electrode in another bath it is called 'unipolar'. It may be noted that adding salt to a

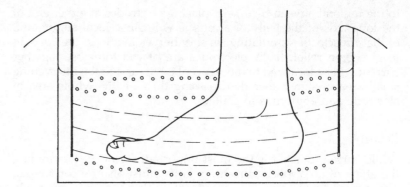

Fig. 3.23 Bipolar bath. Dashed lines = current through tissues; dotted lines = current through water.

unipolar bath results in a greater current passing through the tissues because it lowers the resistance in series thus reducing the total resistance. Adding salt to a bipolar bath will decrease the current through the tissues since greater current will now pass in the parallel water pathway due to its lowered resistance. In some publications, e.g. Alon (1987), bipolar treatments are described as those in which both electrodes or pads are applied to the area being treated, whereas unipolar are those involving a (usually) larger indifferent electrode applied at some distance from the active electrode which is sited over the target tissue. However, it must be emphasized that all these treatments involving a flow of current in the tissues are essentially bipolar in the sense that there must be two connections to the tissues. The use of the terms 'unipolar' and 'bipolar' sometimes creates confusion.

Summary

Methods of application:

- electrodes – carbon rubber or metal
- coupling to skin – by water: wet pad/sponge
                              – by gel or solution
- secured – by bandage, tape, adhesive, gel or suction.

Factors influencing current flow in tissues:

- impedance of pathway – electrode/tissue junction
                                  – skin and superficial tissues
- current density – size of pad/gelled electrode in contact with skin
- nature of applied currents – pulse length
                                       – pulse polarity.

Lowering the electrical resistance at the skin surface

As has been noted already, the electrical resistance of the epidermis is high. It can be reduced by washing the surface to remove some of the keratin and sebum and leaving the skin wet. Warming the skin also helps to lower its resistance by increasing the rate of particle and ionic movement, also perhaps increasing the activity of the sweat glands and blood flow. Thus warming, washing and wetting the skin will allow larger currents to flow for the same applied voltage.

In all cases it must be realized that maintaining the same skin–electrode junction throughout treatment is essential. If the adhesion of the electrode to the skin surface alters, or the pressure of sponge or pad decreases, this can lead to a higher resistance; consequently the fixation of the electrodes to the body surface is very important in keeping a constant uniform low resistance at this junction.

Checking for areas of abnormal resistance

The skin should be inspected before treatment to check for any low resistance areas, such as cuts or abrasions, or any other circumstances which might lead to uneven distribution of the current. Sometimes the pad/electrode can be conveniently moved to avoid this area but, if not, and the area of low resistance is small enough, it can be protected with a layer of petroleum jelly covered with cotton wool. Abnormal epidermal tissue, such as warts or scars, may present areas of higher resistance, which could alter current distribution if they are extensive. Similarly, grease from emollients may need to be removed.

Practical point
To record small currents generated by the tissues, such as the electrocardiogram or surface electromyogram, it is sometimes necessary to reduce the skin surface resistance still further by gently scraping or sandpapering some of the surface epidermis off – removing some of the dead cells that form the outer epidermis – before fixing the electrodes.

Safety recommendations

Electrical apparatus should be energized *before* connecting the patient to the circuit. Likewise, the patient should be disconnected from the equipment before it is switched off. This is because, on some equipment, there is a spike of output before the machine stabilizes.

Thermal damage due to excess current density can occur. For this reason it is recommended (BS5724, Section 2:10, 1988) that special attention be paid to average current densities beyond 2 mA r.m.s./cm^2. The effective (r.m.s.) value of an alternating current is the same as the intensity of direct current that gives the same power. For sine waveforms (a.c.):

$$\text{Effective current} = \frac{\text{Peak current}}{\sqrt{2}}$$

$$= 0.7 \times \text{peak current}$$

$$1.4 \times \text{r.m.s. current} = \text{peak current}$$

Such high current densities are more likely to occur with medium-frequency currents than the short-pulse, low-frequency currents of most muscle stimulators.

Electrically induced thermal burns can occur with very high-current densities beneath or between TENS electrodes (Gersh, 1992), also as a consequence of defective skin–electrode contact. Such events are extremely rare; in fact, no detailed reports seem to be available (see later discussion on Safety with electrical currents).

It is important to recognize that electrochemical damage – as opposed to thermal damage – due to d.c. can occur at low current densities ($0.33 \, mA/cm^2$ is the usual recommended maximum).

APPLICATION AND USES OF SPECIFIC CURRENTS

Pulsed currents for muscle stimulation – faradic-type currents

Electrical muscle stimulation is usually achieved by 0.1–1 ms pulses at frequencies between 30 and 100 Hz (faradic-type pulses). In order to localize the current to individual muscles a small active electrode, i.e. a small pad or button electrode, is applied to the motor point of the muscle, the circuit being completed with a larger dispersive electrode sited in some convenient, usually proximal, area. The motor points of some superficial muscles are often indicated on charts (Fig. 3.24). Such charts act as a guide but a knowledge of the relevant anatomy coupled with a little trial and error will locate the precise point at which the muscle is most effectively stimulated. The usual site is in the lower part of the proximal third of the muscle belly but there are many exceptions. It is obvious that deeply placed muscles can only be successfully stimulated where their fleshy belly becomes superficial, for example, the extensor hallucis longus emerging in the lower part of the leg between tibialis anterior and extensor digitorum longus (Fig. 3.24).

Constant current pulses have sometimes been suggested as the preferred option for techniques in which the electrodes are fixed, because they are reputed to give a more consistent level of stimulation (Alon, 1987). In this case, fluctuation of the skin/electrode resistance causes voltage changes that maintain a nearly constant current. However, for labile techniques involving electrode movement, constant voltage is preferable. In these applications, the effective area (i.e. the area in contact with the skin) of the pad/electrode changes, which alters the current density. If the area of the pad in contact with the tissues becomes smaller, the resistance increases. However, if the voltage remains constant, the current intensity will fall so that the current *density* will remain approximately the same.

Technique of application

Preparation of patient.
Explanation: The nature of the treatment and the sensations to be expected – a tingling sensation and muscle contraction – should be explained to the patient with reassurance that no damage can be caused by this treatment.

Examination and testing.
The skin surfaces to which the current will be applied must be examined and any cuts, abrasions or other

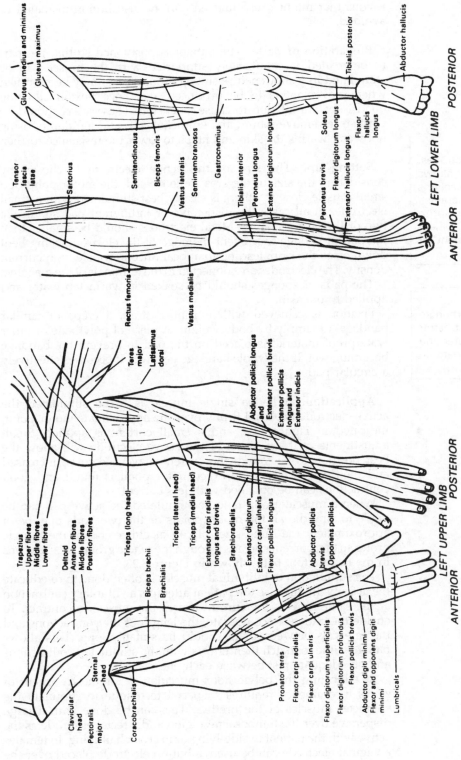

Fig. 3.24 Guide to motor points.

lesions that might cause uneven current distribution insulated or avoided.

Preparation of part. The patient is positioned so that the part to be treated is comfortably supported with the muscles to be stimulated in a shortened position, although this may be modified when movement is to be produced, e.g. knee flexion allowing quadriceps stimulation to cause extension. These areas should be washed to remove sebum and epithelial cells and left damp; using hot water warms the skin and helps to lower the resistance further.

Setting up. The size of the active electrode is chosen by considering the size of the area to be treated; the motor point of a small muscle close to others is clearly best stimulated with a small electrode. In all cases the dispersive or indifferent pad should be two or three times larger. Metal electrodes should be smaller than the pad or sponge to prevent the edge of the electrode being bent down on to the skin, leading to a local uncomfortable high current density. The electrodes are connected to the terminals of the machine.

The pads or sponges should be soaked in warm tap water and applied to the skin.

Fixation is achieved with a rubber strap, a crêpe or similar bandage, or simply by body weight. A piece of polythene or other waterproof material is placed on the pad to prevent the bandage becoming wet. If the whole bandage gets wet, it becomes effectively a circular pad.

Application. When a single muscle is to be stimulated the active electrode is placed firmly over the approximate motor point, indicated in Figure 3.24, and a small current is applied. Small adjustments of the position of the active electrode will allow the best position to be found; the current may need to be increased and then decreased as the exact motor point is found and good contractions can be obtained with less current.

When a muscle group is to be stimulated the active pad can be made to straddle all the motor points or the two pads may be of approximately the same size, placed at either end of the muscle group so that current spreads through the whole group: this happens in the faradic foot bath, shown in Figure 3.23.

The stimulation of individual muscles is often done to re-educate the activity. In this case the patient attempts a voluntary contraction at the same time as the current causes the muscle to contract. To enable the patient to co-operate, the length of the contractions and the intervals between them should be suitably long. This allows patients time to match their efforts with the stimulated contractions and an adequate rest between each one.

Re-educating the pelvic floor musculature for the treatment of stress incontinence requires a special technique to stimulate the sphincter muscles of the urethra. This can be done with a large dispersive over the lumbosacral region and a rectal electrode as the active with the patient in side-lying or in crook half-lying. In females a vaginal electrode can be used; a button electrode placed over the

---

Practical point
Holding the two electrodes, separated, in one hand allows the machine and connections to be tested by the therapist. Observing this may help to allay the anxiety of a patient experiencing this treatment for the first time.

Practical point
Saline or sodium bicarbonate solutions are somewhat better conductors than tap water and may be more appropriate in soft-water areas.

perineal body can be used as the active electrode in either sex (Wadsworth and Chanmugan, 1980). Voluntary contraction is attempted with the electrical stimulation. Faradic-type currents have been used in the successful treatment of this condition (Montgomery and Shepherd, 1983) as well as interferential currents (see later discussion on effects of interferential).

Reduction of oedema. Muscle groups in the limbs can be stimulated rhythmically to provide a muscle-pumping action, enhancing the venous and lymphatic flow to assist the reduction of oedema. This is combined with elevation of the limb and the application of a pressure bandage. The largest volume of muscle that can be stimulated is required, so the quadriceps and plantarflexors of the lower limb and flexors of the elbow and hand in the upper limb are usually chosen. Large pads are applied over these muscle groups, or on the sole of the foot and quadriceps; there are numerous other pad positions to achieve the strong generalized muscle contractions needed. The compression bandage, applied over the pads, should give firm pressure against which the contracting musculature can press but should not be constrictive. Strong slow muscle contractions should be produced with a long period of relaxation (several seconds) to allow vessel filling.

Termination.   The equipment applied to the patient is removed and the skin cleaned, dried and inspected.

Recording.   The parameters of treatment and any immediate resulting effects are recorded.

Long-duration and accommodation pulses

When these pulses are used for the stimulation of denervated muscle, the electrodes should be applied in the long axis of the muscle belly in order to activate the maximum number of muscle fibres.

TENS

It is customary, as already noted, to limit the acronym 'TENS' to low-intensity, short impulses applied largely for pain relief. As local areas are usually treated and self-treatment is common, small carbon-rubber electrodes are usually employed. Since both the intention and effect of the treatment are to relieve pain it is important to be certain that this is appropriate and does not lead to the neglect of the underlying causes of the pain. It is also very important that the pain should be evaluated both initially and during the course of the treatment. This serves both to monitor the effectiveness of the particular treatment parameters used, such as the position of the electrodes, and to measure the progress of the treatment. Any objective methods that are appropriate, such as measuring the range of movement, should be used but often subjective pain assessment is the principal means used. A 10 cm horizontal visual analogue scale (on which the patient marks the intensity of pain between one end marked 'no pain' and the other end 'worst pain ever') and pain behaviour analysis have been recommended (Frampton, 1988).

To be effective it is necessary for TENS to be able to affect conducting afferent nerves. It is thus appropriate to ensure that there is some cutaneous sensation and that this is sufficient to provide protection against the application of excessive current.

The application of TENS requires decisions about where to place the electrodes and what current parameters to use.

Electrode placement

There are several approaches:

- The most usual is to site electrodes close to where the pain is perceived to be; often one electrode is sited over the place where the most intense pain is felt or the greatest tenderness elicited.
- The electrodes may be placed within the same dermatome, myotome or sclerotome. They may be placed to pass current through the long axis of the dermatome. In many, but not all, circumstances the dermatome, myotome and sclerotome overlap.
- Trigger or acupuncture points may be the preferred sites of current application. It is considered (Klein and Pariser, 1987) that acupuncture points can be located by their lower resistance compared with the surrounding skin (due to active sweat glands and/or local vasodilation); they can be found by using an electronic probe. Jones *et al.* (1990) found no difference in pain relief whether the electrodes were placed over the acupuncture point or para-incisionally for post-cholecystectomy patients. A trigger point is an area that is tender on palpation with referred pain.
- Stimulation of peripheral nerves is used. Electrodes are placed in the line of the nerve and where it is particularly superficial. This method is used principally for the treatment of neurogenic pain such as postherpetic neuralgia.
- Over the spinal nerve roots close to the vertebral column.

It is evident from a clinical point of view that these approaches are by no means mutually exclusive. Thus trigger points, peripheral nerves and the painful area all lie in a dermatome. The choice of electrode position is often dictated by an effective result, i.e. relief of pain. Several positions may be tried before success is achieved. Johnson *et al.* (1991a,b) found that most patients in a sample of long-term TENS users applied electrodes over, or immediately proximal to, the site of pain.

Walsh (1997) states that since the cathode is the active electrode, in stimulation of a nerve fibre it should be applied nearest to the desired destination of the action potential. Thus for stimulation of sensory nerves it is proximal to the anode, i.e. nearer the spinal cord.

Current parameters

- TENS is most often applied as short pulses of around 50 µs at 40–150 Hz; this is called conventional TENS (see Fig. 3.25), and is high-frequency, low-intensity stimulation. The intensity is turned up gradually until a prickling or tingling sensation is felt. It should be neither painful nor should it cause a muscle contraction. It is presumed that these low-intensity short pulses will selectively stimulate the large low-threshold A beta fibres to produce pain inhibition by the pain gate mechanism, as described earlier. This conventional mode is the most usual method for self-treatment. The recommended duration and timing of such treatments varies from 30 to 60 min sessions once or twice a day (Klein and Pariser, 1987) to continuous TENS for a minimum of 8 h/day or even a full 24 h/day (Frampton, 1988). Walsh (1997) advises a maximum treatment period of 1 h at a time, repeated as often as required but with half hour breaks between applications to reduce the likelihood of skin irritation.
- High-intensity, low-frequency (acupuncture-like) TENS (Fig. 3.25) is another approach that is often used. Pulses of around 0.2 ms at about 2 Hz are given at intensities that provoke visible muscle contractions. This stimulates the high-threshold A delta and C fibres which leads to the release of endogenous opioids and provides further sensory input from muscle spindle afferents. This kind of stimulation is often applied to acupuncture points but is sometimes applied to the motor points of muscle in the segmentally related myotome. In contrast to conventional TENS it is usually applied once per day for 20 or 30 min (Klein and Pariser, 1987). Mannheimer and Lampe (1984) suggest that acute pain of a superficial nature, including causalgia, responds best to conventional TENS, whereas longstanding, deep, aching pain responds best to low-frequency TENS. However, Johnson *et al.* (1991a,b) found that there was no relation between the cause of pain and the pulse frequency or pattern used by their patients.
- 'Burst TENS' (Fig. 3.25) is a series of pulses (i.e. a train), repeated 1–5 times a second, commonly twice. Each train or burst consists of a number of individual pulses at the usual conventional TENS frequencies of 40–150 Hz but at higher intensity. The benefit claimed for this latter method is that it combines both the conventional and acupuncture-like TENS and therefore provides pain relief by both routes. These modes of stimulation are illustrated in Figure 3.25.
- Brief, intense TENS involves the use of longer duration, around 0.2 ms, pulses at higher frequencies around 100 Hz and the highest tolerable intensity. The application is made for no longer than 15 min at a time. Mannheimer and Lampe (1984) suggest this is an appropriate method for local painful conditions.
- In modulated TENS the pulse length, frequency and amplitudes can be constantly and automatically varied. Some machines provide this facility for all three parameters, some for one or

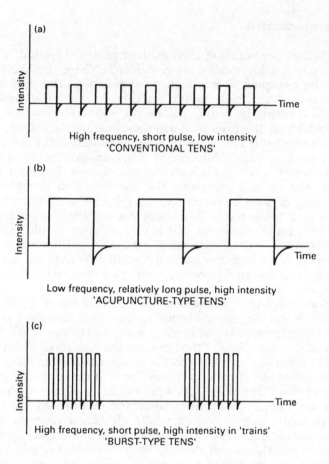

Fig. 3.25 Different forms of TENS.

two of them. This cyclical variation is believed to prevent adaptation of the nerves to the current and is particularly appropriate as a variant of conventional TENS used over long periods.

It should be noted that the figures and names used above are generalizations and do not necessarily conform to all other writers. Mannheimer and Lampe (1984) consider 'high-frequency TENS' to be between 75 and 150 Hz, for example. It must also be recognized that the output from commercially available TENS equipment does not always accurately match the dial settings and on some, a very small change in the setting leads to a large change in output (see Johnson *et al.*, 1989; Walsh, 1997).

Electrode fixation

Electrodes are fixed to the skin with adhesive tape or bandaged into place. A conducting gel is applied between electrode and skin. The leads from the TENS unit are concealed and fixed in the clothing if continuous home treatment is being given. Convenient ready-gelled adhesive electrodes are available.

Summary

Positioning of electrodes over:

- the site of pain
- a point just proximal to the site of pain
- the dermatome, myotome or sclerotome
- the trigger point, acupuncture or motor point
- a peripheral nerve, either locally or over the spinal nerve roots.

Stimulus parameters:

- conventional TENS
  - high frequency, short pulse duration, low intensity
- acupuncture-like TENS
  - low frequency, long pulse duration, high intensity
- burst TENS
  - low frequency trains consisting of high frequency, high intensity, short duration pulses
- brief, intense TENS
  - high frequency, long pulse duration, maximum tolerable intensity applied for limited (<15 min) periods
- modulated TENS
  - continually varying frequency, pulse duration or intensity, singly or in combination.

H-wave therapy

As noted earlier, H-wave comprises a series of exponentially decaying biphasic pulses of fixed form applied at frequencies between 2 and 60 Hz (see Fig. 3.8). It thus might be considered a special form of TENS. While the whole pulse would be described as of fairly long duration – around 11 ms – because it rises rapidly and falls exponentially the 'spike' at highest amplitude would be relatively short and thus similar to TENS pulses.

H-wave has been recommended as treatment for wound healing and the reduction of oedema as well as the relief of pain. As far as the latter is concerned, a series of studies have shown that mechanical pain thresholds were raised by 2 and 60 Hz H-wave therapy, but only a marginal, non-significant effect on ischaemic pain could be found. A further valuable study in this series found a significant increase in local blood flow after H-wave therapy applied at 2 Hz see Walsh *et al.* (1992) and McDowell *et al.* (1994).

Contraindications to TENS

These are mainly the avoidance of potentially hazardous situations; there seems to be no reported incidents of significant damage done due to TENS. TENS should not be applied:

- over the carotid sinus, as this might lead to cardiac arrhythmias
- to patients with demand-type pacemakers, although fixed-rate pacemakers are apparently safe (Eriksson and Schuller, 1978)

- over the pharyngeal region, in case it causes interference with breathing and swallowing co-ordination
- over insensitive skin (this is particularly dangerous when unidirectional TENS is used)
- when unidirectional TENS is being used for prolonged duration or at very high intensities, because of the risk of electrochemical damage
- pregnancy is often given as a contraindication which is for medico-legal reasons; it would seem unlikely that adverse effects could result unless possibly the electrodes are placed over the uterus.

Electroacupuncture

Electroacupuncture consists of two aspects. First, the acupuncture point may be found on the surface by testing the electrical resistance. Second, stimulation of the point may be given with an electric pulse rather than the traditional needle penetrating the skin. Some machines allow both testing and stimulation through the same electrode. Acupuncture points and trigger points (which appear to correspond to each other (Melzack *et al.*, 1977)), apparently have a lower electrical impedance than the surrounding area, as noted above (Klein and Pariser, 1987). These points are located with a point electrode (probe) on the skin and a small applied current is then measured; thus the circuit impedance (or conductance) can be displayed on a meter. The electric pulses used for treatment are usually some form of low-frequency, high-intensity TENS stimulating A delta nerve fibres to achieve encephalinergic pain relief (see earlier). TENS applied to traditional acupuncture points for specific therapies is also used. For example, low-frequency 0.1 ms pulses given over the P6 acupuncture point proximal to the wrist have been successfully used for controlling sickness after chemotherapy (McMillan and Dundee, 1991).

When inserted needles are used these can be connected to a purpose-built electrical stimulator to deliver low-frequency electrical pulses.

Ryodu-Raku (from Japan) is an example of such a system. The device is called a neurometer and can be used to test the tissue resistance between a point electrode applied to the skin and a dispersive held in the hand. Where large differences of conductivity are found treatment is applied. This consists of a few seconds of direct current from the same device given either by means of a small surface electrode or a fine needle into the skin.

Transcutaneous spinal electroanaesthesia (TSE)

This consists of the application of 4 μs pulses of high voltage, 120 V or so, at 600 Hz over the spinal column. It is claimed that such currents applied through electrodes over the spinous processes of T1 and T12 will elicit a 'spinal cord sensation' which differs from the normal tingling of peripheral nerve stimulation. This approach appears to be effective in relieving long-standing chronic pain, but has no effect on acute pain (see Macdonald and Cotes, 1995, for a detailed account).

High-voltage pulsed galvanic stimulation (HVPGS)

Such pulsed currents will pass easily through the tissues (in common with TSE) because they are so brief (see earlier) and will be relatively comfortable due to their wide discrimination between sensory, motor and nociceptor nerve fibres (see Fig. 3.13).

As well as the frequency the intensity can be varied (0–500 V) and the polarity altered. The pattern of current can be changed by a mode switch. In continuous mode the train of twin pulses is delivered continuously. Reciprocate mode refers to the alternate application of trains of pulses to one or other of two active pads and does not mean that the current direction is reversed. Surge mode gives a train of pulses whose intensity is gradually increased, as indicated with square wave pulses in Figure 3.1(e). A meter to indicate peak current may be provided. On some machines the interval between the two peaks may be altered; this is called the intrapulse interval. The current is applied by flexible electrodes and sponges. The electrodes are usually small and are sometimes mounted on a handle. Various special electrodes are available.

Uses of HVPGS

Wound healing.   Since a direct current, albeit of very low total intensity, is being applied, the discussion on this subject in Chapter 2 is relevant. There seems to be evidence that low-intensity currents lead to tissue healing.

Pain modulation.   How pain may be controlled by electrical stimulation has already been discussed. Since both the frequency and intensity of HVPGS can be controlled it is possible to apply both high-frequency, low-intensity stimulation for pain gate control and low-frequency, high-intensity stimulation for encephalin-type pain control. HVPGS has been recommended for controlling all kinds of pain – acute, chronic, neurogenic and pain from many sources (Newton, 1987).

Muscle stimulation.   HVPGS is used for the stimulation of innervated muscle and, due to the short pulses and hence good transmission in the tissues, it is an efficient way of doing so. Consider the strength–duration curve (Fig. 3.13) which shows that short pulses at high intensities will be more selective in stimulating motor rather than pain nerves. HVPGS has therefore been used for muscle strengthening and the reduction of disuse atrophy of innervated muscle. A frequency of around 30 Hz has been suggested with long intervals between bouts of tetanic contraction as the optimum schedule.

Other uses. Effects on the vascular system are claimed in that rhythmical muscle contraction and relaxation due to HVPGS of motor nerves will have a pumping effect, increasing blood flow in muscle and surrounding tissues, as considered earlier. This effect can aid in the reduction of tissue oedema. Fish *et al.* (1991) found that anodal high voltage pulsed current did not curb oedema formation in frog hind limbs. This contrasts markedly with significant treatment effects found with cathodal HVPGS (Taylor *et al.*, 1991). Direct effects on autonomic nerves leading to local vasodilation, increased fluid exchange in the tissues and other beneficial effects have been claimed (Wadsworth and Chanmugan, 1980; see earlier discussion on oedema reduction). Consequent upon its ability to stimulate innervated muscle HVPGS has been recommended in the treatment of muscle spasm and to increase joint mobility (Newton, 1987).

Some uncertainty exists over the advantages of the twin peaks waveform, which is what makes this current unique. It has been suggested that a single pulse could be just as effective (Alon, 1987).

Sinusoidal currents

Effects

If a sinusoidal current is applied continuously it will cause a tetanic muscle contraction and a tingling sensation due to stimulation of motor and sensory nerves. It is usually surged to cause rhythmical muscle contractions. The sensory stimulations can lead to pain relief by some of the mechanisms described in connection with TENS. The rhythmical muscle contractions induced can help reduction of oedema by muscle pumping action. Intramuscular metabolism and blood flow are also increased. Various specific effects have been claimed, such as increased blood flow in the treated region suggested by the marked cutaneous erythema that can develop. Similarly it is claimed that unsurged sinusoidal current will help the absorption of oedema or inflammatory exudate (Wadsworth and Chanmugan, 1980). There seems to be no clear evidence to support these latter claims.

Application

Sinusoidal current can be applied in the same way as other low-frequency currents by means of electrodes and pads. However, because of the marked sensory stimulation this current is often applied to large areas and rarely used for local muscle stimulation. Thus it is applied either through large pads or water baths or both. For pain control continuous sinusoidal current at intensities close to the limit of tolerance is recommended, increasing the current as the patient accommodates. This is applied for about 5 min and repeated if there is insufficient immediate effect. For reduction of oedema and to increase the limb circulation surged sinusoidal current is suggested, causing regular rhythmical muscle pumping actions.

Sinusoidal current is rarely used in modern physiotherapy departments. It is interesting, however, to note that the series of 10 ms phases gives marked sensory nerve stimulation in the skin, acting in part like modern TENS stimulators. Recent understanding of pain control may account for some of the benefits that were claimed for this treatment (Wadsworth and Chanmugan, 1980).

Diadynamic currents

Therapeutic effects

The effects claimed (Rennie, 1988) include:

- pain relief due to the mechanisms described already, i.e. pain gate mechanism, pain suppression by neurologically stimulated endorphins and encephalins, removal of irritants from the area by the increased circulation, and the placebo effect
- decreased inflammation and swelling due to the increased muscle pumping action and increased local circulation; changes in cell membrane permeability are also claimed
- muscle re-education and strengthening are considered to occur due to the stimulation of muscles
- increased local circulation due, it is claimed, both to the altered autonomic activity such as reduced sympathetic tone leading to vasodilation and the release of histamine-like substances due to the unidirectional effects
- facilitation of tissue-healing due to local circulatory changes noted above and to the polar effects leading to increased cell activity (see Chapter 2).

Application of electrodes

Either metal plate or carbon-rubber electrodes may be used with pads. Two equal-sized electrodes on either side of the area to be treated may be used or a small electrode may be placed over a trigger or motor point with a larger electrode placed proximally. Various treatment parameters are suggested. For pain relief and most other effects, an initial minute or so of DF followed by up to 5 min of CP or LP (Rennie, 1988) (see Fig. 3.9). The reasons for preferring these or any other particular regimens are not provided in commentary on this subject.

It is suggested for all treatments that the current intensity should be perceptible but not painful. The major danger with such currents is tissue damage due to the polar effects. These may be avoided by current reversal during treatment.

Rebox

When applied to normal tissue the current rises over a period of about 1 s giving a characteristic displacement of the meter, of sound in the earphone, and of the shape of the graph. When applied to damaged or abnormal tissue a different pattern is said to occur in which the rise of current is slower, taking 3 or 4 s, and may occur in a series of steps. These differences do not seem to have supporting experimental evidence nor is there a clear theoretical basis for them.

Repeated application of this current for a few seconds at a time (up to 20 V leading to a maximum current of 0.3 mA proximal to the injured area), using the device as a treatment is claimed to lead to a normal response when the same area is subsequently tested, and to therapeutic benefit. It has been used in the treatment of musculoskeletal pains, recent trauma and a number of other conditions. In a controlled double-blind cross-over study, Johannsen *et al.* (1993) found a minor but significant beneficial effect of Rebox in the treatment of lateral epicondylitis. The benefits have been accounted for by postulating that the current causes increased ionic movement in the tissue fluid, and that monitoring rate of change of current in the tissues helps to localize the area of abnormality (Hervik, 1989).

Russian currents

In the 1970s claims were published that the 2500 Hz medium-frequency interrupted current could be used to generate greater muscle force than a maximal voluntary muscle contraction. This current, described earlier, is called 'Russian' because its use was first investigated by Dr Y. M. Kots in the Russian literature. It provoked much interest because the very successful Russian Olympic team were using it in addition to their usual training methods and it was suggested that its use led to significant (30–40%) gains in muscle strength.

Although it is a medium-frequency current the nerves are stimulated because it is interrupted to give a low-frequency stimulation of 50 Hz. Due to the short pulses (of 0.2 ms phase) it will pass fairly easily through the skin and be effective in stimulating motor nerves, but the stimulus is due to the initial electrical pulse, thus the purpose of the rest of the 10 ms train is not clear. It is, in fact, like a short-duration faradic-type pulse at 50 Hz.

The theoretical basis for its use is that maximum electrical stimulation can cause nearly all the motor units in a muscle to contract synchronously: something that cannot be achieved in voluntary contraction, it was claimed. This would allow stronger muscle contractions to occur with electrical stimulation and hence greater muscle hypertrophy. This has not been found to occur in the subsequent research. Many investigations have determined that electrical muscle stimulation leads to muscle hypertrophy but not to any greater degree than voluntary activity (Currier, 1987).

Not only was it claimed that the electrically generated force was greater than that generated voluntarily but also that this occurred without producing pain. This claim has not been entirely supported either; in one careful study which assessed torque values and pain scores (Gilles and Bélanger, 1987) the assertions were definitely refuted.

This current can be applied in the usual way with electrodes applied over the muscle belly. To achieve muscle hypertrophy, which is the usual purpose, currents of high intensity producing maximum tolerable muscle contraction are given in spells of a few seconds separated by somewhat longer rest periods.

Interferential currents

The principle of interferential therapy, as explained, is to pass two medium-frequency alternating currents which are slightly out of phase through the tissues. Where the currents intersect a new current is set up (Fig. 3.10).

Medium-frequency currents will pass much more easily through the skin than low-frequency currents due to the lower impedance offered to very short electrical pulses. Such currents will pass easily through the tissues because they are medium-frequency but stimulate nerves because of the amplitude modulation.

Although the spread of medium-frequency current in the tissues is more uniform than a low-frequency current it is still at greater intensity close to the electrodes (Fig. 3.26(a),(b)). The effects thus occur deeper in the tissues.

About 50 years ago this idea was developed by Hans Nemec in Vienna and although used quite widely in the intervening years, it has become much better known recently with the development of cheaper electronic circuitry. A later development involves the use of a third current in a path at right angles to the other two; this is called stereodynamic interference current (Kloth, 1987). Thus the tissues are stimulated in a three-dimensional system; however, the usefulness of such a system is not clearly established.

Most interferential machines allow a constant beat frequency to be selected, e.g. 10, 50 or 100 Hz – in fact any frequency from 1 to 250 Hz – called the constant or static mode. They also have an arrangement that allows the beat frequency to change automatically and regularly between some pre-set pair of frequencies over a specified time period. This is variously called a frequency modulation, swing or sweep. Thus the machine could be set to sweep, for example, between 20 and 80 Hz over a period of 6 s and back over the next 6 s. The pattern and timing of this modulation is usually adjustable and is sometimes called the spectrum. Such an arrangement is believed to be useful to prevent nerve habituation and may also extend the range of nerve types that can be stimulated.

Figure 3.26(c) shows the theoretical distribution of current in a homogeneous medium. The clover-leaf shape of maximum current modulation is due to the fact that both the current amplitudes and their directions need to be summated, i.e. vector addition. The distribution shown for four equally spaced electrodes is unlikely to be realized in real tissue, since variations in tissue resistance and electrode distances would prevent this neat uniformity. The real pattern is likely to be much more irregular and diffuse in all tissues between and around the electrodes. None the less the pattern shown

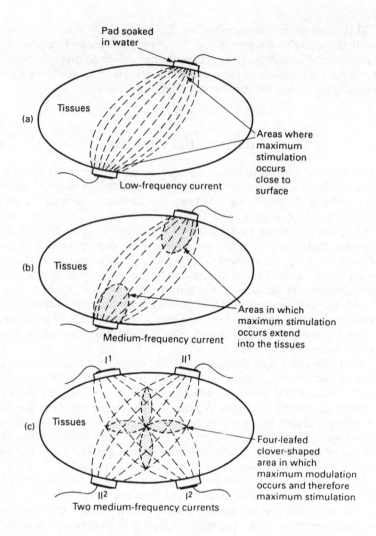

Pad soaked in water

(a) Tissues

Areas where maximum stimulation occurs close to surface

Low-frequency current

(b) Tissues

Areas in which maximum stimulation occurs extend into the tissues

Medium-frequency current

(c) Tissues

I^1 II^1

Four-leafed clover-shaped area in which maximum modulation occurs and therefore maximum stimulation

II^2 I^2

Two medium-frequency currents

Fig. 3.26 Areas of maximum stimulation.

is a valid concept and a useful guide. This is a static pattern but, by varying the current amplitude in the two circuits with respect to each other, it is possible to move the clover-leaf pattern of maximum modulation to and fro through 45°, thus giving a more uniform total distribution of the interferential current in the tissues. There are various names for such a mechanism, including 'vector sweep', 'scanning', 'rotating vector system' or 'dynamic interference field system'. It serves to increase the area of effective treatment.

Control of the current amplitude is provided to allow more or less stimulation as needed. There is also usually automatic timing control for the timing of treatment. Thus, in summary, controls on the interferential machine are:

- settings for constant beat frequency, e.g. 80 Hz
- settings for variable beat frequencies, e.g. 20–80 Hz
- control for time of variable beat frequencies cycle, e.g. 6 s
- intensity control

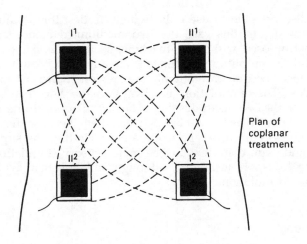

Plan of coplanar treatment

Fig. 3.27 Electrode arrangement for interferential therapy. Plan for coplanar treatment.

- control for using rotating vector mechanisms, e.g. on or off
- control for total treatment time, e.g. 10 min.

Currents are applied by metal or carbon-rubber electrodes with water-soaked sponges or lint. Carbon-rubber electrodes may be used with conducting gel, as already described. Since two circuits are involved, four electrodes, i.e. a quadripolar technique, are usually used. These electrodes may be secured by rubber straps or bandages; alternatively they may be secured by suction. Suction units can be connected to the interferential machine. Flexible rubber cups are connected by tubes to a pump that can provide a negative pressure. This suction may be continuous or variable. Metal electrodes mounted inside the cups are connected by wires carried within the tubes to the interferential source. Contact is made by moistened sponges placed inside the cups between the metal electrode and the skin. The negative pressure is set to vary rhythmically during treatment, which diminishes the risk of skin damage. It should be adjusted to maintain good electrical contact without causing discomfort. As well as maintaining electrical contact the suction has a mild massaging effect on the skin, stimulating cutaneous sensory nerves and causing slight vasodilation, both of which may contribute to the effectiveness of treatment. It is inadvisable to use suction on skin of poor quality which may break down; for example, due to severe oedema or in the elderly.

The electrodes must be placed so that the currents cross one another in the target tissue. In Figure 3.27 the current of the first circuit is carried via electrodes I^1 and I^2 and that of the second circuit by electrodes II^1 and II^2, thus generating the interferential field in the deep tissue. The electrodes are positioned in a coplanar arrangement to treat a flat surface such as the back. It is normally recommended to use the largest electrode sizes that can conveniently be applied (Savage, 1984) in order to ensure a comfortable current of sufficient intensity throughout the treated area. The leads (and suction tubes) are colour-coded to ensure correct arrangement of the circuit.

It is also possible to use only two electrodes; this is called the bipolar mode. In this case the two medium-frequency currents are superimposed within the machine, so that the single current produced is amplitude-modulated already. The result is that interference occurs throughout the region between the two electrodes. The modulation is always 100%. For this type of application the two electrodes should be placed opposite one another so that the part to be treated lies between them. Because the current modulation occurs throughout the area, including the superficial tissues and skin, there tends to be more sensory stimulation than with the four-pole technique, although still less than with low-frequency stimulation.

Precautions

It would seem wise to wash the skin before treatment to reduce skin impedance and to use large enough (sponge) pads to ensure that neither the electrodes nor their connections touch the patient's skin. This obviates any risk which could occur with high current densities.

It has been estimated that interferential currents of 50 mA applied to the thorax could induce currents of sufficient intensity to cause ventricular fibrillation (Health Protection Board of Health and Welfare Canada, 1988). It is considered inadvisable, therefore, to apply high-intensity interferential currents to the thorax.

Comments on the effects

Different frequencies and ranges of frequencies are recommended, often for the treatment of similar problems. The appropriate dosage parameters are not universally agreed. Some researchers (Laycock and Green, 1988) have found that 2 kHz is preferable for muscle strengthening to a 4 or 5 kHz carrier frequency.

A definitive and valuable study (Ward and Robertson, 1998) using 50 Hz modulation found that discrimination between pain and sensory nerve fibre thresholds increased with increasing carrier frequency and that the optimum for pain and motor fibre discrimination was around 10 Hz. This indicated that higher carrier frequencies are clinically preferable.

Most commentators suggest a range of amplitude modulation frequencies for different effects (see De Domenico, 1982; Goats, 1990; Savage, 1984). Hogenkamp *et al.* (1987) however postulate that amplitude modulation frequency has no effect on the selective stimulation of thick nerve fibres, but only determines the frequency with which nerve fibres depolarize. They suggest using a high AMF (70–150 Hz) for acute problems and pain, and frequencies below 50 Hz for chronic and subacute conditions and where muscle contraction is required.

Interferential currents are frequently employed for pain relief by means of mechanisms already described.

A placebo effect, which occurs in all treatments, is likely, especially since interferential machines are technically impressive and produce a distinct, somewhat unusual but not unpleasant sensation.

While there are many claims that interferential current is effective as a pain-relieving treatment there is little objective evidence in support. A rise in the pain threshold, based on the time taken to elicit ischaemic pain, and changes in the strength–duration curves of muscle were found after interferential therapy in one study (Pärtan *et al.*, 1953). A more recent study (Scott and Purves, 1991) did not find any increase in the time to tolerance for ischaemic pain due to interferential current at a beat frequency of 130 Hz. However, Stephenson and Johnson (1995) found that a fixed beat frequency of 100 Hz significantly elevated the cold-induced pain threshold of healthy subjects. Subsequently, Johnson and Wilson (1997) were able to show that a particular swing pattern (beat frequency modulated from 90 Hz to 130 Hz over 6 s and back again over 6 s) was also able to raise the cold-induced pain threshold in normal subjects. Other studies have found no change in nerve conduction velocities after interferential and no significant difference between interferential and placebo treatments (Taylor *et al.*, 1987).

Muscle contraction can also be achieved at higher current amplitude. Strong muscle contractions can be achieved without any significantly uncomfortable skin sensation. It is sometimes used in the treatment of stress incontinence. In 1988, Laycock and Green suggested a bipolar technique, placing one electrode under both ischial tuberosities and one over the anterior perineum immediately inferior to the symphysis pubis for females. Male patients were treated with two electrodes placed either side of the gluteal cleft, under the ischial tuberosities, anterior to the anus. Subsequently, Laycock and Jerwood (1993) reported using a medium electrode over the perineal body and a small electrode immediately inferior to the symphysis pubis. They used three specific frequencies for 10 min each, and found a significant increase in strength in the interferential therapy group; however, there was also improvement in a number of patients receiving placebo treatment, showing a strong placebo effect for interferential procedures.

A study of stress incontinence in the UK (Mantle, 1991) found that, after pelvic floor exercises, interferential was the most widely preferred treatment, but the methods and parameters of application varied widely.

SAFETY WITH ELECTRICAL CURRENTS

Primum non nocere – firstly do no harm – is a central tenet of every therapy but is especially applicable where damage can easily occur. Damage to the tissues as a result of the passage of electrical currents can occur in three ways:

- direct or uniphasic currents can cause electrochemical damage, often called a chemical burn (see Chapter 2)

- currents varying at rates that will stimulate nerve or muscle, that is, all those currents discussed in this chapter, could cause damage by provoking excessively powerful or prolonged muscle contractions or more seriously the heart muscle, thus stopping the circulation
- currents of sufficient amplitude can cause heating in the tissues leading to a heat burn.

All these kinds of damage could occur together but serious shocks or fatalities are usually confined to the last two points. If large currents are passed it is called an electric shock. In all cases what matters is the electric charge, that is, the current amplitude and the length of time for which it flows.

Damage due to the therapeutic use of electricity is, in fact, extremely rare and most damage that does occur is due to the mains current and is of the kind that may equally well take place in the home with ordinary domestic equipment.

It is usual to distinguish *macroshock*, in which current passes through the skin, from *microshock* which refers to the very small currents which are applied directly to, say, the heart as an external pacemaker; in this situation quite small current increases can be fatal. This latter will not be considered further.

It will be apparent from what has been described earlier in this chapter that quite high currents can be passed through the body without ill effects provided they are applied as very short pulses (Fig. 3.13). As a general observation electrotherapeutic equipment is designed so that it cannot deliver pulses of sufficient charge to be seriously damaging to the tissues, except as considered below (maximum recommended 300 mJ per pulse).

Electric shock due to mains-type current

If an electric current is passed through the whole body it tends to spread throughout the low-resistance subcutaneous tissues. It will be recalled that the skin resistance here is very much greater than that of the internal tissues. Normal skin resistance is many thousands of Ω, but wet skin can be as little as 1000 Ω; the internal tissues have resistances of only a few hundred Ω; for instance, the resistance between hand and foot excluding the skin resistance is about 500 Ω (Ward, 1986).

The current through the body – it is the current which is the critical factor – will depend directly on the voltage (240 V root mean square (RMS) in the UK) and inversely on the resistance ($I = V/R$), where I = intensity, V = voltage and R = resistance. Thus very much larger currents will flow if the skin is wet, because wetting greatly lowers its resistance; this explains why serious domestic accidents involving electrocution often occur in the bathroom or laundry. Applying Ohm's law the current through a 1000 Ω resistance due to 240 V would be 240 mA which is enough to cause ventricular fibrillation in the heart muscle and could well be fatal. With dry skin having a resistance of, say, 100 000 Ω the current would be

2.4 mA, causing tingling sensations. Most of the therapeutic currents described in this chapter are applied to wetted, hence low-resistance, skin but are driven by voltages much lower than that of the mains; the maximum output from many muscle stimulating units is around 40 or 50 V.

At 50 Hz (mains frequency) current densities around 0.5–1 mA/cm^2 are just detectable and at 10–20 times this value become uncomfortable or painful. Higher currents lead to muscle contractions and currents through the body of 50–250 mA may lead to ventricular fibrillation and hence may be fatal. Currents of still higher intensities tend to provoke complete cardiac arrest and severe heat burns (Ward, 1986). Thus it can be seen why the nature of the electrical contact with the skin is so critical; anything that lowers skin resistance allows larger currents to pass. Voltages higher than that of the mains are proportionally more dangerous because they will cause larger currents; for this reason areas in which high voltages are found, such as transformer substations, are specially protected. It must also be understood that the consequences of electrocution depend on the path the current follows in the body. Thus if the current passes from, say, a hand touching the live wire through the body to earth via the feet standing on the ground, the current then passes through the heart, lungs and abdomen and may well cause cardiac arrest and/or the cessation of respiration and thus prove fatal. Touching both contacts of a lighting socket with one finger would be likely to cause a painful shock and burns to the fingertip.

Immediate treatment of mains current shock

Firstly, the circuit must be disconnected to stop the flow of current through the victim. This may be simply a matter of switching off and unplugging, but it is important to ensure that disconnection has been made before touching the victim otherwise the rescuer may form another path to earth and also receive a shock.

Secondly, the carotid pulse and respiration should be checked. If absent the airway must be cleared, mouth-to-mouth resuscitation and external cardiac massage immediately started and assistance summoned. In all cases the victim should be medically examined as soon as possible – urgently if there has been any loss of consciousness. Musculoskeletal damage can occur as a result of abrupt muscle contraction due to the electric shock as well as cutaneous burns, which are usually evident.

Safety features of electrical apparatus supplied from the mains

The safety of electrical apparatus connected to the mains is ensured in several ways. The metal casing of the apparatus is connected to the large earth terminal of the three-pin plug and socket. Thus if the live wire were to touch the casing of the machine a large current would flow to earth causing the protective fuse to 'blow' and interrupting the circuit. If an earth wire is not present, or if it is broken, and the casing becomes live, anyone touching the machine may provide a low-resistance pathway to earth.

Small portable pieces of electrical equipment such as radios and hair-driers are often double-insulated and connected to the mains by only two terminals, live and neutral. In these the casing is made of some non-conducting plastic material and the electrical conducting parts are separately insulated. Any exposed metal, such as the cutters of electric razors, is again separately insulated. All mains equipment is protected in one of these ways.

Two further safety measures are of consequence: the use of isolating transformers and core-balance relays.

The safety of electromedical equipment is subject to recommendations made by the British Standards Institution (BSI) and the International Electrotechnical Commission (IEC). These bodies specify certain safety conditions such as the maximum permissible leakage current both normally and under fault conditions and designate the equipment accordingly. Most of the electrical stimulators referred to in this chapter (designated type BF) would have more stringent protection against delivering an electric shock than equipment to which the patient is not directly connected, electric heating pads for example, but less than the very strict precautions taken for equipment directly connected to the heart such as external cardiac pacemakers (designated type CF). The regulations are covered by BS5724 and its amendments and supplements (Section 2:10, 1988).

The CE mark is the European symbol of safety and compliance with agreed international standards. All electromedical products which are intended for sale in any EU country must be CE marked.

Electric shock or damage due to therapeutic nerve and muscle-stimulating currents

As already noted, these do not usually cause damage because the output of the machine will not permit a sufficiently high current. However, certain situations could lead to pain, alarm and possibly tissue damage or other adverse effects, see Partridge and Kitchen (1999).

If current is applied at high amplitude very abruptly, the sensation and pain caused are likely to frighten the patient. It will be recalled that the sensory nerves are stimulated by lower intensities than the pain nerve endings, so that high currents are more painful. Some pain may well be an appropriate part of treatment, but it should never provoke anxiety or fear. It has already been emphasized that the major resistance to current flow is the skin so that any break in the skin provides a low-resistance pathway and therefore a high local current density, which may be painful. Subjects become accustomed or adapt to electrical stimulation so that high intensities are easily tolerated if the current is increased gradually over a few minutes. The term 'shock' is often used confusingly; any sudden sensory stimulation may be described as a 'shock' (psychological); this would include electric 'shock' which refers specifically to electrical injury.

There is quite widespread apprehension about contact of the body with electricity. This is doubtless partly a fear of the ill understood. However, it is also culturally engendered in many places to suggest fear (and vitalize monsters!) in old films and new videos. There are even allusions to it in literature; for example, in Shelley's *Epipyschidion*:

> 'Her touch was as electric poison.'

These anxieties may, at first, cause the sensations due to electric currents to be perceived as painful. As current flows so the feelings become familiar and toleration rises. When applying treatment such fears must be taken into account; the patient must be carefully reassured and treatment applied initially at low intensity which can be gradually increased. It has been noted already that the current density is important in determining the strength of the effects, so the area of skin/electrode contact must be carefully considered. Furthermore, there appear to be very wide differences in sensory responsiveness to electrical stimulation. It has been found that, in general, women appear to have lower thresholds for 'detection, pain and tolerance to cutaneous electrical stimulation than men' (Lautenbacher and Rollman, 1993). This is presumably associated with the fact that women are more sensitive to pressure pain than men (Fischer, 1987), although there are no differences between the sexes for thermal thresholds or heat pain. These factors account for the wide discrepancies found among patients and therapists concerning the painfulness or otherwise of particular intensities of therapeutic current. It may be emphasized that the pain due to electrical stimulation is not associated with, or due to, any tissue damage (except as noted below) but is the result of sensory, including pain, nerve stimulation and is thus harmless.

As these currents can cause strong muscle contraction it is possible that exceptionally vigorous artificially produced contraction might cause mechanical muscle or joint damage. However, such damage seems unlikely in normal tissues because of the protective mechanism of the Golgi tendon organs, and the fact that electrical muscle stimulation rarely produces a greater contraction than can be produced voluntarily. Further, there seems to be no recorded instance of such injuries happening to normal muscles and joints. With tissues that are already diseased or injured, such as partial muscle rupture, overstrong muscle contraction could be damaging. It is also possible that muscle contraction could dislodge the attachment of a deep vein thrombus, causing an embolus. Prolonged and intensive electrical muscle stimulation can lead to muscle soreness like that due to voluntary activity (Hon Sun Lai *et al.*, 1988).

It is recommended (Wadsworth and Chanmugan, 1980) that infected or inflamed areas should not be treated with low-frequency currents because there is a risk of spreading the infection. This is presumably due to the muscle-pumping effect; there seems no other reason why infection should spread. Certainly, as far as acute inflammation is concerned, any increased activity would be undesirable.

Since these currents provoke nerve impulses it is often recommended that areas in which autonomic nerves might be inappropriately stimulated should be avoided; for example, the region of the carotid sinus (Frampton, 1988). Similarly, treatment close to the pregnant uterus might provide undesirable uterine movements. While neither circumstance appears to have been reported it would seem proper to be cautious.

If haemorrhage, either on the surface or in the tissues, is occurring or likely to occur then electrical stimulation by causing muscle movement and vasodilation could prevent or disrupt clotting; it should therefore be avoided.

Although there appears to be no evidence for this effect it is usual and reasonable to avoid direct treatment of neoplastic tissue in case metastasis is provoked, or growth encouraged.

Currents applied in the region of an implanted cardiac pacemaker could alter the stimulus leading to cardiac arrhythmia. A separate slight risk is of the electromagnetic field generated by the therapeutic stimulator interfering with demand-type pacemakers, this is a remote possibility with almost any piece of electrical equipment.

A significant danger arises from failure to recognize when the current applied is a direct current, or has a direct current component: with sufficient charge an electrochemical burn can result. Even extremely low current densities, such as that from some TENS machines, can have this effect given sufficient time. In most circumstances the patient's sensation warns of this danger and nothing more than skin irritation occurs. Electrochemical burns seem to develop because the sensations of burning and pain experienced by the patient due to the current are not particularly sharp. There may also be a gradual increase of current, due to falling skin resistance, to which the patient adapts. It is therefore important that adequate explanation and warning should be given to the patient before treatment and careful checks made during treatment. It is essential that the physiotherapist knows if there is any direct current component in the treatment being applied, since treatment of insensitive skin or of a particularly tolerant and tough-minded patient could lead to damage (see Chapter 2).

CONTRAINDICATIONS

Contraindications to electrical stimulation may be summarized as circumstances in which:

- strong muscle contraction might cause joint or muscle damage; detachment of a thrombus; spread of infection; and haemorrhage

- stimulation of autonomic nerves might cause altered cardiac rhythm or other autonomic effects
- currents might be unduly localized due to open wounds or skin lesions, e.g. eczema
- currents might provoke undesirable metabolic activity in neoplasms or in healed tuberculous infections
- current is not evenly biphasic, leading to possible skin damage or irritation, especially if there is loss of sensation.

REFERENCES

Alon G. (1987). Principles of electrical stimulation. In *Clinical Electrotherapy* (Nelson R. M., Currier D. P., eds) Norwalk, Connecticut, USA: Appleton and Lange, pp. 29–80.

Axelgaard J., Brown J. C. (1983). Lateral electrical surface stimulation for the treatment of progressive idiopathic scoliosis. *Spine*, **8**, 242.

Baker L. L. (1981). Neuromuscular electrical stimulation in the restoration of purposeful limb movements. In *Electrotherapy* (Wolf S., ed.) Edinburgh: Churchill Livingstone, pp. 25–48.

Baker L. L. (1987). Clinical uses of neuromuscular electrical stimulation. In *Clinical Electrotherapy* (Nelson R. M., Currier D. P., eds) Norwalk, Connecticut, USA: Appleton and Lange, pp. 115–39.

Baker L. L., Parker K. (1986). Neuromuscular electrical stimulation of the muscles surrounding the shoulder. *Phys. Ther.*, **66**, 1930–7.

Baker L. L., Bowman B. R., McNeal D. R. (1987). Effects of waveform on comfort during neuromuscular electrical stimulation. *Clin Orthop.*, **233**, 75–85.

Baker L. L., Yeh C., Wilson D. *et al.* (1979). Electrical stimulation of wrist and fingers for hemiplegic patients. *Phys. Ther.*, **59**, 1495–9.

Balogun J. A., Onilari O. O., Akeju O. A., Marzouk D. K. (1993). High voltage electrical stimulation in the augmentation of muscle strength: effects of pulse frequency. *Arch Phys. Med. Rehabil.*, **74**, 910–16.

Barr J. O., Nielson D. H., Soderberg G. L. (1986). Transcutaneous electrical nerve stimulation characteristics for altering pain perception. *Phys. Ther.*, **66**, 1515–21.

Bélanger A. Y. (1991). Neuromuscular electrostimulation in physiotherapy: a critical appraisal of controversial issues. *Physiother. Theory Pract.*, **7**, 83–9.

Bending J. (1993). TENS relief of discomfort 'like worms wriggling under the skin'. *Physiotherapy*, **79**, 773–4.

Berger R. A. (1982). Applied exercise physiology. Philadelphia: Lea and Febiger.

Bettany J. A., Fish D. R., Mendel F. C. (1990). Influence of high voltage pulsed direct current on edema formation following impact injury. *Phys. Ther.*, **70**, 219–24.

Binder-Macleod S. A., Lee S. C. K., Baadt S. A. (1997). Reduction of the fatigue-induced force decline in human skeletal muscle by optimised stimulation trains. *Arch. Phys. Med. Rehab.*, **78**, 1129–37.

Blowman C., Pickles C., Emery S. *et al.* (1991). Prospective double blind controlled trial of intensive physiotherapy with and without stimulation of the pelvic floor in treatment of genuine stress incontinence. *Physiotherapy*, **77**, 661–4.

Bowsher D. (1988). Modulation of nociceptive input. In *Pain: Management and Control in Physiotherapy* (Wells P. E., Frampton V., Bowsher D., eds) London: Heinemann Medical Books, pp. 30–6.

Bowsher D. (1994). (a) Central pain mechanisms, (b) Modulation of nociceptive input. In *Pain Management by Physiotherapy*, 2nd edn (Wells P. E., Frampton V., Bowsher D., eds) Oxford: Butterworth-Heinemann, pp. 47–53, 54–8.

Brown M. D., Cole M. A., Jeal S., Anderson S. I. (1998). *Chronic Low Frequency Stimulation of Normal and Ischaemic Human Skeletal Muscles: Vascular Effects and*

Muscle Fatigue. Abstract from Scientific Meeting Human Motor Performance. The Interaction between Science and Therapy. University of East London. 21–23 July 1998.

Buller A. J., Eccles J. C., Eccles E. W. (1960). Differentiation of fast and slow muscles in the cat hind limb. *J. Physiol.*, **150**, 399–416.

Burridge J. H., Taylor P. N., Hagan S. A., Wood D. E., Swain F. D. (1997). The effects of common peroneal stimulation on the effort and speed of walking. A randomised controlled trial with chronic hemiplegic patients. *Clin. Rehab.*, **11**, 201–10.

Callaghan M. J., Oldham J. A. (1997). A critical review of electrical stimulation of the quadriceps muscles. *Crit. Rev. Phys. Rehab. Med.*, **9**, 301–14.

Carmick J. (1993). Clinical use of neuromuscular electrical stimulation for children with C.P. *Phys. Ther.*, **73**, 505–22.

Cassella M. C., Hall J. E. (1991). Current treatment approaches in the non-operative and operative management of adolescent idiopathic scoliosis. *Phys. Ther.*, **71**, 897–909.

Cawley D. M., Hendriks O. (1992). Evaluation of the Endomed CV405 as a treatment for urinary incontinence. *Physiotherapy*, **78**, 495–8.

Ciba Foundation. (1988). *Plasticity of the neuromuscular system*, Ciba Foundation Symposium 138.

Cosgrove K. A., Alon G., Bell S. F. *et al.* (1992). The electrical effects of two commonly used clinical stimulators on traumatic edema in rats. *Phys. Ther.*, **72**, 227–33.

Cramp M. C. (1998). *Alterations in Human Muscle and Central Control Mechanisms*. PhD Thesis. University of East London.

Cramp M. C., Manuel J. M., Scott O. M. (1995). Effects of different patterns of long-term electrical stimulation of human quadriceps femoris muscle. *J. Physiol.*, **483**, 82.

Currier D. P. (1987). Electrical stimulation for improving strength and blood flow. In *Clinical Electrotherapy* (Nelson R. M., Currier D. P., eds) Norwalk, Connecticut, USA: Appleton and Lange, pp. 141–64.

Currier D. P., Mann R. (1983). Muscle strength development by electrical stimulation in healthy individuals. *Phys. Ther.*, **63**, 915.

Currier D. P., Petrilli C. R., Threlkeld A. J. (1986). Effects of medium frequency electrical stimulation on local blood circulation to healthy muscle. *Phys. Ther.*, **66**, 937–43.

Davis H. L. (1983). Is electrostimulation beneficial to denervated muscle? A review of results from basic research. *Physiotherapy* (Canada), **35**, 306–10.

De Domenico G. (1982). Pain relief with interferential current. *Aust. J. Physiother.*, **28**, 14–18.

De Domenico G., Strauss G. R. (1986). Maximum torque production in the quadriceps femoris muscle group using a variety of electrical stimulators. *Aust. J. Physiother.*, **32**, 51–6.

Delitto A., Robinson A. J. (1989). Electrical stimulation of muscle: techniques and applications. In *Clinical Electrophysiology, Electrotherapy and Electrophysiological Testing*. (Synder-Mackler Z., Robinson A. J., eds) Baltimore: Williams and Wilkins.

Delitto A., Strube M. J., Shulman A. D. *et al.* (1992). A study of discomfort with electrical stimulation. *Phys. Ther.*, **72**, 410–21.

Deyo R. A., Walsh N. E., Martin D. C. *et al.* (1990). A controlled trial of TENS and exercise for chronic low back pain. *N. Engl. J. Med.*, **322**, 1627–34.

Dimitriyević M. M., Soroker N., Pollo F. E. (1996). Mesh glove electrical stimulation. *Sci. Med.*, May/June, 54–63.

Domaille M., Reeves B. (1997). TENS and pain control after coronary artery bypass surgery. *Physiotherapy*, **83**, 510–16.

Eckerson L. F., Axelgaard J. (1984). Lateral electrical surface stimulation as an alternative to bracing in the treatment of idiopathic scoliosis: treatment protocol and patient acceptance. *Phys. Ther.*, **64**, 483.

Electrotherapy Standards Committee (1990). *Electrotherapeutic Terminology in Physical Therapy*, Report by the Electrotherapy Standards Committee of Section on Clinical Electrophysiology. American Physical Therapy Association.

Eriksson M., Schuller H. (1978). Hazard from transcutaneous nerve stimulation in patients with pacemakers. *Lancet*, **i**, 1219.

Fahrer H. (1991). Analgesic low-frequency electrotherapy. In *Physiotherapy: Controlled Trials and Facts. Rheumatology: The Interdisciplinary Concept, Vol. 14* (Schlapbach S., Gerber N. J., eds) Basel: Karger.

Farragher D. J., Kidd G. L., Tallis R. G. (1987). Eutrophic electrical stimulation for Bells palsy. *Clin. Rehab.*, **1**, 256–71.

Ferguson A. C. B., Granat M. H. (1992). Evaluation of functional electrical stimulation for an incomplete spinal cord injured patient. *Physiotherapy*, **78**, 253–6.

Fish D. R., Mendel F. C., Schultz A. M. *et al.* (1991). Effect of anodal high voltage pulsed current on edema formation in frog hind limbs. *Physical Therapy*, **71**, 724–30.

Fischer A. A. (1987). Pressure algometry over normal muscle: standard values, validity and reproducibility of pressure threshold. *Pain*, **30**, 115–26.

Forster E. L., Kramer J. F., Lucy S. D., Scudds R. A., Novick R. J. (1994). Effect of TENS on pain, medications and pulmonary function following coronary artery bypass graft surgery. *Chest*, **106**, 1343–8.

Frampton V. (1988). Transcutaneous electrical nerve stimulation and chronic pain. In *Pain: Management and Control in Physiotherapy* (Wells P. E., Frampton V., Bowsher D., eds) London: Heinemann Medical Books, pp. 89–112.

Garnett R., Stephens J. A. (1981). Changes in the recruitment threshold of motor units produced by cutaneous stimulation in man. *J. Physiol.*, **311**, 463–73.

Gersh M. R. (1992). Transcutaneous electrical nerve stimulation (TENS) for management of pain and sensory pathology. In *Electrotherapy in Rehabilitation* (Gersh M. R., ed.) F. A. Davis, pp. 149–96.

Gibson J. N. A., Smith K., Rennie M. J. (1988). Prevention of disuse muscle atrophy by means of electrical stimulation: maintenance of protein synthesis. *Lancet*, **ii**, 767–9.

Gilles N., Bélanger A. Y. (1987). Rélation entre la force maximale volontaire, force tatanique et douleur lors de l'éléctrostimulation du quadriceps fémoris. *Physiother. Canada*, **39**, 377–82.

Goats G. C. (1990). Interferential current therapy. *Br. J. Sports Med.*, **24**, 87–92.

Gordon T. (1998). Adaptability of paralysed muscles after spinal cord injury. Proceedings of Human Motor Performance Congress, University of East London.

Grisogono V. (1989). Physiotherapy treatment for Achilles tendon injuries. *Physiotherapy*, **75**, 562–72.

Hanegan J. L. (1992). Principles of nociception. In *Electrotherapy in Rehabilitation* (Gersh M. R., ed.) F. A. Davis, pp. 26–48.

Herman E., Williams R., Stratford P., Fargas-Babjak A., Trott M. (1994). A randomised controlled trial of transcutaneous electrical nerve stimulation (CODETRON) to determine its benefits in a rehabilitation program for acute occupational low back pain. *Spine*, **19**, 561–8.

Hervik J. B. (1989). Rebox II. *Physiotherapy*, **75**, 417.

Health Protection Branch of Health and Welfare Canada (1988). *Physiother. Canada*, **40**, 205–6.

Hogenkamp M., Mittelmeijer E., Smits I. *et al.* (1987). *Interferential Therapy*. Delft: Enraf-Nonius.

Hon Sun Lai, De Domenico G., Strauss G. R. (1988). The effect of different electromotor stimulation training intensities on strength improvement. *Aust. J. Physiother.*, **34**, 151–64.

Hnik P. (1962). Rate of denervation muscle atrophy. In *The Denervated Muscle* (Gutman E. ed.) pp. 341–75. Prague: Publishing House of Czechoslovakia.

Isakov E., Mizrahi J. (1993). FES system for self-activation, an electrical stimulator and instrumental walker. *Clin. Rehabil.*, **7**, 39–44.

Johannsen F., Gam A., Hauschild B., Mathresen B., Jensen L. (1993). Rebox: an adjunct in physical medicine? *Arch. Phys. Med. Rehabil*, **74**, 438–40.

Johnson D. H., Thurston P., Ashcroft P. J. (1977). The Russian technique of faradism in the treatment of chondromalacia patellae. *Physiother. Canada*, **29**, 266–8.

Johnson M. I. (1997). The physiology of the sensory dimension of clinical pain. *Physiotherapy*, **83**, 526–36.

Johnson M. I. (1999) The mystique of interferential currents when used to manage pain. *Physiotherapy*, **85**, 294–7.

Johnson M. I., Ashton C. H., Bousfield D. R., Thompson J. W. (1989). Analgesic effects of different frequencies of transcutaneous electrical nerve stimulation on cold-induced pain in normal subjects. *Pain*, **39**, 231–6.

Johnson M. I., Ashton C. H., Thomson J. W. (1991a). An in-depth study of long-term uses of transcutaneous electrical stimulation (TENS). Implications for clinical use of TENS. *Pain*, **44**, 221–9.

Johnson M. I., Ashton C. H., Thomson J. W. (1991b). The consistency of pulse frequencies and pulse patterns of transcutaneous electrical nerve stimulation (TENS) used by chronic pain patients. *Pain*, **44**, 231–4.

Johnson M. I., Penny P., Sajawal M. A. (1977). An examination of the analgesic effects of microcurrent electrical stimulation (MES) on cold-induced pain in healthy subjects. *Physiother. Theory Pract.*, **13**, 293–301.

Johnson M. I., Wilson H. (1997). The analgesic effects of 6^6 and 1]∭ swing patterns of interferential current (IFC) on cold-induced pain in healthy subjects. A preliminary study. *Physiotherapy*, **83**, 461–7.

Jones A. Y. M., Hutchinson R. C. (1991). A comparison of the analgesic effect of transcutaneous electrical nerve stimulation and Entonox. *Physiotherapy*, **77**, 526–29.

Jones A. Y. M., Lee R., Holzberger D. *et al.* (1990). A comparison of different electrode placements on the effectiveness of TENS in pain relief for post-cholecystectomy patients. *Physiotherapy*, **76**, 567–9.

Kantor G., Alon G., Ho H. S. (1994). The effects of selected stimulus wave forms on pulse and phase characteristics at sensory and motor thresholds. *Phys. Ther.*, **74**, 951–62.

Kidd G. L., Oldham J. A. (1988a) Motor unit action potential (MUAP) sequence and electrotherapy. *Clin. Rehab.*, **2**, 23–33.

Kidd G. L., Oldham J. A. (1988b). An electrotherapy based on the natural sequence of motor unit action potential; a laboratory trial. *Clin. Rehab.*, **2**, 125–38.

Kidd G. L., Oldham J. A., Stanley J. K. (1988c). Eutrophic electrotherapy and atrophied muscle: a pilot clinical trial. *Clin. Rehab.*, **2**, 219–30.

Kidd G. L., Oldham J. A., Stanley J. K. (1989). A comparison of uniform and eutrophic electrotherapies in a procedure of clinical rehabilitation of some hand movements in arthritics. *Clin. Rehab.*, **3**, 27–39.

Klein J., Pariser D. (1987). Transcutaneous electrical nerve stimulation. In *Clinical Electrotherapy* (Nelson R. M., Currier P. D., eds) Norwalk, Connecticut: Appleton and Lange, pp. 209–30.

Kloth L. (1987). Interference current. In *Clinical Electrotherapy* (Nelson R. M., Currier P. D., eds) Norwalk, Connecticut: Appleton and Lange, pp. 183–207.

Lagassé P. P., Roy M. A. (1989). Functional electrical stimulation and the reduction of co-contraction in spastic biceps brachii. *Clin. Rehab.*, **3**, 111–16.

Lautenbacher S., Rollman G. B. (1993). Sex differences in responsiveness to painful and non-painful stimuli are dependent upon the stimulation method. *Pain*, **53**, 255–64.

Laycock J., Green R. J. (1988). Interferential therapy in the treatment of incontinence. *Physiotherapy*, **74**, 161–8.

Laycock J., Jerwood D. (1993). Does pre-modulated interferential therapy cure genuine stress incontinence? *Physiotherapy*, **79**, 553–60.

Levin M. F., Hui-Chan C. W. Y. (1993). Conventional and acupuncture-like transcutaneous electrical nerve stimulation excite similar afferent fibres. *Arch. Phys. Med. Rehabil.*, **74**, 54–60.

Livesley E. (1992). Effects of electrical neuromuscular stimulation on functional performance in patients with multiple sclerosis. *Physiotherapy*, **78**, 914–17.

Lloyd T., De Domenico G., Strauss G. R. *et al.* (1986). A review of the use of the electro-motor stimulation in human muscle. *Aust. J. Physiother.*, **32**, 18–30.

Macdonald A. J. R., Coates T. W. (1995). The discovery of transcutaneous spinal electroanalgesia and its relief of chronic pain. *Physiotherapy*, **81**, 653–61.

McDowell B. C., McCory M., Baxter G. D., Allen J. M., Walsh D. M. (1994). A double-blind investigation of the hypoalgesic effects of low pulse repetition rate H-wave therapy (2–16 Hz) upon experimentally induced ischaemic pain. *Irish J. Med. Sci.*, **163**, 101.

McMillan C. (1994). Transcutaneous electrical stimulation of Neiguan anti-emetic acupuncture point in controlling sickness following opioid analgesia in major orthopaedic surgery. *Physiotherapy*, **80**, 5–9.

McMillan C. M., Dundee J. W. (1991). The role of cutaneous electrical stimulation of Neiguan anti-emetic acupuncture point in controlling sickness after cancer chemotherapy. *Physiotherapy*, **77**, 499–502.

McQuire W. A. (1975). Electrotherapy and exercises for stress incontinence and urinary frequency. *Physiotherapy*, **61**, 305–7.

Mannheimer J. S., Lampe G. N. (1984). Electrode placement technique. In *Clinical Transcutaneous Electrical Nerve Stimulation* (Mannheimer J. S. and Lampe G. N.) Philadelphia: Davis, 331–495.

Mantle J. (1991). Stress incontinence: physiotherapy management in the UK. *WCPT 11th International Congress Proceedings, Book II*, London: World Federation for Physical Therapy, 884–6.

Marchand S., Charest J., Li J. *et al.* (1993). Is TENS purely a placebo effect? A controlled study on chronic low back pain. *Pain*, **54**, 99–106.

Melzack R., Wall P. D. (1965). Pain mechanisms: a new theory. *Science*, **150**, 971.

Melzack R., Stillwell R. M., Fox E. J. (1977). Trigger points and acupuncture points for pain: correlations and implications. *Pain*, **3**, 3–23.

Mendel F. C., Wylegala J. A., Fish D. R. (1992). Influence of high voltage pulsed current on edema formation following impact injury in rats. *Phys. Ther.*, **72**, 668–73.

Merskey H. (1991). The definition of pain. *Eur. J. Psychiat.*, **6**, 153–9.

Meyer G. A., Fields H. L. (1972). Causalgia treated by selective large fiber stimulation of peripheral nerves. *Brain*, **95**, 163–8.

Mills P. M., Deakin M., Kiff E. S. (1990). Percutaneous electrical stimulation for ano-rectal incontinence. *Physiotherapy*, **76**, 433–8.

Milner-Brown H. S., Stein B. B. (1975). The relation between the surface electromyogram and muscular force. *J. Physiol.*, **246**, 549.

Mizrahi J. (1997). Fatigue in muscles activated by functional electrical stimulation. *Crit. Rev. Phys. Rehab. Med.*, **9**, 93–129.

Montgomery E., Shepherd A. M. (1983). Electrical stimulation and graded pelvic exercise for genuine stress incontinence. *Physiotherapy*, **68**, 112.

Nelson H., Smith M., Bowman B. *et al.* (1980). Electrode effectiveness during transcutaneous motor stimulation. *Arch. Phys. Med. Rehab.*, **61**, 73–7.

Newham D. J. (1991). Skeletal muscle pain and exercise. *Physiotherapy*, **77**, 66–70.

Newton R. (1987). High voltage pulsed galvanic stimulation: theoretical bases and clinical applications. In *Clinical Electrotherapy* (Nelson R. M., Currier D. P., eds) Norwalk, Connecticut: Appleton and Lange, 165–82.

Nolan M. F. (1991). Conductive differences in electrodes used with transcutaneous electrical nerve stimulation devices. *Phys. Ther.*, **71**, 746–51.

Noling L. B., Clelland J. A., Jackson J. R., Knowles C. J. (1988). Effect of transcutaneous electrical nerve stimulation of auricular points on experimental cutaneous pain threshold. *Phys. Ther.*, **68**, 328–32.

Nussbaum E., Rush P., Disenhaus L. (1990). The effects of interferential therapy on peripheral blood flow. *Physiotherapy*, **76**, 803–7.

Obajuluwa V. A. (1991). Effect of electrical stimulation for ten weeks on quadriceps femoris muscle strength and thigh circumference in healthy young men. *Physiother. Theory Pract.*, **71**, 191–7.

Pandyan A. D., Granat M. H., Powell J., Stott D. J., Fuller C. (1996). Effects of electrical stimulation on the wrist of hemiplegic patients. *Physiotherapy*, **82**, 184–8.

Pärtan J., Schmid J., Warum F. (1953). The treatment of inflammatory and degenerative joint conditions with interferential alternating currents of medium frequency. *Wien. Klin. Wochenschr.*, **31**, 624–8.

Partridge C. J., Kitchen S. S. (1999). Adverse effects of electrotherapy used by physiotherapists. *Physiotherapy*, **85**, 298–303.

Patterson R. P. (1983). Instrumentation for electrotherapy. In *Therapeutic Electricity and Ultra-violet Radiation* (Stillwell K., ed.) Baltimore: Williams & Wilkins, pp. 65–108.

Pette D., Vrbova G. (1985). Neural control of phenotype expression in mammalian muscle fibres. *Muscle Nerve*, **8**, 294–7.

Pfeifer A. M., Cranfield T., Wagner S., Craik R. L. (1997). Muscle strength: a comparison of electrical stimulation and volitional isometric contractions in adults over 65 years. *Physiotherapy* (Canada), Winter, 32–9.

Quirk A. S., Newman R. J., Newman K. J. (1985). An evaluation of interferential therapy, shortwave diathermy and exercise in the treatment of osteoarthrosis of the knee. *Physiotherapy*, **71**, 55–7.

Rankin R. R., Stokes M. J. (1992). Fatigue effects of rest intervals during electrical stimulation of the human quadriceps muscle. *Clin. Rehabil.*, **6**, 195–201.

Reed B. V. (1988). Effect of high voltage pulsed electrical stimulation on microvascular permeability to plasma proteins: a possible mechanism in minimising edema. *Phys. Ther.*, **68**, 491–5.

Rennie S. (1988). Diadynamic current therapy. In *Current Physical Therapy* (Peat M., ed.) Toronto: B. C. Decker, pp. 207–11.

Rieb L., Pomeranz B. (1992). Alterations in electrical pain thresholds by use of acupuncture-like transcutaneous electrical nerve stimulation in pain-free subjects. *Phys. Ther.*, **72**, 658–67.

Roche P. A., Gijsers K. K., Belch J. J. F. *et al.* (1984). Modification of induced ischaemic pain by transcutaneous nerve stimulation. *Pain*, **20**, 45–52.

Rutherford O. M., Jones D. A. (1988). Contractile properties and fatiguability of the human adductor pollicis and first dorsal interosseous: a comparison of the effects of two chronic stimulation patterns. *J. Neurol. Sci.*, **85**, 319–31.

Salmons S., Vbrova G. (1969). The influence of activity on some contractile characteristics of mammalian fast and slow muscles. *J. Physiol.*, **210**, 535–49.

Santiesteban A. J. (1981). Application of transcutaneous electrical nerve stimulation for post-operative, cardiopulmonary and obstetric patients. In *Electrotherapy* (Wolf S. L., ed.) London: Churchill Livingstone, pp. 179–97.

Scott O. M. (1996). Sensory and motor nerve activation. In *Clayton's Electrotherapy*, 10th edn (Kitchen S., Bazin S., eds) Philadelphia: WB Saunders, pp. 61–82.

Scott O. M., Purves C. E. (1991). The effect of interferential therapy in the relief of experimentally induced pain: a pilot study. *WCPT International Congress, London. Proceedings Book II*, **67**, 346–50.

Scott O. M., Vrbova G., Hyde S. A. *et al.* (1985). Effects of chronic low frequency electrical stimulation on normal tibial anterior muscle. *J. Neuro. Psych. Psychiatry*, **48**, 774–81.

Scudds R. J., Helewa A., Scudds R. A. (1995). The effects of transcutaneous nerve stimulation on skin temperature in asymptomatic subjects. *Phys. Ther.*, **75**, 621–8.

Shindo N., Jones R. (1987). Reciprocal patterned electrical stimulation of the lower limbs in severe spasticity. *Physiotherapy*, **72**, 579–82.

Sim D. T. (1991). Effectiveness of transcutaneous electrical nerve stimulation following cholecystectomy. *Physiotherapy*, **77**, 715–22.

Simmonds M., Weissel J., Scudds R. (1992). The effect of pain quality on the efficacy of conventional TENS. *Physiotherapy* (Canada), **44**, 35–40.

Singer K. P. (1986). The influence of unilateral electrical muscle stimulation on motor unit activity patterns in atrophic human quadriceps. *Aust. J. Physiother.*, **32**, 31–37.

Singer K. P., De Domenico G., Strauss G. (1987). Electromotor stimulation for research methodology and reporting: a need for standardisation. *Austral. J. Physiother.*, **33**, 43–7.

Sjölund B. H., Eriksson M. B. E. (1979). The influence of naloxone on analgesia produced by peripheral conditioning stimulation. *Brain Res.*, **173**, 295–301.

Sluka K. A., Bailey K., Bogush J., Olson R., Ricketts A. (1998). Treatment with either high or low frequency TENS reduces the secondary hyperalgesia observed after injection of kaolin and carrageenan into the knee joint. *Pain*, **77**, 97–102.

Snyder-Mackler L., Robinson A. J. (1989). *Clinical Electrophysiology.* Baltimore: Williams and Wilkins.

Snyder-Mackler L. S., Ladin Z., Schepsis A. A., Young J. C. (1991). Electrical stimulation of the thigh muscles after reconstruction of the anterior cruciate ligament. *J. Bone Joint Surg.*, **73**, 1025.

Soo C. L., Currier D. P., Threlkeld J. A. (1988). Augmenting voluntary torque of healthy muscles by optimization of electrical stimulation. *Phys. Ther.*, **68**, 3.

Spielholz N. (1987). Electrical stimulation of denervated muscle. In *Clinical Electrotherapy* (Nelson R. M., Currier D. P., eds) Norwalk, Connecticut: Appleton and Lange, pp. 97–113.

St Pierre D., Gardiner P. F. (1987). The effect of immobilization and exercise on muscle function: a review. *Physiotherapy* (Canada), **39**, 24–36.

Stephens W. G. S. (1965). The user of triangular pulses in electrotherapy. *Physiotherapy*, **51**, 147–50.

Stephenson R., Johnson M. (1995). The analgesic effects of interferential therapy on cold-induced pain in healthy subjects – a preliminary report. *Physiother. Theory Pract.*, **11**, 89–95.

Stokes M., Cooper R. (1989). Muscle fatigue as a limiting factor in functional electrical stimulation: a review. *Physiother. Pract.*, **5**, 83–90.

Strauss G. R., De Domenico G. (1986). Torque production in human upper and lower limb muscles with voluntary and electrically stimulated contractions. *Aust. J. Physiother.*, **32**, 38–49.

Sunderland D. S. (1978). *Nerves and Nerve Injuries*, 2nd edn. Edinburgh: Churchill Livingstone.

Taylor K., Newton R., Personius W. *et al.* (1987). Effect of interferential current stimulation for treatment of subjects with recurrent jaw pain. *Phys. Ther.*, **67**, 346–50.

Taylor K., Fish D. R., Mendel F. C. *et al.* (1991). Effect of a single thirty minute treatment of high voltage pulsed current on edema formation in frog hind limbs. *Phys. Ther.*, **72**, 63–8.

Tekeodlu Y., Adak B., Góksoy T. (1998). Effect of transcutaneous electrical nerve stimulation (TENS) in Barthel activities of daily living (ADL) index score following stroke. *Clin. Rehab.*, **12**, 277–80.

Thompson J. W. (1994). Neuropharmacology of the pain pathway. In *Pain Management by Physiotherapy*, 2nd edn (Wells P. E., Frampton V., Bowsher D., eds) Oxford: Butterworth-Heinemann, pp. 59–67.

Thornsteinsson G. (1983). Electrical stimulation for analgesia. In *Therapeutic Electricity and Ultra-violet Radiation* (Stillwell K., ed.) Baltimore: Williams & Wilkins, pp. 109–23.

Thorsteinsson G., Stonnington H. H., Stillwell G. K. *et al.* (1977). Transcutaneous electrical stimulation: a double blind trial of its efficacy for pain. *Arch. Phys. Med. Rehab.*, **58**, 8–13.

Tracy J. E., Currier D. P., Threlkeld A. J. (1988). Comparison of selected pulse frequencies from two different electrical stimulators on blood flow in healthy subjects. *Phys. Ther.*, **68**, 1526–32.

Wadsworth H., Chanmugan A. P. P. (1980). *Electrophysical Agents in Physiotherapy*, 2nd edn. Marrickville, NSW, Australia: Science Press.

Walsh D. M. (1997). *TENS: Clinical Applications and Related Theory.* Edinburgh: Churchill Livingstone.

Walsh D. M., Baxter G. D., Allen J. M., Bell A. J., Mokhtar B. (1992). An assessment of the analgesic effects of H-wave therapy upon experimentally induced ischaemic pain. *Irish J. Med. Sci.*, **161**, 472.

Walsh M., Baxter G. D., Allen J. M. (1993). The effect of transcutaneous electrical nerve stimulation (TENS) upon conduction latencies in the human superficial radial nerve in vivo. *Journal of Physiology,* **467**, 95.

Walsh D. M., Foster N. E., Baxter G. D., Allen J. M. (1995a). Transcutaneous electrical nerve stimulation (TENS): relevance of stimulation parameters to neuro-physiological and hypoanalgesic effects. *Am. J. Phys. Med. Rehab.,* **74**, 199–206.

Walsh D. M., Greer K., Baxter G. D. (1995b). Relevance of transcutaneous electrical nerve stimulation parameters to neurophysiological effects. Proceedings, 12th International Congress of the World Confederation for Physical Therapy, p. 576.

Walsh D. M., Liggett H. C., Baxter D., Allen J. M. (1995c). A double-blind investigation of the hypoanalgesic effects of transcutaneous electrical nerve stimulation upon experimentally induced ischaemic pain. *Pain,* **61**, 39–45.

Ward A. (1986). *Electricity Fields and Waves in Therapy.* Marrickville, NSW, Australia: Science Press.

Ward A. R., Robertson V. J. (1998). Sensory, motor and pain thresholds for stimulation with medium frequency alternating current. *Arch. Phys. Med. Rehab.,* **79**, 273–8.

Woolf C. J. (1979). Transcutaneous electrical nerve stimulation and the reaction to experimental pain in human subjects. *Pain,* **7**, 115–27.

4 Electrophysiological evaluation

In this chapter, electrophysiology is considered in its role of investigating the functional integrity of the neuromuscular system. First, briefly outlined are the ways in which electric charges are utilized in evaluation and diagnosis, followed by some consideration of the pathology that may arise in peripheral nerves. Electromyography is considered and is followed by a description and explanation of strength–duration testing. Finally, evoked potentials, including nerve conduction velocity studies, are briefly considered.

THE USE OF ELECTRIC CHARGES IN EVALUATION AND DIAGNOSIS

- Assessment of nerve and muscle potentials:
  - voluntary and involuntary EMG used for both diagnosis and rehabilitation
- Assessment of results of stimulating nerve and muscle with an electric charge
  - Observing muscle contraction:
    - establish presence of muscle contraction
    - establish nerve continuity
    - establish degree of muscle innervation by strength–duration test
    - establish changes in muscle innervation over time with strength–duration test
  - Evoked potentials
    - conduction velocity tests, motor and sensory
    - reflex tests (e.g. H reflex)
    - centrally evoked responses.

PATHOLOGICAL CHANGES IN PERIPHERAL NERVES

There are many different ways in which the peripheral nerve may be damaged by injury or disease but conduction in the nerve fibre can only be affected in three ways:

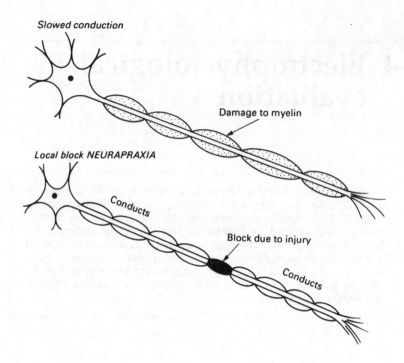

Fig. 4.1 Peripheral nerve lesions without fibre degeneration.

- it can be slowed, which is usually due to the myelin sheath being affected
- it can be stopped over a small section of the nerve fibre – a local block – so that conduction above and below is normal
- it can be stopped over the whole distal length of the nerve from the site of injury to skin and muscle.

Temporary mild compression of the nerve will lead to a conduction block, called a *neurapraxia* (see Fig. 4.1), due simply to displacement of the myelin sheath and local oedema of the nerve fibre itself. As there is no permanent damage recovery occurs rapidly in a few days or weeks. Since only a section of the nerve fibre is affected conduction beyond the blockage is normal; thus electrical stimulation of motor nerve fibres beyond (distal to) the block will cause muscle contraction. Nerve impulses, however, cannot pass across the block so that electrical stimulation applied proximal to the block does not result in muscle contraction. It must be realized that in an affected mixed peripheral nerve only a proportion of the fibres may be involved; the large-diameter fast-conducting fibres are most susceptible to disruption. Clinically, therefore, a neurapraxia can be a partial block with some conduction across the affected region; the more severe lesions will leave a larger number of nerve fibres affected. Thus the severity of the damage can be quantified, to some extent, by measuring the current needed to provoke a given muscle contraction, as more current is needed to stimulate sufficient of the remaining conduction fibres. This is described below as a nerve excitability test.

More severe compression injury may cause sufficient damage to the nerve axon so that it is unable to support the metabolic processes of its distal part, resulting in degeneration of the whole length of the nerve fibre, including the myelin sheath, distal to the lesion. This process is called Wallerian degeneration. It takes some days to extend throughout the distal part of the nerve so that for perhaps 3 or 4 days or more the distal section of the nerve remains excitable and can conduct impulses. The fibrous framework of the bundle of nerve fibres remains intact and fills with a chain of Schwann cells so that ultimately nerve fibrils sprouting from the intact proximal part of the nerve are guided in their proper channels to reform the complete nerve processes. This kind of injury is called an *axonotmesis*. The length of time needed for full recovery to occur will depend on the site of the lesion and the length of nerve that has to regrow. The rate of regrowth is somewhat variable, being more rapid at first, up to 5 mm/day, but is usually considered to be on average 1–2 mm/day.

If, instead of compression, the injury is such as to disrupt all tissues of the nerve fibre – such as a cut through the nerve – then the distal segment will degenerate completely, as described already. Since the tissues are totally disrupted the axon filaments will not readily find correct channels down which to regrow so that recovery is at best imperfect. This lesion is called a *neurotmesis*. Such lesions often require surgery to ensure that the two cut ends are sufficiently approximated to allow successful regrowth.

If the nerve cell is damaged by injury or disease all its processes, including the peripheral nerve, will suffer and may completely degenerate – an axonotmesis. If the cell dies so will its processes. These points are illustrated in Figure 4.2.

Various toxins, some produced by bacteria or viruses, some due to ingested or inhaled poisons (alcohol or heavy metals) may act systemically to cause damage to a large number of peripheral nerves throughout the body. It is often the myelin sheath that is most affected, reducing the conduction velocities of the large-diameter nerves. This occurs in diseases grouped as the polyneurites, of which the most widely recognized is the Guillain–Barré syndrome.

It can be seen that some nerve lesions may be mixtures, with some fibres being completely interrupted while others suffer only a neurapraxia which leads to different effects on nerve conduction. Electrical tests can elucidate these differences and contribute to making decisions about the prognosis.

ASSESSMENT OF NERVE AND MUSCLE POTENTIALS

Electromyography

Electromyography involves detecting, amplifying and displaying the electrical changes that occur when a muscle contracts. The

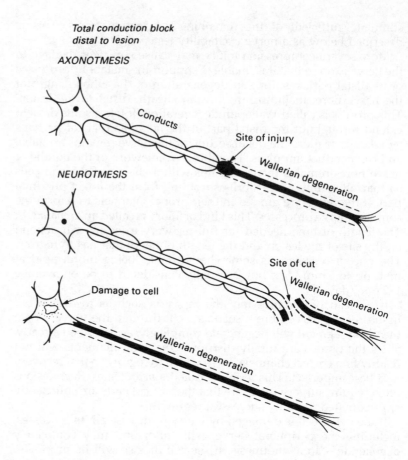

Total conduction block
distal to lesion

AXONOTMESIS

Conducts

Site of injury

Wallerian degeneration

NEUROTMESIS

Site of cut

Wallerian degeneration

Damage to cell

Wallerian degeneration

Fig. 4.2 Peripheral nerve lesions involving degeneration.

signals are tiny, a few microvolts, but are amplified about a thousand times to give millivolt values that can be displayed on an oscilloscope, operate a loudspeaker and be recorded on a chart.

The alpha motor neuron from each anterior horn cell branches at its termination in the muscle to supply a number of individual muscle fibres scattered throughout the muscle. This whole arrangement of neuron and muscle fibres is called a motor unit (Fig. 4.3) (see Chapter 3).

When a normal muscle contracts all the individual muscle fibres of the motor unit depolarize (and then repolarize) at the same time causing a local electrical disturbance in the muscle. This can be detected either by electrodes on the skin or by a needle electrode inserted into the muscle. Surface electrodes are often silver/silver chloride, coated with a suitable conducting gel, and can be taped on to the skin. Light, malleable, self-adhesive electrodes are also available. Needle electrodes consist of fine wires, insulated save at the tip, which are inserted into the chosen muscle by means of a hypodermic needle. In both cases the electrical disturbance recorded is the sum of the potentials due to all the muscle fibres activated. Thus activation of a single motor unit can be recognized because the many muscle fibres contract at nearly the same time producing

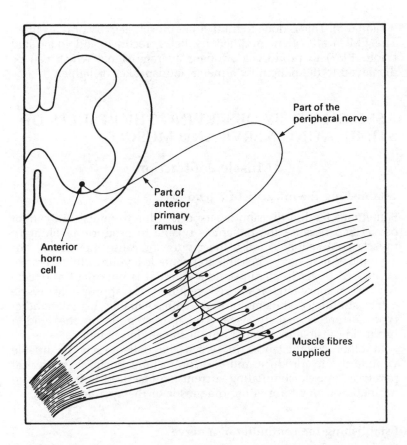

Fig. 4.3. A single motor unit.

a single characteristic trace, called an action potential, on the recording. Since skeletal muscles are under voluntary control, action potentials can be recorded from muscles during different degrees of contraction. If no muscle contraction is occurring then no electrical activity is detectable. However, in abnormal conditions potentials may be recorded when the muscle is at rest and these can be used in the diagnosis of nerve and muscle pathologies. Denervated muscle membrane becomes hypersensitive to acetylcholine causing spontaneous potentials. These show on the electromyographic record as 1 ms potentials of low amplitude, called fibrillation potentials, the consequence of depolarization of individual muscle fibres. Various other forms of spontaneous activity, such as positive potentials and fasciculation, the spontaneous discharge of whole motor units, also occur in denervated muscle; still other forms are characteristic of muscle disease. Voluntary contraction of disordered muscle may also give a characteristic abnormal EMG record. Thus records taken during reinnervation show large polyphasic potentials. Needle electrodes are generally employed for diagnostic EMG because better localization can be achieved and deeper muscle can be reached.

The normal EMG can be employed by physiotherapists, using surface electrodes, for muscle training – a process called biofeedback

(Chapter 5). This is done to train either muscle activity or relaxation. The EMGs are often modified by being rectified and integrated (Wolf, 1987) to produce a stronger average signal which can be displayed to the patient by a meter, loudspeaker or lights.

ASSESSMENT BY OBSERVING THE RESULTS OF STIMULATING NERVE AND MUSCLE

Muscle contraction

Establishing the integrity of a tendon

Sometimes tendon division is suspected due to injury, but cannot be verified because the patient is unable to produce a voluntary muscle contraction to tense the tendon or cause movement. For example, it may not be possible to persuade a young child to move an injured finger in circumstances where it is important to decide whether primary tendon suture is required. The appropriate muscle can be stimulated at its motor point with a suitable current; faradic-type current is usually used. The muscle pulls on the tendon producing visible movement only if the tendon is intact.

In other circumstances in which the patient may be unable voluntarily to produce muscle contraction, such as hysterical paralysis, muscle-stimulating current may be used to demonstrate normal movement, for either diagnostic or therapeutic reasons.

Establishing the continuity of a nerve

If a peripheral motor nerve is stimulated with a suitable electrical pulse at some point and the muscles that it supplies distally are seen to contract then it can be concluded that the nerve is able to conduct impulses. This is sometimes called a nerve conduction test but should not be confused with a nerve conduction velocity test (see below), which is also sometimes referred to as a nerve conduction test. For example, the ulnar nerve may be stimulated behind the medial epicondyle of the humerus to cause contraction of the hypothenar and intrinsic hand muscles as well as the flexor carpi ulnaris and part of flexor digitorum profundus. Similarly the facial (VII) nerve can be stimulated to cause all the facial muscles to contract. To some extent this can be used as a quantitative test, called a nerve excitability test, since the voltage or current needed to stimulate the normal side can be compared to that needed to give a similar contraction on the affected side. Single 0.1 or 1 ms rectangular pulses with a 1 or 2 s interval between each pulse are used so that the resulting muscle twitch can be assessed. The threshold intensity (or voltage) needed to elicit a minimal muscle contraction is noted for each side. The normal difference in current intensity between the two sides (due to variations in soft tissue thickness, differences in electrode positioning, as well as natural variations in nerve excitability) is considered to lie within 2 mA (Wadsworth and Chanmugan, 1980) and is certanly less than 4 mA

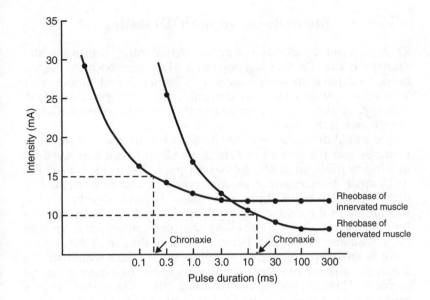

(Nash, 1979) for the facial nerve. This should be repeated a few times to check the consistency of the result.

The technique used for a facial nerve lesion (Bell's palsy) assessment involves placing a dispersive electrode behind the neck with the patient lying down and applying a small stimulating electrode to the skin below the tragus of the ear just in front of the mastoid process to stimulate the facial nerve as it emerges from the stylomastoid foramen. The three trunks of the facial nerve may be assessed separately.

If a neurapraxia is present the difference between the two sides is within the normal variation, i.e. about 2 mA, because stimulation is applied to normally conducting nerve beyond the conduction block. If some axonotmesis is present larger currents, 4–8 mA, will be needed to stimulate sufficient of the remaining conducting fibres to produce a contraction equivalent to that on the normal side. If there is axonotmesis of all the nerve fibres then no muscle contraction will occur unless very high currents, of 10, 20 or more times that of the normal side, are used which would directly stimulate the muscle (Fig. 4.4). Several tests may be done on successive days.

The value of these tests lies in their ability to determine easily the changes in conduction in the early stages of this lesion. Thus a simple neurapraxia will show no conduction loss at any time. The need for a higher current on the affected side indicates conduction loss, hence some degree of axonotmesis, which worsens during the first few days as nerve degeneration occurs. This information would be helpful in deciding whether active decompression measures should be applied (Nash, 1979) and for determining the prognosis of the particular case.

Strength–duration (S–D) testing

This is a more sensitive way of determining neuromuscular excitability than the tests just described. The principles have already been considered to some extent in Chapter 3 and Figure 3.13. Strength–duration tests are used mainly for motor nerve assessment, although similar methods can be employed in sensory nerve testing (Smith and Mott, 1986).

A minimal detectable muscle contraction is used as the standard response and the current or voltage needed to elicit that response at different pulse lengths is plotted on a graph. As already considered in Chapter 3, a certain minimal amount of charge is needed to depolarize the nerve fibre membrane beyond threshold. The magnitude of the charge is a product of current intensity and the time for which it flows. Thus with shorter-duration pulses greater current intensity is needed. However, even if the stimulating pulses were to last a very long time – infinite time – there would still be a minimal amount of energy (charge) necessary to trigger the nerve impulse. Thus, for any given situation (tissue resistance, rate of pulse rise, etc.) there is a minimal current or voltage required and this is known as the *rheobase* (Fig. 4.4).

Long electrical pulses will stimulate excitable tissue, muscle and nerve at the appropriate rheobase current. Using a constant voltage stimulator in which the voltage remains a constant value throughout the pulse duration, the rheobase is often between 10 and 20 V. Using a constant current stimulator the rheobase is approximately 2–10 mA. For muscle tissue, electrical pulses of approximately 30 ms duration have insufficient charge at the rheobase current and must be increased to depolarize the muscle membrane; pulses of about 10 ms may need twice as much current and the current needed increases exponentially with shorter and shorter pulses. Nerve tissue, on the other hand, is much more excitable so that pulses as short as 1 ms are still an effective stimulus at rheobase currents; shorter pulses, however, need the same exponential current increase as muscle tissue. Therefore if the strength–duration graphs of nerve and muscle are plotted on the same scales they have the same shape but appear on different parts of the abscissa. The graph of current against pulse duration is characteristic but quantitatively different for nerve and muscle tissue. When muscles are made to contract by nerve impulses, as happens when innervated muscle is stimulated, the response will be characteristic of nerve tissue. A typical graph for innervated and denervated muscle is shown in Figure 4.4. Denervation appears to lower the rheobase value (Stephens, 1973; Wadsworth and Chanmugan, 1980; Ward, 1986). This is probably associated with the acetylcholine hypersensitivity that develops in muscle tissues when they are denervated (Spielholz, 1987). It should be noted that such graphs differ slightly depending on whether the electrical pulses are of constant current or constant voltage. With constant-voltage machines, stimuli of somewhat shorter duration can be used before the voltage needs to be increased compared to constant-current machines. This makes constant-voltage machines more comfortable because less electrical energy is being used and hence they are safer (Cywinski and Gobelet, 1998). Constant-current graphs are said to be more accurate, although the difference is trivial.

Technique for performing strength–duration tests

The part to be tested needs to be firmly supported and the patient reassured by adequate explanation of what is to happen.

One electrode and pad is fixed near the end of the muscle to be tested and the other is moved until a good muscle contraction is obtained using a long duration pulse of 100 or 300 ms. Small electrodes are used to localize the current to the muscle being tested. A hand-held button electrode with dispersive may be used but fixed electrodes, both suction and adhesive, which free the physiotherapist's hand are recommended. However, this is a matter of preference since there is little evidence for inconsistency within a single test (see below). The muscle contraction is identified visually or by palpation, or both. The pulses are applied at a rate of 1/s, or one every 2 s to allow plenty of time for muscle recovery between contractions. The intensity or voltage is then reduced until the contraction can only just be detected and this value is recorded. A shorter pulse, say 30 ms, is then applied. If the muscle contraction remains the same the strength of the pulse is recorded and a still shorter pulse is applied and so on. If the muscle contraction disappears the current is increased until the contraction returns and is just detectable again. It is usual to take 8 or 10 points from 100 ms to 0.01 ms for constant-voltage machines and from 300 ms to 0.1 ms for constant-current stimulators. It is important to maintain constant position and constant pressure of the electrodes during the test. The current intensities that have been noted, or stored in the memory of the stimulator, are plotted against the appropriate pulse duration on a suitable piece of graph paper. This test does not take very long; perhaps 2–3 min.

Interpretation

The graphs produced will do more than discriminate between innervated and denervated muscle. To some extent they can quantify the state of innervation of a muscle. If only a few fibres are innervated amongst a mass of denervated fibres the first part of the graph will be typical for those denervated fibres, but at higher current intensities with shorter pulses the few innervated fibres are unmasked because the denervated fibres are no longer able to contract. Thus two curves result; one with a low rheobase due to the mass of denervated fibres and a few (masked) innervated fibres, and a second with a high rheobase due to the scattered innervated fibres – the rheobase must be high to provide enough current to reach all the innervated fibres. The typical 'kinked' curve is shown in Figure 4.5. Now the amplitude of the higher rheobase is a function of the number of innervated fibres so that if more fibres become innervated the 'kink' will shift downwards and vice versa.

> **Practical point**
> Warming and wetting the skin through which current is to pass helps to lower its resistance.

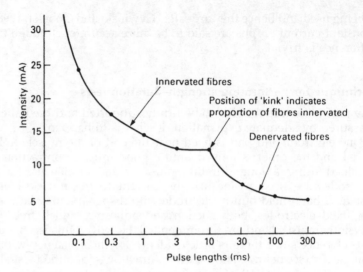

Fig. 4.5. A 'kinked' curve showing partial denervation.

Comparison of a series of S–D curves taken at intervals can indicate progressive denervation or reinnervation.

Chronaxie

The chronaxie is an index of nerve and muscle excitability. It is the pulse duration in milliseconds needed to cause a minimal perceptible muscle contraction with a current (or voltage) of twice the rheobase. It is a very different value, i.e. longer time, for muscle compared to nerve tissue (Fig. 4.4). It is therefore a simple method of discriminating between innervated and denervated muscle. Normal innervated values vary somewhat from one muscle to another (Wadsworth and Chanmugan, 1980) but are well below 1 ms for constant-current and below 0.1 ms for constant-voltage stimulators. Denervated muscle values are around 10 ms or more.

Pulse ratio is occasionally mentioned. This is the ratio of the current or voltage required at 100 ms pulse duration, to that required at 1 ms duration. A value greater than 2.2 indicates abnormality.

Reliability of strength–duration curves

Since the usefulness of these curves depends on the comparison of one curve with another, it is essential that the variability and what is within normal limits can be recognized. When successive S–D curves are made by different testers on the same subject almost identical figures are obtained. Remarkably high inter-rater reliability has been demonstrated in a careful study (Nelson and Hunt, 1981), which found an average correlation coefficient between testers of 0.945. This quantifies the previously expressed view of one of us (Low, 1979) regarding the impressive consistency of repeated curves made by different testers during training sessions. It has also been shown that two testers making S–D curves for 20 different subjects achieved very similar results (Alexander, 1974). All this evidence

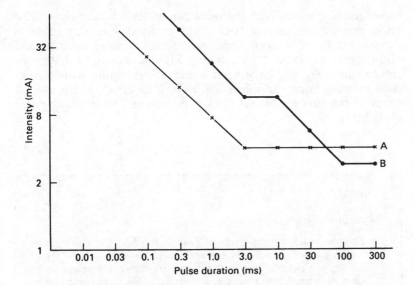

Fig. 4.6 Strength–duration graph plotted on log log scale. A = Normally innervated; B = denervated muscles.

indicates that different testers are able to make very much the same S–D curve, contrary to opinions sometimes expressed.

The repeatability of curves made on different occasions is not nearly as consistent. A coefficient of correlation of 0.541 has been found (Nelson and Hunt, 1981). The shape of the curve remains consistent but the absolute values vary. All the sources quoted above note that the variations in rheobase are minimal with longer stimuli but become greater with the higher intensities required at shorter pulse lengths. Different electrode sizes and polarity affect the numerical values and shape of the curve (Arsenault and Stevens, 1979) but these differences are not large and allow the plot to fall within a normal composite curve.

It is easy to increase the reliability of S–D curves by plotting all the curves to be compared on a standard rheobase. Since the rheobase will vary with skin resistance, electrode pressure, the presence of oedema and other factors, this is an important correction to make. All that needs to be done is to divide all readings by the rheobase, thus expressing them all as a function of the rheobase, which is taken as one. This is simple to do by hand, but some machines have a facility that allows the readings to be taken directly as multiples of the rheobase.

Another way of improving the usefulness of these readings is to plot the graph with the ordinate (i.e. the strength of pulse) as a logarithmic scale. This has the effect of converting the typical exponential curve into two straight lines. The point at which the graph starts to rise is therefore precisely defined. If two curves are evident, as occurs in partial denervation, the three angles – the kinks – and their positions become exactly defined. This is valuable in assessing changes in innervation, as described above (Fig. 4.6).

Comparisons are also more reliable if a constant technique is applied, that is the electrodes are of the same size and placed in the same position for each test. Constancy is more important than technique employed. With the most careful technique there will be variations in the normal S–D curve from day to day. This is considered to be a normal physiological variation (Nelson and Hunt, 1981) and is hardly surprising when it is realized that nerve conduction velocities have been found to vary quite widely from time to time. Such variations will have little effect on the overall shape of the curve, which is the key parameter in describing nerve excitability.

Summary

Strength–duration curves can:

- *Demonstrate the presence of innervated fibres in the muscle being tested.* If all fibres are denervated a typical denervated curve will result. This is then said to show 'the reaction of degeneration' or RD. If a small number of fibres are innervated amongst a mass of denervated fibres a 'kinked' curve may be evident; the position of the kink is a reflection of the number of innervated fibres. If a large number, or all, of the fibres are innervated then a normal curve will result.
- *Demonstrate changes in innervation by means of successive graphs.* This information is often critically important in the clinical situation where it may be essential to know if reinnervation is occurring. Progressive reinnervation (and denervation) is indicated by changes in the position of the kink. The appearance and movement of a kink towards the normal form in successive plots of the curve can herald reinnervation before any voluntary recovery can be detected.
- *Indicate the value of the rheobase, chronaxie and utilization time.* As already discussed, the rheobase varies with a number of factors, such as skin resistance, position and size of stimulating electrodes, skin temperature, presence of oedema or skin atrophy and other factors. The rheobase, therefore, has limited value as an indicator of nerve excitability except when the two sides can be directly compared, as in the nerve excitability tests considered above. The chronaxie has already been described as the pulse duration at which a current of twice the rheobase is required to elicit a twitch (Stephens, 1973); it can simply be read off the graph. It provides a single number to indicate the state of innervation. The utilization or effective time is the duration of the shortest pulse that causes a muscle contraction with the rheobase current. If therapeutic stimulation of the muscle is to be performed it is the appropriate pulse length to use.

Strength–duration testing can also be done with accommodation pulses (see Stephens, 1973).

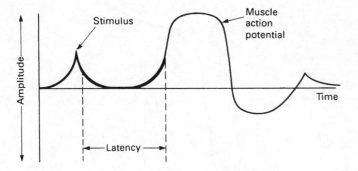

Fig. 4.7 Evoked muscle action potential.

EVOKED POTENTIALS

In these tests the peripheral nerve is electrically stimulated and the resulting nerve impulse or muscle potential is measured. These tests can provide a measurement of the velocity of the nerve impulse and information about its amplitude and nature.

Nerve conduction velocity studies

Nerve conduction velocity studies are performed on peripheral nerves only, as opposed to reflex testing or centrally recorded evoked responses which involve the central nervous system. Both motor and sensory conduction velocities can be recorded. The stimulus is applied to the nerve by two small electrodes fixed on the skin about 2 cm apart. The pulse duration used can be varied from 0.05 to 2 ms; at a frequency of 1 or 2 Hz. The recording is made from a different set of electrodes which are placed over the stimulated muscle or sensory nerve. Both the stimulating and response signals are displayed on an oscilloscope; some method of making a permanent record, whether photographic or pen and chart, is included. From this permanent trace conduction velocity and other measurements can be made. More sophisticated equipment is able to display such measures automatically and almost instantly.

To determine motor conduction velocity the nerve is stimulated with single pulses which will initiate impulses in many axons to activate the motor end-plates of many thousands of muscle fibres, causing a brisk muscle contraction called the M wave. This can be displayed with the stimulus to show the conduction time between stimulus and the start of muscle contraction, which is called latency (Fig. 4.7). This includes the time it takes the impulse to cross the motor end-plate and provoke muscle contraction. To measure the time that is due to nerve conduction only, stimulation is given at two points along the course of a nerve. The linear distance between these two points is measured on the body surface. The latency is then found from each of the two points so that the time difference between them can be divided into the distance. This will give a reasonably accurate conduction velocity (Fig. 4.8). For example, if

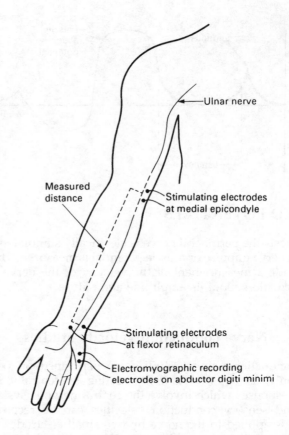

Ulnar nerve

Measured
distance

Stimulating electrodes
at medial epicondyle

Stimulating electrodes
at flexor retinaculum

Electromyographic recording
electrodes on abductor digiti minimi

Fig. 4.8 Nerve conduction velocity calculation.

stimulation of two sites 20 cm apart were to give latencies of 7 ms from the proximal and 3 ms from the distal site then the velocity would be found by:

$$\frac{20\,\text{cm}}{7-3\,\text{ms}} = 5\,\text{cm/ms}$$

Thus velocity = 50 m/s.

Conduction velocities of the two sides can be compared and checked against published normal values. Conduction velocities are often reduced in compression lesions, such as carpal tunnel syndrome, and may indicate the diagnosis.

Sensory nerve conduction tests are performed in a similar way except that the recording is made from the nerve itself, i.e. the nerve impulses. This can be done either by stimulating at the periphery and recording from the proximal nerve trunk – the orthodromic direction – or it can be done antidromically. The nerve impulse is, of course, a much smaller electrical disturbance than the action potential of many muscle fibres acting together but with modern equipment it can easily be recorded and gives a direct measure of the conduction velocity.

Not only are the latency and velocity of nerve impulses measured but also the shape and amplitude of the impulses which may vary in some disease processes.

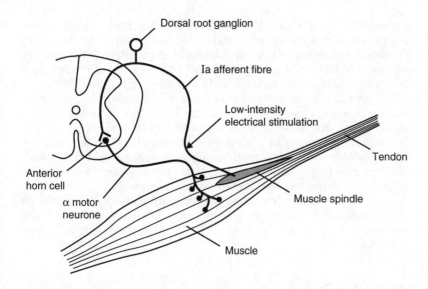

Fig. 4.9 The H reflex. The stretch reflex may be stimulated via Ia fibre by either (a) a tap on the tendon via the muscle spindle, or (b) electrical stimulation of the fibre.

Electrical reflex testing

The H reflex

The H reflex (Fig. 4.9) refers to testing a stretch reflex, such as the ankle jerk, by electrically stimulating the afferent (Ia) fibres from the muscle spindles. A tap on the tendon causes stretch of the muscle and hence muscle spindles, which send impulses through a monosynaptic reflex in the spinal cord to cause a muscle twitch. If the nerve proximal to the muscle, e.g. the posterior tibial nerve for tendocalcaneous reflex, is stimulated with a low-intensity short (say 0.1 ms) pulse the Ia afferent nerves can be selectively stimulated. The current must be kept below the threshold for the alpha motor neuron fibres, otherwise these will directly initiate a muscle twitch and the reflex will be lost. Thus the afferent side of the stretch reflex is stimulated beyond the spindles, leading to a muscle twitch which is recorded electromyographically and appears after a delay of approximately 30 ms (Nelson, 1987).

The reflex is most evident in those muscles that have many muscle spindles. It can be used to assess conduction rates. This is useful if nerve compression in the intervertebral foramen is suspected since peripheral nerve conduction velocity through this region cannot otherwise be assessed. The H of this reflex refers to Hoffman who first suggested the test; it should not be confused with the Hoffman reflex. The blink reflex has also been examined by electrical stimulation in a somewhat similar way.

Evoked potentials in the CNS

Electrical potentials can be recorded with the use of modern sensitive electronic equipment from sites over the spinal cord, brainstem and cortex. The impulses passing in nerve tracts produce an electrical disturbance which can be measured at the body surface. The amplitude of this measured signal is due to the sum of all the action potentials occurring at that time. It has been calculated that changes of around 100 mV in a nerve fibre would result in a change of a few microvolts on the nearest body surface (Lehmkuhl, 1981).

A stimulus is applied outside the CNS, either by electrical stimulation of a peripheral nerve or by direct stimulation of a sense organ, and this stimulus is exactly timed and repeated. The consequent responses of a series of such stimuli are added together electronically so that the random noise signals cancel one another out but any response repeated at exactly the same time after the stimulus is enhanced and becomes clearly evident.

In general, diseases involving demyelination are characterized by lower conduction velocities, hence longer latencies, whereas those involving loss of neurons are associated with a lower signal amplitude.

REFERENCES

Alexander J. (1974). Reproducibility of strength–duration curves. *Arch. Phys. Med. Rehab.*, **55**, 56–60.

Arsenault A. B., Stevens J. (1979). A study of the variability of the strength–duration curve parameters. *Physiother. Canada*, **31**, 125–30.

Cywinski J., Gobelet C. (1998). Transcutaneous EMS stimulation therapy: relativity of chronaxie. Proceedings of Human Motor Performance Congress, University of East London.

Lehmkuhl L. D. (1981). Evoked spinal, brainstem and cerebral potentials. In *Electrotherapy* (Wolf S. L., ed.) London: Churchill Livingstone, pp. 123–54.

Low J. (1979). A review of the uses and reliability of strength–duration curves. *N.Z. J. Physiother.*, **13**, 16–20.

Nash J. D. (1979). Prognostic nerve conduction test. *Physiotherapy*, **65**, 82.

Nelson R. M. (1987). Electrophysiologic evaluation: an overview. In *Clinical Electrotherapy* (Nelson R. M., Currier D. P., eds) Norwalk, Connecticut: Appleton and Lange, pp. 243–57.

Nelson R. M., Hunt G. C. (1981). Strength–duration curve: intrarater and interrater reliability. *Phys. Ther.*, **61**, 894–7.

Richardson A. T., Wynn-Parry C. B. (1957). The theory and practice of electrodiagnosis. *Am. Phys. Med.*, **4**, 3–16.

Smith P. J., Mott G. (1986). Sensory threshold and conductance testing in nerve injuries. *J. Hand. Surg.*, **11B**, 157–62.

Spielholz N. (1987). Electrical stimulation of denervated muscle. In *Clinical Electrotherapy* (Nelson R. M., Currier D. P., eds) Norwalk, Connecticut: Appleton and Lange, pp. 97–113.

Stephens W. G. S. (1973). The assessment of muscle denervation by electrical stimulation. *Physiotherapy*, **59**, 292–4.

Wadsworth H., Chanmugan A. P. P. (1980). Electrophysical agents in physiotherapy. Marrickville, NSW, Australia: Science Press.

Ward A. R. (1986). *Electricity Fields and Waves in Therapy.* Marrickville, NSW, Australia: Science Press.

Wolf D. (1987). Electromyographic biofeedback: an overview. In *Clinical Electrotherapy* (Nelson R. M., Currier D. P., eds) Norwalk, Connecticut: Appleton and Lange, pp. 259–78.

5 Biofeedback

Feedback is the coupling of the output of a process to the input. The word has been defined (Wiener, 1948) as 'a method of controlling the system by re-inserting into it the results of its past performance'. This idea is involved in many physiological systems.

This chapter opens with a consideration of the general concepts of feedback and the two major uses of biofeedback; first, the control of muscle activity and body movement, and second, the treatment of stress-related conditions. This is followed by a description of the application of temperature biofeedback to provide an example.

The concept of feedback is widely recognized in engineering and physiological mechanisms as 'negative feedback', in which a deviation of the system in one direction leads to a correction of this deviation. 'Positive feedback' occurs when the deviation leads to further deviation in the same direction to the limits of the system. Biofeedback refers to the application of negative feedback to biological systems and specifically to the conscious control of some of those systems which are usually considered to be autonomically (automatically) regulated.

As an example, the temperature of the skin of the fingers is under sympathetic regulation which is largely dependent on the local and general environmental temperature, as described in Chapter 7. If a sensitive skin thermometer is applied to the skin of the finger most people are able to make a small alteration of the skin temperature at will (Fig. 5.1). This may take a little time and some practice but can be done providing the subject can see the thermometer reading and thus has immediate information of any change in skin temperature; this is the 'feedback'.

Many physiological changes of which people are normally unaware can be made visible or audible with suitable electronic instruments. This has enabled biofeedback control to be practised for a whole range of activities such as the control of blood pressure, heart rate, skin temperature but principally for the contraction and relaxation of voluntary muscle electromyographically. This effect can also be demonstrated in animals. Experiments have shown that the heart rate in rats and dogs can be controlled, in some cases, by operant conditioning.

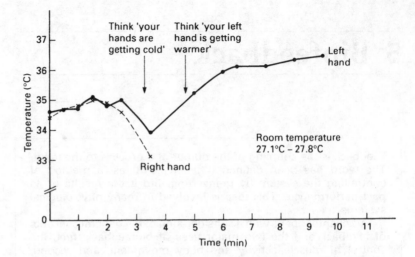

Fig. 5.1 Skin temperature as recorded over 10 min for the left and right middle fingers of a 58-year-old normal subject.

The concept can be expressed in principle by the feedback loop shown in Figure 5.2. The physiological change is detected or measured by some device, e.g. the skin temperature alters the resistance of the thermistor. The output of this measurement is displayed on a digital indicator, the subject perceives this information about the temperature and he or she now makes conscious attempts to alter it, i.e. to warm or cool the finger (Fig. 5.1). Exactly which neuronal pathways are involved in this last part of the loop is not understood, but the fact that it is possible to exert some control, albeit to a limited extent, indicates that such pathways exist.

This is not different in principle from the re-education given by physiotherapists in providing feedback for the correction of posture or the initiation of a muscle contraction. All human movement is controlled by feedback. Information from muscle spindles, joint motion and position sensors, the vestibular apparatus, skin sensors and visual cues all contribute. These are sometimes collectively referred to as intrinsic feedback to distinguish them from the extrinsic (augmented) feedback provided by the physiotherapist or some outside source. The development of relatively cheap electronic circuitry allows electromyography with surface electrodes to record motor unit action potentials reasonably easily. Similarly, suitable instruments are available to record body movement, blood pressure, heart rate (electrocardiograph) and electric potentials developed in the central nervous system (electroencephalograph).

USES OF BIOFEEDBACK

Biofeedback is used for two broad purposes:

- for conditions in which control over some defective muscle action or movement is attempted
- for control of stress-related conditions.

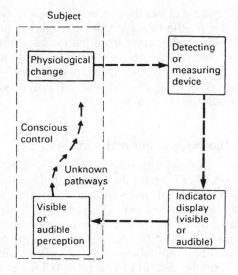

Fig. 5.2 Feedback loop.

The latter often applies to circumstances in which some control over the autonomic nervous system is attempted. There is overlap between these purposes in that muscle relaxation may be used for both.

Biofeedback for the control of muscle activity and movement

Electromyographic biofeedback

It will be recalled from Chapter 4 that diagnostic use can be made of the electrical signals generated when a motor unit fires. When one of these fires, the muscle fibres it supplies all contract together causing an electrical disturbance called the motor unit action potential. When a muscle contracts normally many hundreds of these motor units fire asynchronously, producing electrical potentials which can be detected either by needle electrodes in the muscle tissue or from surface electrodes. These signals can be displayed on an oscilloscope screen or recorded on a strip of paper (chart recorder) as well as being fed to a loudspeaker to generate a series of audible clicks, as explained in Chapter 4.

The electromyographic display bears an approximate relationship to the magnitude of the muscle contraction causing it. The relationship is quite complicated because the motor unit action potentials that occur will not all be equally detected and recorded. However, for biofeedback purposes, the overall effect of stronger contractions leading to more and louder clicks, merging into a roar, and a large display on the screen are adequate.

Electromyographic machines specifically built for biofeedback usually provide both audible and visual outputs, the latter often as a moving meter needle rather than an oscilloscope trace. The smooth movement of the needle is achieved by rectifying and averaging the motor unit electrical activity from the muscles, thus producing an output which varies smoothly with the average muscle activity. Surface electrodes are usually used so that localization of the electromyogram (EMG) signal is not exact. It is also only applicable for reasonably superficial muscles.

Uses of EMG biofeedback for motor control

Hemiplegia.   The majority of published accounts of the use of EMG biofeedback have been for the treatment of hemiplegic patients most commonly as attempts to re-educate controlled dorsiflexion of the foot and thus improve the gait. This can involve two approaches: encouraging activity in the tibialis anterior and other dorsiflexors and/or discouraging the unwanted spasticity of the plantarflexors. Biofeedback can be applied to any superficial muscle of the hemiplegic patient; the deltoid has been treated in order to improve shoulder control, for example.

Most studies have found biofeedback to be a successful method of treatment; some found it more successful than conventional treatment (e.g. Basmajian *et al.*, 1975). However, not all patients appear able to improve with biofeedback and it is difficult to separate any specific gain from that due to the enthusiasm engendered by any new treatment.

Spinal cord injury.   Biofeedback techniques have been recommended (Basmajian, 1981) and applied in the rehabilitation of spinal cord injury. A comparison between treatments involving physical exercise and electrical muscle stimulation with and without EMG feedback in spinal cord injury (Klose *et al.*, 1993) showed no significant advantage for biofeedback. (Patients had defects involving C5–7 and had at least some active contraction.) However, this study noted marked differences between individuals. Some patients benefited particularly with biofeedback, suggesting that a particular subset of spinal cord injury patients responded. This may conform with the conclusion at the end of this chapter that biofeedback is especially beneficial if other feedback is lacking. One striking point that emerged from several studies was the extent to which improvement occurred with any treatment in patients who had been selected on the assumption that further improvement was unlikely (Marcer, 1986).

Spasticity.   Attempts have been made to reduce and control spasticity from causes other than cerebrovascular accidents, e.g. head injury, multiple sclerosis or cerebral palsy. In the case of cerebral palsied children teaching the technique of biofeedback may be difficult and any improvement may be particularly hard to distinguish from that due to growth and maturation. It should be noted that in all neurological disorders treated by biofeedback it is assumed that there are some intact neuronal pathways available to suppress the spasticity. If this is known not to be the case – in a complete transection of the spinal cord, for example – biofeedback would be pointless.

Dystonic conditions.   Dystonic conditions in which the patient suffers uncontrollable movements or postures have also been treated by EMG biofeedback (Moon, 1980). Spasmodic torticollis is the most widely known of these conditions and has been treated by biofeedback to the sternocleidomastoid muscles. This has enabled patients voluntarily to inhibit the forceful inappropriate neck movements and proved to be a successful treatment given the intractable nature of the condition.

Writer's cramp and blepharospasm are other dystonias which have been treated with biofeedback (Marcer, 1986).

Recovering peripheral nerve injuries.   As might be expected, biofeedback has been used in the treatment of recovering peripheral nerve injuries. Once motor unit activity has been detected on the electromyograph voluntary repetition can be encouraged. This use nicely illustrates the point that the principle of biofeedback is used in physiotherapy without its being described as such. Once a trivial muscle contraction or a flicker can be detected manually the physiotherapist encourages the patient to further effort, thus providing the feedback by recognizing the muscle contraction and informing the patient. What EMG biofeedback provides is a means of extending the recognition to the least possible motor activity (single motor unit) and of quantifying it to some extent.

A study of biofeedback for long-standing facial muscle paresis found it to be clinically efficacious (Ross *et al.*, 1991). This study also compared a group of patients who were taught exercises with a mirror (visual feedback) with a group treated similarly, but with the addition of EMG biofeedback. There was no statistically significant difference between these groups.

In cases of nerve transplant, biofeedback can be used to help the patient learn the new muscle action. Notice that this contrasts with and complements the use of muscle-stimulating currents (see Chapter 3) to provoke artificial muscle contraction of the newly innervated muscle which the patient attempts to copy. Biofeedback informs the patient when he or she is making the correct response.

Training specific muscle activity. After trauma to a muscle or its attachments or after a tendon or muscle transplant it may not be possible for the patient to perform a particular voluntary movement. Similarly some voluntary movements which are therapeutically useful, such as abduction of the great toe, are not easy for some patients to perform at will. In all these circumstances biofeedback can be used provided the muscle is sufficiently superficial to give a reasonably isolated output. In all cases the patient is able to detect from the EMG output when the voluntary effort is producing a contraction in the appropriate muscle. Knight and Laycock (1994) have described the use of biofeedback as an adjunct to pelvic floor exercises in the conservative management of incontinence caused by pelvic laxity.

Summary

Uses of electromyographic biofeedback for motor control:

- hemiplegia
  - encourage muscle action
  - discourage spasticity
- head injuries, multiple sclerosis, cerebral palsy
  - control spasticity
- dystonic conditions (spasmodic torticollis, etc.)
  - control unwanted movement
- peripheral nerve lesions
  - encourage motor activity
- specific muscles
  - training activity.

Application of EMG biofeedback

Instruments for providing EMG biofeedback vary in complexity. The simplest give only averaged motor unit responses on a meter. The more complex machines allow changes in sensitivity from showing a single motor unit response to those coupled to computing facilities and chart recorders which provide a permanent record of each training session and printouts of measures such as the average EMG activity during each minute of the session. The action potentials are only a few microvolts so essentially the EMG instrument is simply a very powerful amplifier. This means that any extraneous electrical signals will also be amplified and tend to interfere with the output. It is therefore important that good electrical contact be maintained with the skin and that other sources of electric fields be kept away. In the physiotherapy department pulsed shortwave is a likely source of interference, but any electrical field can have an effect. Several types of electrodes are available to make the good electrical contact with the skin surface that is essential for biofeedback. Silver/silver chloride electrodes are electrically the most suitable (Hurrell, 1980) but others, e.g. steel, are quite satisfactory.

It is important that the electrode be fixed firmly in place with sticky tape because movement over the skin will lead to interference.

The position and support of the patient must be carefully chosen for this treatment. If relaxation is to be attempted then the whole body must be fully supported lying or half-lying so that all postural muscles will be relaxed. If a movement is to be attempted then it is essential to position the patient so that this particular movement can occur unhindered and be visible to the patient; further, the need for fixator or synergistic activity in other muscles should be diminished. For example, if the deltoid is to be re-educated the upper limb should be supported in about 60° abduction and slight flexion at the shoulder. Most importantly the patient must be able to see the biofeedback meter or other signal. A full explanation of

Practical point
To make good electrical contact the skin can be cleaned with an alcohol wipe (gentle rubbing with pumice is also recommended) and saline gel smeared between electrode and skin.

Practical point
De Weerdt and Harrison (1986) recommend taping the signal wires to the patient to reduce movement.

the purpose of the treatment and what is expected of the patient is given and the electrodes are fixed in place as described above. The positioning of the electrodes depends on the muscles involved and requires a knowledge of muscle anatomy. Generally the strongest signals will be had from electrodes placed close to the belly of the muscle and where it is most superficial. It may be helpful for the initial treatment if the working of the EMG biofeedback machine is shown to the patient and trials made by taking signals from a muscle which can easily be controlled by the patient.

The need to remain still to prevent unwanted potentials from other muscles interfering is explained to the patient. The sensitivity of the instrument can be altered by adjusting a dial to give an appropriate signal. Some muscles will generate strong outputs because many motor units are active and are close to the surface. In other circumstances, such as recovering nerve lesions, only a few isolated spike potentials may be present and the sensitivity must be increased to recognize them.

The training session consists of a series of attempts by the patient to increase the signal, or decrease it if relaxation is the objective. The physiotherapist encourages the patient verbally and suggests attempting activities which may lead to the desired muscle contraction, such as trying the activity on the opposing normal limb. Other ways of facilitating muscle contraction such as passive stretching may be used providing they do not create unwanted EMG signals. As voluntary control of a muscle contraction improves, the sensitivity of the device can be deliberately reduced to provide the patient with a new goal. If relaxation is the aim then the sensitivity would be increased as the patient improves. In the treatment of spasticity it is suggested that once the motor unit activity in the muscle at rest is under control, the physiotherapist stretches the muscle and the patient attempts to reduce the electrical activity in the muscle during various degrees and rates of stretch (Currier, 1988). Since the patient has to concentrate hard during all biofeedback treatments it is important to judge the length of time for which the patient can make the best effort. Overlong treatments may be unsuccessful and thus unrewarding and frustrating.

Other forms of biofeedback for control of activity

Posture control.   Monitors are worn which signal tilt away from the vertical. The inclination monitor is worn on the trunk and the head-position trainer is worn as a helmet. A trunk inclination monitor has also been used for the treatment of low back pain. Such a device, fitted with audio feedback, has been compared with the use of a corset to limit trunk flexion. A study involving a series of tasks (Haig *et al.*, 1991) found that biofeedback was more effective at preventing flexion than the corset.

Functional breathing disorder.   Biofeedback has been utilized in the treatment of patients with disorders such as hyperventilation or shallow breathing (Moon, 1981). A medical gas analyser (mass spectrometer) was used to measure the partial pressure of carbon dioxide in the expired air. The patient was shown how varying the respiration rate altered the amount of expired carbon dioxide and was encouraged to slow the rate in order to increase the carbon dioxide to bring it nearer to the normal level of 40 mm Hg. Others have used biofeedback in the teaching of diaphragmatic breathing (Johnston and Kyu-ha Lee, 1976).

Control of incontinence.   The pressure of balloon-like devices in the rectum can be measured and used for biofeedback treatment for the control of incontinence. As far as urinary incontinence is concerned the method was no more successful than simple bladder training (Marcer, 1986) or, probably, electrical stimulation of the perineal muscles. Vaginismus has been successfully treated with biofeedback.

Muscle training control.   Muscle-strengthening and endurance-training devices have electronic displays which indicate the strength or power developed which can, in a sense, act as biofeedback devices as the subject can exercise at a predetermined rate, for example at 50% of maximum, thus learning to maintain a particular training schedule.

Weight-bearing control.   The amount of weight taken through one foot can be monitored with a pressure-sensitive pad in the shoe. This is connected to a circuit and battery carried in a small box (some are about 40 by 80 mm) which is attached either to the leg or at the waist. The circuit generates an audible signal when a pre-set pressure is reached. This can be used to encourage weight-bearing with, for example, hemiplegic patients (Triptree and Harrison, 1980) or in training patients in partial weight-bearing. In the former case the sound occurs when the patient takes sufficient weight and the sensitivity of the device can be decreased as he or she improves. In the latter the signal is set to sound when too much weight is taken on the leg (see Betts and Watson, 1992). In both cases the patient is receiving feedback to show how to modify the activity, in this case walking. The pad can also be used to re-educate sitting or kneeling posture or the proportion of weight taken through the heel compared to that through the forefoot.

Joint angle control.   The use of a monitor which gave an audible signal when knee hyperextension first occurred in patients with hemiplegia was investigated by Morris *et al.* (1991). The pitch of the signal increased with greater angles of hyperextension. It was found that the use of this device significantly enhanced the effect of treatment. Feedback of the knee angle during gait has also been used (Olney *et al.*, 1989).

Balance control.   Standing balance training using a force plate connected to a visual display has been reported as a successful approach to improving control of postural sway in hemiplegic patients (Shumway-Cook *et al.*, 1988; Winstein, 1989).

Movement practice. Feedback through computer-generated displays has been developed using a number of sensing devices such as pressure pads and switches. These can be arranged in various ways to encourage the repeated practice of a particular movement, for example a switch operated by extension of the wrist. Since the output can be linked to available computer games, such systems may be especially useful in the treatment of children with movement disorders (see Hartveld *et al.*, 1996).

Summary

Forms of non-electromyographic feedback for the control of:

- posture
- functional breathing disorders
- incontinence
- muscle training
- weight-bearing
- joint angles
- balance
- practising movement.

Biofeedback for the treatment of stress-related conditions

In these conditions some form of relaxation is found to be beneficial and biofeedback may well provide the means and motivation for the continued practice of relaxation. The electrical resistance of the hands can be measured and displayed visually or as an audible signal. Increased or decreased stress is reflected in the amount of sweating that occurs, which in turn determines the skin resistance. Such devices have been recommended and used for teaching relaxation. Conversely, as a means of measuring stress, they form the basis of one form of 'lie-detector'.

Essential hypertension. The blood pressure is monitored and displayed to the patient who ultimately learns some voluntary control. Harvey (1978) reports that subjects can learn to reduce blood pressure by anything up to 35 mm Hg.

Cardiac arrhythmias. The heart rate is monitored and displayed to the patient who can learn to gain some control mainly by slowing the heart rate. Schwartz (1977) suggests that it can be more helpful to train patients to reduce heart rate and blood pressure simultaneously.

Raynaud's disease. Biofeedback is appropriate for idiopathic Raynaud's disease, not the disorder due to arterial disease or vibration trauma. The temperature of the fingers is monitored using a suitable skin thermometer and the patient attempts voluntarily to increase the temperature, as described later.

Migraine.   Hand-warming has also been used for the treatment of migraine with some success but with much less obvious connection (Marcer, 1986).

Tension headache.   Relaxation of the occipitofrontalis muscle and posterior neck muscles is taught with biofeedback displaying the EMGs of these muscles. This has been a widely used treatment based on the hypothesis that tension in these muscles is the cause of the headaches. Chronic pain associated with muscle tension at other sites, notably chronic back pain, has also been treated with biofeedback.

Epilepsy.   Sterman *et al.* (1974) discovered it was possible for patients to reduce the frequency of epileptic fits by producing a special rhythm in the electroencephalogram – the sensory motor rhythm.

Technique of application of temperature biofeedback

Although the instruments monitoring blood pressure or heart rate will differ from the thermometer measuring skin temperature the principles of application are the same. The physiotherapist first explains the rationale of the biofeedback treatment emphasizing its harmless and painless nature. It should also be stressed that it may take some time, perhaps several sessions, to achieve control. The patient is supported in a comfortable sitting or half-lying position in a room which remains at a comfortable constant temperature and where interruptions will not occur. The thermistor is attached to the skin of any fingertip (the middle finger of the dominant hand is recommended) with sticky tape. After a few seconds the reading on the thermometer is taken and recorded as the baseline. The patient is then asked to close the eyes, relax, and imagine circumstances in which his or her hands and fingers are being warmed. Various situations can be suggested to the patient, such as holding the hands in front of a warm fire or washing them in warm water. It is often helpful to ask the patient to repeat phrases such as: 'I feel relaxed and my hands are getting warmer'. The thermometer reading should be recorded every 30 s and the attention of the patient drawn to any slight temperature increase (Fig. 5.1).

Once the patient is accustomed to the treatment he or she is encouraged to watch the thermometer. The physiotherapist must ensure that relaxation is maintained with the patient's eyes open. The kind of imagery that is used will clearly depend on social, geographical and cultural factors.

In the early stages, short, 10 min or so, treatment sessions are advised. Once control is achieved, longer sessions may be used. At first, the 30 s temperature record can show the small amounts of successful warming as it occurs. With successful control only the initial and final temperatures are noted and the frequency of treatment is reduced. The patient is encouraged to practise hand warming at home, especially in situations in which digital

---

Practical point
It may be helpful to warm the opposite hand with hot water or an infrared lamp to provide the patient with a warm sensation to aim for, but it must be remembered that this will lead to some reflex heating of the treated hand which may be mistaken for voluntary control.

vasospasm may occur. Some patients with Raynaud's disease (and some migraine sufferers) have a marked reduction in the number of their attacks. Others have less or only short-lived relief.

Mechanisms of biofeedback

It is sometimes considered that biofeedback works by making the patient aware of his or her own sensations when the dysfunction occurs, e.g. the spasticity, and then consciously preventing it from occurring. Thus, once learned, control can be maintained. In many patients, however, control is gradually lost when the immediate feedback is stopped. It has been suggested by Colgan (1980) that EMG biofeedback works by operant (behavioural) conditioning because it has been found that the motor response can be conditioned without awareness on the part of the patient. In order to maintain control the feedback must be withdrawn from some of the trials so that the patient gradually learns the response with progressively fewer feedback reinforcements; this is called generalization training.

It is also considered that feedback should be proportional to the response. Thus a strong muscle contraction should produce a strong signal. Further, visual signals such as a digital meter are better than auditory feedback because direct comparisons can be made from one trial to another. Colgan (1980) also pointed out that direct sensory information from the muscle is needed for control and without it, it seems unlikely that significant therapeutic benefits can occur. This conforms with the successful effects of muscle practice and artificial stimulation considered below.

EFFECTIVENESS OF BIOFEEDBACK

The division of biofeedback strategies into those associated with control of the autonomic system and those concerned with control of movement has been deliberately followed in the belief that the mechanisms and pathways of the central nervous system involved in control are different. It must be recognized, however, that there is no evident difference in success between these two groups.

Many conditions associated with autonomic control have been found to benefit from relaxation training; indeed several exponents have combined biofeedback and relaxation training and found this to be the most successful treatment. It is arguable that biofeedback acts in the same way in all these conditions by encouraging and rewarding relaxation (see Marcer, 1986 for discussion).

In all studies the successful outcomes occur in some, but not all, patients treated and the success that does occur is often modest. This happens in most therapeutic situations and is quite appropriate. It only needs to be noted to counter previously made claims that biofeedback was a universally successful, powerful panacea for all problems. It has been pointed out that biofeedback has been largely reported as an independent therapy, but that it is more beneficial as an integrated part of an appropriate treatment programme (Wolf,

1987). What is, perhaps, different and important about biofeedback is that it sets out to teach patients control of their own body, be it movement control or autonomic, thus giving long-term benefits in both psychological and economic terms. A recent careful meta-analysis of 8 selected separate studies using electromyographic biofeedback in the treatment of hemiplegic patients (Schleenbaker and Mainous, 1993) concluded that it was an effective therapy and should be included in the therapeutic regimen of these patients. This analysis used statistical techniques to compare and combine the degree to which biofeedback altered function (the effect size) in the different studies. The average effect size was relatively large at 0.81 (0.5 is usually considered to be of practical importance) and this result was highly significant ($p > 0.00001$).

EVALUATION OF EMG BIOFEEDBACK FOR MUSCLE CONTROL

Using EMG, subjects can be taught to contract a single motor unit and to control the rate of firing of that unit at will (Basmajian, 1963). The subject is only consciously aware of this contraction through the feedback of the oscilloscope and loudspeaker. Single motor units can be identified because each causes a single spike potential. Almost all normal subjects are able to control a single motor unit and many can control two or more (Basmajian, 1974). With practice some especially able subjects can apparently follow complex rhythms with the firing of a single motor unit and even, amazingly, continue to control the unit from memory, with no visual or audible feedback.

Superficially EMG biofeedback would seem appropriate as a means of training skilled muscle action since activity in the desired muscle can be quantified. Two points must be recognized in this connection: first, it is not easy to be certain that the EMG signals are arising entirely in the muscle intended unless intramuscular electrodes are used. Second, training in skilled repetitive movements involves inhibition of unwanted activity in antagonistic muscles (Basmajian *et al.*, 1975), thus it is more a matter of decreasing unwanted muscular contractions than increasing the activity. It is reasonable to suppose that what applied to training in normal healthy neuromuscular systems would also apply to re-education of the damaged systems.

Control of abduction of the great toe was used to compare the effectiveness of EMG biofeedback with other methods of training normal subjects (Middaugh, 1978). The range of voluntary abduction of the hallux was measured and four different treatment groups arranged, each of 10 subjects:

- EMG feedback
- manually applied sensory stimulation and practised muscle contractions
- unassisted practised muscle contractions
- no activity, control group.

Table 5.1 Range of motion of abduction before and after electrical stimulation and practice ($n = 102$)

	Pretest		Post-test	
	Left toe	*Right toe*	*Left toe*	*Right toe*
Mean	8.67°	8.98°	10.35°	11.05°
Range	0–20°	0–17°	0–22°	0–24°
Standard deviation		3.98°		4.12°

All of these, including the control group, had an increased range of voluntary abduction when a post-treatment measurement was made. The mean initial range of movement in this study was 7° with considerable differences between subjects (1–14°). This conforms with data collected by one of us (JL), using the same method of measurement in 102 young adults. After the pretest the abductor hallucis was electrically stimulated and voluntary abduction attempted. The post-test measurement was made one week later without further training.

As shown, in Table 5.1 the average range of right, big toe abduction increased by 2° (about 22%) and this difference is statistically (*t*-test) highly significant ($p > 0.001$). It is, however, largely accounted for by those subjects who had the least movement initially, which again conforms with the results of Middaugh (1978). This is hardly surprising since training would not be expected to increase an already large range of movement.

Thus it seems that movement control can be developed by voluntary practice, sensory stimulation, electrical muscle stimulation and biofeedback, all of which provide conscious proprioceptive feedback (feeling the toe move) and visual feedback (seeing it move), but the biofeedback adds further information of muscle contraction.

As well as evaluating the range of movement Middaugh also measured the EMG activity in the muscle and was thus able to monitor changes in total muscle activity. From this, it was concluded that EMG biofeedback was very effective in increasing the electrical response (muscle activity) in subjects who had little ability to use the abductor hallucis initially, i.e. those who had a poor range of movement on the pretest. However as training for a relatively brief contraction, such as that needed to measure the range of movement, EMG biofeedback was no better than unassisted practice of the contraction. In those subjects who had considerable control already, i.e. those with a good range of movement on the pretest, unassisted practice was most effective; in fact it was suggested that EMG biofeedback may interfere with training in this group.

It is suggested that EMG biofeedback is likely to be most effective when feedback from other sources is at a minimum, which would accord with these results. If there was little or no movement to start with there will be little feedback either from the joint or from seeing the toe move so any additional feedback helps. A sustained muscle contraction leads to less sensory feedback than brief (phasic) movement so that EMG biofeedback is an effective teaching method for a sustained contraction. On the other hand, when good movement already exists feedback can add little, so voluntary practice works better.

The therapeutic implications of this would seem to be that EMG biofeedback is a valuable additional method of movement training for those situations in which other feedback is lacking – in many neurological conditions, some hemiplegic patients and recovering nerve lesions. If normal sources of feedback are present EMG seems to have no advantage.

REFERENCES

Basmajian J. V. (1963). Control and training of individual motor units. *Science*, **141**, 440–1.

Basmajian J. V. (1974). *Muscles Alive: Their Function Revealed by Electromyography*, 3rd edn. Baltimore: Williams and Wilkins.

Basmajian J. V. (1981). Biofeedback in rehabilitation: a review of principles and practices. *Arch. Phys. Med Rehabil.*, **62**, 469–74.

Basmajian J. V., Kukulka C. G., Narayan M. G., Takebe K. (1975). Biofeedback treatment of foot-drop after stroke compared with standard rehabilitation technique effects on voluntary control and strength. *Arch. Phys. Med. Rehabil.*, **56**, 231–6.

Betts R. P., Watson A. G. (1992). Leg load monitor for rehabilitation. *Physiotherapy*, **78**, 172–3.

Colgan M. (1980). Biofeedback treatment of neuro-muscular dysfunction. *N.Z. J. Physiother.*, **8**, 12–15.

Currier D. P. (1988). Nerve and muscle stimulating currents – biofeedback. In *Physical Agents for Physical Therapists* (Griffin J. E., Karselis T. C., eds) Springfield, Illinois: Charles C. Thomas, pp. 132–166.

De Weerdt W., Harrison M. A. (1986). Electromyographic feedback for stroke patients: some practical considerations. *Physiotherapy*, **72**, 106–8.

Haig A. J., Grobler L. J., Pope M. *et al.* (1991). The relative effectiveness of lumbosacral corset and trunk inclination audio biofeedback on trunk flexion. *Eur. J. Phys. Med. Rehabil.*, **2**, 29–37.

Hartveld A., Hegarty J. R., Burton A. W. (1996). Tools to give computer feedback to movement. *Physiotherapy*, **82**, 509–13.

Harvey P. G. (1978). Biofeedback – trick or treatment? *Physiotherapy*, **64**, 333–5.

Hurrell M. (1980). Electromyographic feedback in rehabilitation. *Physiotherapy*, **66**, 293–8.

Johnston R., Kyu-ha Lee (1976). Myofeedback: a new method of teaching breathing exercises in emphysematous patients. *Phys. Ther.*, **56**, 826–9.

Klose K. J., Needham B. M., Schmidt D. *et al.* (1993). An assessment of the contribution of electromyographic feedback as an adjunct therapy in the physical training of spinal cord injured persons. *Arch. Phys. Med. Rehabil.*, **74**, 453–6.

Knight S. J., Laycock J. (1994). The role of biofeedback in pelvic floor re-education. *Physiotheraphy*, **80**, 145–8.

Marcer D. (1986). *Biofeedback and Related Therapies in Clinical Practice*. London: Croom Helm.

Middaugh S. J. (1978). EMG feedback as a muscle re-education technique. *Phys. Ther.*, **58**, 15–22.

Moon M. H. (1980). The therapist and EMG: biofeedback training for spasmodic torticollis. *N.Z. J. Physiother.*, **8**, 21–4.

Moon M. H. (1981). Biofeedback using a respiratory parameter in the treatment of behavioural breathing disorders. *N.Z. J. Physiother.*, **9**, 19–20.

Morris M. E., Matyas T. A., Bach T. *et al.* (1991). The effect of electromyographic feedback on knee hyperextension following stroke. *WCPT 11th International Congress Proceedings, Book I,* London: World Conference for Physical Therapy, 469–71.

Olney S. J., Colborne G. R., Martin C. S. (1989). Joint angle feedback and biomechanical gait analysis in stroke patients: a case report. *Phys. Ther.,* **69,** 863–70.

Ross B. R., Nedzelski J. M., McLean J. A. (1991). Efficacy of feedback training in long-standing facial nerve paresis. *WCPT 11th International Congress Proceedings, Book II,* London: World Confederation for Physical Therapy, 1034–36.

Schleenbaker R. E., Mainous A. G. (1993). Electromyographic biofeedback for neuromuscular re-education in the hemiplegic stroke patient: a meta-analysis. *Arch. Phys. Med. Rehabil.,* **74,** 1301–4.

Schwartz G. E. (1977). Biofeedback and the self-management of disregulation disorders. In *Behavioural Self-management* (Stuart R. B., ed.) New York: Brunner/Mazel.

Shumway-Cook A., Anson D., Haller S. (1988). Postural sway biofeedback: its effects on re-establishing stance stability in hemiplegic patients. *Arch. Phys. Med. Rehabil.,* **69,** 395–400.

Sterman M. B., MacDonald L. R., Stone R. K. (1974). Biofeedback training of the sensorimotor electroencephalogram rhythm in man: effects on epilepsy. *Epilepsia,* **15,** 393–416.

Triptree V. J., Harrison M. A. (1980). The use of sensor pads in the treatment of adult hemiplegia. *Physiotherapy,* **66,** 299.

Wiener N. (1948). *Cybernetics or Control and Communication in the Animal and the Machine.* New York: Wiley.

Winstein C. J. (1989). Standing balance training: effects on balance and locomotion in hemiplegic adults. *Arch. Phys. Med. Rehabil.,* **70,** 755–62.

Wolf S. L. (1987). Electromyographic biofeedback: an overview. In *Clinical Electrotherapy* (Nelson R. M., Currier D. P., eds) Norwalk, Connecticut: Appleton and Lange, pp. 259–78.

6 Therapeutic ultrasound

Ultrasound is not strictly electrotherapy because it is mechanical vibration, albeit produced electrically. It has sometimes been described as micro-massage.

This chapter deals first with the nature and, briefly, the production of ultrasound. Attention is given to the important matter of the way in which a beam of sonic energy behaves in the tissues. The physiological and therapeutic effects of this therapy are considered and some uses, including phonophoresis, discussed. The principles of application are described and this is followed by a description of the appropriate dosage parameters.

The chapter concludes with some discussion on the possible dangers and contraindications.

Ultrasound refers to mechanical vibrations which are essentially the same as sound waves but of a higher frequency. Such waves are beyond the range of human hearing and can therefore also be called ultrasonic. Vibration merges with sound at frequencies around 20 Hz; vibration below this frequency is often called infrasound or infrasonic. The upper limit of frequency for human hearing, and hence the range of frequencies defined as sound, varies considerably. It is higher in children and lower in old age; it is about 16–20 kHz. Most of the frequencies involved in speech and music lie in the range of 30 to 4000 Hz. Ultrasonic energy or ultrasound describes any vibration at a frequency above the sound range but it is frequencies of a few megahertz that are typically used in physiotherapy: several different frequencies are employed in the range from 0.5 to 5 MHz (Table 6.1). The terms 'sonic' and 'sound' are often used interchangeably, a course followed here, but strictly sound refers to audible frequencies.

THE NATURE OF SONIC WAVES

Sonic waves are a series of mechanical compressions and rarefactions in the direction of travel of the wave, hence they are called longitudinal waves (Fig. 6.1). They can occur in solids, liquids and gases and are due to regular compression and separation of molecules. (In solids, but not fluids, transverse waves can also occur; ter Haar, 1987.) The passage of these waves of compression through

Table 6.1 Frequency and wavelength of ultrasound at 1500 m/s

Frequency (MHz)	Wavelength (mm)	Period (μs)
0.5	3.0	2
0.75	2.0	1.33
0.87	1.724	1.15
1.0	1.5	1
1.5	1.0	0.66
2.0	0.75	0.5
3.0	0.5	0.35
5.0	0.3	0.2

matter is, of course, invisible because it is the molecules that vibrate about their average position as a result of the sonic wave. It is important to understand that it is energy that travels as the wave, not matter: this is true of any waves, not just sonic waves.

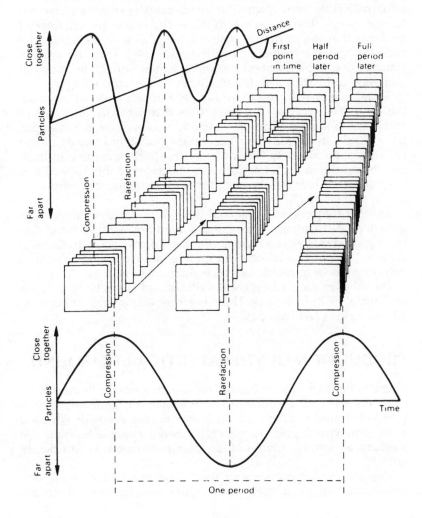

Fig. 6.1 Longitudinal wave.

As sound waves pass through any material their energy is dissipated or attenuated. Sometimes all the energy is absorbed at once; sometimes the sound wave passes with almost no loss. The molecules of all matter are in constant random motion; the amount of molecular agitation is what is measured as heat – the greater the molecular movement, the greater the heat (see Chapter 7). This motion is oscillatory, for instance the whole molecule may move or rotate to and fro, or it may change shape in an oscillatory way and this may occur at many different frequencies.

As the molecules jostle one another energy will be transferred from one to another so that some will oscillate at higher frequencies and with greater amplitude because they have gained energy while others will be at lower frequencies and amplitudes because their energy has been transferred by collision. When sonic vibration is applied to a material it is superimposed on the existing motions and will add to them. The ultimate result is that the regular sonic wave energy tends to become randomized as the energy it gives to particular molecular motions becomes spread out in collisions with other molecules. In this way the sonic energy is steadily converted to heat energy. The rate at which this exchange occurs will depend on both the nature of the material, i.e. the way the molecules oscillate, and the frequency of the sonic wave. Thus the ratio of transmission to absorption of sonic waves differs in different materials and varies with the frequency of the sonic energy.

Sound waves will pass more rapidly through material in which the molecules are close together, thus their velocity is higher in solids and liquids than in gases. Sound waves in air, for example, have a velocity of 343 m/s. The velocity of sound waves in salt water is approximately 1500 m/s and is almost the same in most soft tissues. From the relationship, as described in the Appendix, it is simple to deduce the wavelengths of those frequencies employed in physiotherapy (Table 6.1).

At other frequencies ultrasound is used for various purposes. In industry low-frequency ultrasound is used for many cleaning and mixing processes since efficient vibration of very small particles is achieved. It can also be used for cutting and engraving as well as detecting cracks in metal such as welding defects.

The other major medical uses of ultrasound are in body imaging and dental drills/descalers. These latter usually operate at between 20 and 60 kHz (Williams, 1987).

PRODUCTION OF THERAPEUTIC ULTRASOUND

There is no difficulty in producing low-frequency ultrasound by means of mechanical vibration, an extension of the familiar ways in which sound is produced, such as vibrating reeds or whistles. With somewhat higher frequencies it is not possible to make the mechanical part, or column of air, change its direction sufficiently quickly.

Piezoelectrical transducers are used to achieve the high-frequency ultrasound energy needed for imaging and therapy. These are suitably cut crystals which change shape under the influence of an electric charge.

Many types of crystal can be used but the most favoured are quartz, which occurs naturally, and some synthetic ceramic materials such as barium titanate and lead zirconate titanate (PZT). The crystal must be cut to suitable dimensions – the most important being thickness – so that it will resonate at the chosen frequency and so achieve maximum vibration. In order to apply the electric charges, metal electrodes must be fixed to the crystal. If a suitable metal plate is fixed to one surface of the crystal while the opposite surface is in air, then almost all the vibrational energy is transmitted from the crystal to the plate and thence to any solid or liquid to which it is applied. This is the treatment head which is used to transmit sonic energy to the tissues.

The other essential parts of a therapeutic ultrasound generator are a circuit to produce oscillating voltages to drive the transducer and a controlling circuit, which can turn the oscillator on and off to give a pulsed output.

A suitable circuit can maintain a constantly oscillating electric charge to cause the piezoelectric crystal to change shape at the same frequency and so drive the metal plate backwards and forwards also at the same high frequency, producing a train of sonic compression waves in any medium with which it is in contact.

A suitable resistance circuit is provided to control the amplitude of the electrical oscillations which in turn controls the magnitude of the mechanical vibration of the crystal and hence the amplitude of the sonic wave. This amplitude is referred to as the intensity and is the energy crossing unit area in unit time perpendicular to the sonic beam. It is therefore measured in watts per square centimetre (i.e. joules per sec per cm^2).

Current supplied to the oscillator circuit can be automatically switched on and off to produce a pulsed output, typically giving ratios of 1:1 or 1:4.

A meter is often included which measures the electrical oscillations applied to the crystal but not the vibration of the crystal. The International Electronic Commission (1984) has postulated that acoustic output power, the effective intensity in the transducer and the maximum temporal intensity may fluctuate $\pm 30\%$ from values indicated. Guirro *et al.* (1997) found that in one centre almost all the equipment tested fell outside these specifications independent of age and usage of machines. This conforms with findings of Pye (1996). He stressed the need for careful, documented testing of ultrasound equipment when new and at every stage of its lifetime.

TRANSMISSION OF SONIC WAVES

The metal plate of the treatment head moves backwards and forwards to generate a stream of compression waves that forms the sonic beam. Due to the fact that the wavelength of these waves is much smaller than the transducer face, the sonic beam is roughly cylindrical and of the same diameter as the transducer (Williams,

1987). Even the smallest therapeutic transducers are 2 or 3 cm across and, as can be seen from Table 6.1, wavelengths are only a few millimetres. (For audible sound with wavelengths much larger than the source producing them – about 1.34 m for middle C – the sound waves spread out in all directions so that sound can be heard equally well at all places equidistant from the source.)

This beam of ultrasound emitted from the transducer is by no means uniform even in a homogeneous medium. The beam non-uniformity ratio (BNR) is the ratio between peak intensity and average intensity in the beam. The lower the BNR the more uniform the beam. Waves emitted from the different places on the face of the transducer will travel to the same point in space in front of the transducer face by different paths and hence arrive out of phase. Some waves cancel out, others reinforce so that the net result is a very irregular pattern of sonic waves in the region close to the transducer face, called the near field or Fresnel zone. In the region beyond this, the far field or Fraunhofer zone, the sonic field spreads out somewhat and becomes much more regular because the differing path lengths from points on the transducer become insignificant at greater distances. The length of the near field will depend:

- directly on the square of the radius of the transducer face
- inversely on the wavelength. Thus:

$$\text{Length of Fresnel zone} = r^2/\lambda$$

e.g. a 3 cm diameter transducer working at 1 MHz in water, or soft tissues, would have a near field stretching 15 cm from the treatment head: $r = 15$ mm, $r^2 = 225$, $\lambda = 1.5$ mm (Table 6.1)

$$\frac{225}{1.5} = 150\,\text{mm} = 15\,\text{cm}$$

Table 6.2 shows other examples.

Table 6.2 Length of near (Fresnel) zone in cm for different sized transducers at various frequencies

Transducer size		Frequency (MHz)			
Diameter (cm)	*Radius (cm)*	*0.75*	*1*	*1.5*	*3*
2	1	5 cm	6.7 cm	10 cm	20 cm
3	1.5	11.25 cm	15 cm	22.5 cm	45 cm
5	2.5	31.25 cm	41.16 cm	62.5 cm	125 cm

As can be seen, for all practical purposes therapeutic ultrasound utilizes the near field and hence is irregular. There is relatively more energy on average, carried in the central part of the cross-section of the beam.

These irregularities are illustrated in Figures 6.2 and 6.3. It will be evident that the intensity of such fields cannot be expressed in a simple way because it varies from place to place in the ultrasonic beam. Thus the spatial *peak* intensity or the spatial *average* intensity may be specified – see Figure 6.4.

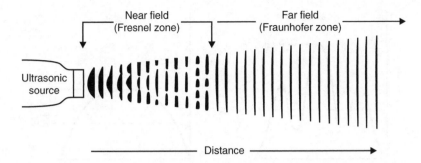

Fig. 6.2 The irregular intensity of an ultrasonic beam in the near field becoming more regular in the far field.

Further, if the output is pulsed the intensity over time varies so it can either be expressed as temporal average or temporal peak. Thus the intensity can be described in four ways: spatial average temporal average (SATA), spatial peak temporal average (SPTA), spatial peak temporal peak (SPTP) or spatial average temporal peak (SATP). It is usual for spatial average to be given, but it is important

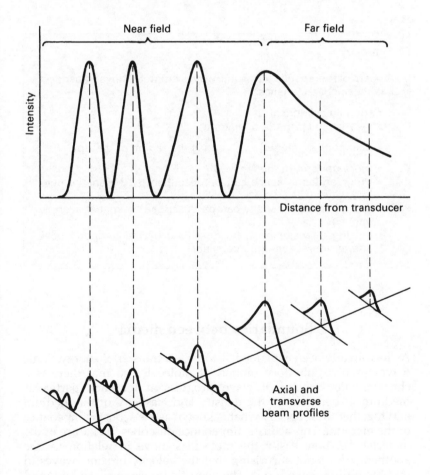

Fig. 6.3 Axial and transverse beam – spatial variation.

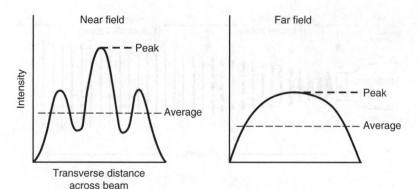

Fig. 6.4 Transverse profile of ultrasound beam – spatial variation.

to ascertain whether the meter is displaying temporal average or temporal peak intensity. This irregularity can be 'ironed out' to some extent by continuous movement of the treatment head during therapy.

Summary

A beam of therapeutic ultrasonic waves emitted from a transducer has these characteristics

- roughly cylindrical
- very irregular in the near zone
- near zone is defined by $\dfrac{r^2}{\lambda}$ and is the region of therapy
- more uniform in the far field
- irregularities in space can be described by the spatial peak intensity
- overall spatial intensity can be described by spatial average intensity
- pulsing intensities can be described by the temporal peak and temporal average intensities.

Boundaries between media

As has already been explained, a wave is a transfer of energy. Sonic waves involve vibratory motion of molecules so that there is a characteristic velocity of wave progression for each particular medium. It depends on the density and elasticity of the medium and together these specify what is known as the acoustic impedance of the medium. This acoustic impedance describes the nature of the material, i.e. how easily the molecules move in relation to one another, so it is not surprising that the velocity of sonic waves in that medium is linked to it. The acoustic impedance can be found by multiplying the density of a medium by the velocity of sonic waves through it.

The energy carried by a wave also depends on its frequency (the higher the frequency, the greater the energy) and its amplitude (the larger the amplitude, the greater the energy). Most of us have experienced this when standing in the sea; the higher and more frequent the waves, the harder it is to keep on our feet!

When sonic waves come to a boundary, various changes occur:

- They must travel in the new medium at a velocity characteristic for that medium and related to its acoustic impedance.
- The frequency remains the same, so the wavelength must change.
- Some of the energy is reflected back. The amount of energy reflected is proportional to the difference in acoustic impedance between the two media. Thus water and glass have rather different acoustic impedances so that over 63% of the original sonic energy is reflected at this interface. Water and soft tissue, on the other hand, have very similar impedance so that only 0.2% is reflected (Williams, 1987). This applies to waves that strike boundaries at right angles.
- If the wave front strikes the boundary at some other angle the reflected wave will travel away from the boundary at the same angle; that is, the angle of incidence of a beam equals the angle of reflection and is in the same plane (see Fig. 11.3).
- If some energy is reflected back, but the frequency remains the same, there must be a decrease in amplitude of the wave.
- Refraction also occurs with sonic waves due to the difference in acoustic impedance. The beam of sonic energy that passes through the second medium does not continue in a straight line but changes direction at the boundary because of the different velocities in the two media. If the boundary between air and water is considered, a sonic wave travelling in air at 343 m/s striking the water surface at an angle of incidence of about 10° would be refracted in water through an angle of about 50° (Fig. 11.3). If the acoustic impedances are closely matched little refraction will occur.
- The turning back of a wave in the same medium has a further consequence. Two waves, the original and the reflected, are travelling in opposite directions so that at some points they will be combined, producing a much greater amplitude and hence wave energy, and at other points they will cancel one another out. This tends to produce a stationary wave pattern, logically called a standing wave. Such waves are certainly generated in the tissues by therapeutic ultrasound and may have significant consequences.

It can be seen that the transmission of ultrasound through differing media, like the tissues, with many boundaries, or interfaces as they are often called, can alter the direction and intensity of the beam by reflection, refraction and the formation of standing waves. For a particularly clear and detailed description of these concepts see Ward (1986).

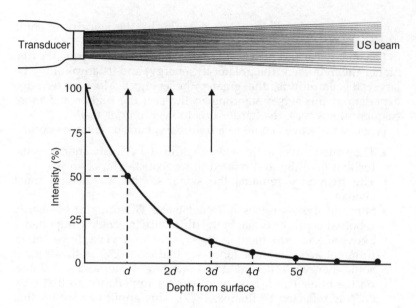

Fig. 6.5 The exponential decrease in ultrasound energy with depth.

Absorption of sonic waves in a parallel beam

It has been seen already that ultrasound will increase the motion of molecules causing more molecular vibration and molecular collisions, resulting in heat. Thus kinetic energy is converted to heat energy as it passes through the material. The energy will decrease exponentially with distance from the source in an homogenous material because a proportion of it is absorbed at each unit distance so that the remaining amount will become a smaller and smaller percentage of the initial energy (see Figs 6.5 and 11.5). There is an inverse relationship between the amount of energy that penetrates a material and the amount that is absorbed. Thus if a beam of ultrasound is passed through the tissues it will be steadily reduced in intensity in the manner shown in Figure 6.5. This can be expressed as the absorption coefficient.

Half-value depth.   There is no depth at which all the energy has been absorbed so it is usual to specify a half-value depth, that is, the depth or distance at which half the initial energy has been absorbed. The half-value depth can be used to describe the exponential curve of energy transmitted against distance penetrated, and is analogous to the half-life of radioactive material. (cf. penetration depth, Chapter 11.)

Since the conversion of sonic energy to heat is due to increased molecular motion it follows that the amount converted will depend on the nature of those molecules and on the frequency/wavelength of the ultrasound. Thus the half-value depth will be different in different tissues for any given ultrasound frequency (Table 6.3). It will be seen that the values given vary considerably, and any value estimated for living tissue has the added uncertainty of differing thickness of each kind of tissue. Wadsworth and Chanmugan (1980)

Table 6.3 (a) Half-value depth of penetration in mm for 1 MHz. (b) Half-value depth of penetration in mm for 3 MHz

Tissue	ter Haar (1978, 1996)	Hoogland (1986)	Ward (1986)	McDiarmid and Burns (1987)
(a)				
Skin	40	11.1	—	—
Fat	50	50	153	48
Muscle	10–20	9 (24.6)*	28	9
Tendon	—	6.2	—	—
Cartilage	—	6	—	—
Bone	15	2.1	0.4	—
(b)				
Skin	25	4	—	—
Fat	16	16.5	26.4	16
Muscle	30–60	3 (8)*	7.7	3
Tendon	—	2	—	—
Cartilage	—	2	—	—
Bone	5	—	0.04	—

* In line of muscle fibres (not the usual direction of clinical application).

give 65 and 30 mm for 1 and 3 MHz, respectively, as an approximate average.

It will be seen in Table 6.4 that absorption of sonic energy is greatest in tissues with the largest amounts of structural protein and lowest water content. Thus tissues can be listed in order of increasing absorption of sonic energy (Frizzel and Dunn, 1982).

Table 6.4 Protein content and absorption of ultrasound in various tissues

Blood	Least protein content	Least absorption of US
Fat		
Nerve		
Muscle		
Skin		
Tendon		
Cartilage		
Bone	Greatest protein content	Greatest absorption of US

Attenuation of ultrasound in the tissues

The loss of energy from the ultrasound beam in the tissues is called attenuation and depends on both absorption and scattering:

- Absorption accounts for some 60–80% of the energy lost from the beam (ter Haar, 1996). Of course, the scattered energy may also be absorbed other than in the region to which the ultrasound beam is applied.
- Scattering is caused by reflections and refractions which occur at interfaces throughout the tissues. This is particularly apparent where there is a large difference in acoustic impedance, e.g. between soft tissue and bone.

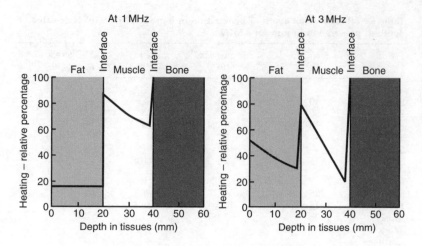

Fig. 6.6 Proportional heating of 1 and 3 MHz ultrasound through tissues. Continuous line represents the heating pattern predicted for a three-layer model of fat–muscle–bone as a percentage of the maximum – the muscle/bone interface. Modified from Ward (1986).

- Shear waves can also be formed (Williams, 1987) which transmit energy along the periosteal surface at right angles to the ultrasound beam. Due to the fact that this reflection is quite large (25%; Ward, 1986) and that sonic energy is absorbed almost immediately in bone, there is marked heating at the bone surface (Fig. 6.6). This mechanism is considered to account for the periosteal pain that can arise with excessive doses of therapeutic ultrasound. Differences of acoustic impedance between other soft tissues are much smaller.

Summary

Attenuation of the ultrasonic beam depends on:

- absorption – which itself depends on:
  - nature of the tissue (protein and water content)
  - frequency/wavelength of ultrasound
- scattering – which itself is due to:
  - reflection at interfaces
  - refraction at interfaces.

Heating in the tissues due to ultrasound

Calculations of the relative rate of heating for a fat–muscle–bone system have been made (Ward, 1986) and these are shown in Figure 6.6. The important factor is the rate of tissue heating which is influenced both by the blood flow, which constantly carries heat away, and by heat conduction. Both of these will reduce the peaks and troughs of the heating rate predicted on absorption and reflection characteristics. In highly vascular tissues such as muscle it is likely that heat would be rapidly dissipated preventing any large temperature rise; on the other hand, less vascular tissue, such as dense connective tissue in the form of tendon or ligament, may experience a relatively greater temperature rise.

It was noted earlier that moving the transducer head during treatment was important to smooth out the irregularities of the near field. It will also reduce some of the irregularities of absorption that might occur due to reflection at interfaces, standing waves, refraction, differences in tissue thermal conduction or blood flow. Thus the resulting heating pattern is likely to be much more evenly distributed than that indicated in Figure 6.6.

It has been estimated that for an output of $1\,\text{W/cm}^2$ there is a temperature rise of $0.8°\text{C/min}$ if vascular cooling effects are ignored (ter Haar, 1987).

Pulsed ultrasound

A circuit in the ultrasonic generator is arranged to turn the ultrasound on in short bursts or pulses. This reduces the time averaged intensity and hence the amount of energy available to heat the tissues while ensuring that the energy available in each pulse (pulse averaged intensity) is high enough for mechanical rather than thermal effects to predominate (see also discussion, Chapter 10).

Many therapeutic ultrasound generators produce 2 ms pulses and vary the intervals between pulses. This can be expressed either as:

- the mark:space ratio, which is the ratio of the pulse length to the interval
- the duty cycle, which is the ratio of the pulse length to the total length of pulse plus interval, expressed as a percentage. Thus:

Pulse	Interval	Mark:space ratio	Ratio of pulse to total period	Duty cycle
2 ms	2 ms	1:1	1 in 2	50%
2 ms	8 ms	1:4	1 in 5	20%

Some ultrasound machines are produced that give a 12.5 ms pulse at a frequency of 16 pulses/s, hence a duty cycle of 20%. Sixteen hertz is thought to be a fundamental frequency of the intracellular calcium system and is therefore claimed to be more effective.

Effects of pulsing

If pulsed ultrasound is applied at a mark:space ratio of 1:4 the amount of introduced energy is one-fifth of that which would be introduced by continuous ultrasound applied for the same length of time and at the same intensity. The same amount of energy could be introduced into the tissues either by extending the treatment for five times the length of time or giving five times the intensity of the continuous treatment. Yet the effect is not the same because with pulsed treatment there is time for the heat to be dissipated by conduction in the tissues and in the circulating blood. Therefore, higher intensities can be safely used in a pulsed treatment because the average heating is reduced.

Ultrasound application can increase rates of ion diffusion across cell membranes (Dyson, 1985); this could be due to increased particle movement on either side of the membrane and, possibly, increased motion of the phospholipids and proteins that form the membrane. It is possible that mild mechanical agitation of the tissues has certain effects which remain the same no matter how long the agitation is continued but that short bursts of more vigorous agitation have different, more significant effects.

PHYSICAL AND PHYSIOLOGICAL EFFECTS

The result of absorption of ultrasound in the tissues, as has already been discussed, is the oscillation of particles about their mean position. This oscillation, or sonic energy, is converted into heat energy which is proportional to the intensity of the ultrasound. If all this heat is not dissipated by the normal physiological means a local rise in temperature will occur and thermal effects will result. If heat dissipation equals heat generation there is no net rise in temperature and any effects are said to be non-thermal. Non-thermal effects are achieved by using low intensities or pulsing the output.

Thermal effects

If local temperature is raised to between 40 and 45°C hyperaemia will result (Lehmann and Guy, 1972). Temperatures above 45°C are destructive. To achieve a useful therapeutic effect the tissue temperature has to be maintained between these values for at least 5 min (Lehmann and deLateur, 1982). Heating fibrous tissue structures such as joint capsules, ligaments, tendons and scar tissue may cause a temporary increase in their extensibility, and hence a decrease in joint stiffness. The advantage of using ultrasound to achieve this heating is due to the preferential heating of collagen tissue and to the effective penetration of this energy to deeply placed structures. However, ultrasound-absorbing structures can prevent the treatment reaching deeply placed target tissues if they intervene in the path of the sonic beam (Dyson, 1987). Mild heating can also have the effect of reducing pain and muscle spasm and promoting healing processes. Kramer (1987), investigating the increase in conduction velocity in motor and sensory nerves following therapeutic ultrasound, concluded that this was likely to be related to the heating effect of ultrasound.

Non-thermal effects

Cavitation

Cavitation is the formation of tiny gas bubbles in the tissues as a result of ultrasound vibration. These bubbles, generally of a micron (10^{-6} m) or so in diameter (ter Haar, 1987), although they can grow much larger under some circumstances, are of two kinds – stable or transient cavitation.

Stable cavitation occurs when the bubbles oscillate to and fro within the ultrasound pressure waves but remain intact.

Transient (or collapse) cavitation occurs when the volume of the bubble changes rapidly and then collapses (implodes) causing high pressure and temperature changes and resulting in gross damage to tissues.

The former kind, associated with acoustic streaming, is considered to have therapeutic value (see below) but the latter, which is only likely to occur at high intensities, can be damaging. Cavitation can be easily demonstrated experimentally and it has now been established that it occurs in the tissues as a result of ultrasound therapy (ter Haar and Daniels, 1981). Pulsing reduces the risk of damage due to cavitation.

Acoustic streaming

This is a steady circulatory flow due to radiation torque. Additionally, as a result of either type of cavitation there is a localized, unidirectional fluid movement around the vibrating bubble. These very small fluid movements also occur around cells, tissue fibres and other boundaries. The effect, called microstreaming, exerts viscous stress on the cell membrane and thus may increase membrane permeability. This may alter the rate of ion diffusion causing therapeutically useful changes. These include increased secretion from mast cells (Fyfe and Chahl, 1982), increased calcium uptake (Mortimer and Dyson, 1988) and greater growth factor production by macrophages (Young and Dyson, 1990).

Standing waves

Standing waves have already been described as being due to reflected waves being superimposed on the incident waves. The result is a set of standing or stationary waves with peaks of high pressure (antinodes), half a wavelength apart, between which are zones of no pressure (nodes). This pressure pattern has been shown to cause stasis of cells in blood vessels at the pressure nodes (Dyson and Pond, 1973). The endothelium of the blood vessels exposed to standing waves can also be damaged leading to thrombus formation (Dyson *et al.*, 1974). There is also the possibility of marked local heating where the amplitude of the combined waves is high. It must be realized that if the transducer is moved during treatment standing waves are unlikely to form.

Micromassage

The waves of compression and rarefaction may produce a form of micromassage which could reduce oedema (Summer and Patrick, 1964).

Summary

Effects of ultrasound on the tissues:

- thermal
- non-thermal:
  - cavitation
  - acoustic streaming
  - standing waves
  - micromassage.

Therapeutic mechanisms

There have been two schools of thought which have developed historically concerning the therapeutic mechanisms of ultrasound. One considers heating to be the only effect. This view is found in much of the American writing on the subject. High doses are recommended and little value is seen in low-intensity and pulsed treatments. The term 'ultrasonic diathermy' is often used and emphasizes the heating effect. The other school of thought, largely European, is more concerned with low-intensity treatments causing mechanical or biological effects and with pulsed treatments. These different views and their historical development are well described by Fyfe and Bullock (1985).

It is evident that many uncertainties remain concerning ultrasound. The part played by heat versus the mechanical effects, ignorance of the distribution of ultrasonic energy in the tissues and inaccurate calibration of ultrasound machines are all areas in which little is known. A lack of clinical research also contributes (Partridge, 1987).

Effects of ultrasound on inflammation and repair processes

The inflammation and repair that occur after tissue injury have been described in Chapter 1 and reference should be made to that section.

Acute stage

The effects of stable cavitation and acoustic streaming appear to increase calcium ion diffusion across the cell membrane. This is of great importance since calcium, as a cellular 'second messenger', can have a marked effect in increasing the production and release of wound-healing factors. These include the release of histamine from mast cells and, importantly, factors released from macrophages (Young and Dyson, 1990). In this way, ultrasound has the potential to accelerate normal resolution of inflammation providing that the inflammatory stimulus is removed (Dyson, 1987). This acceleration could also be due to the gentle agitation of the tissue fluid which may increase the rate of phagocytosis and the movement of particles and cells (Evans, 1980). It should be noted that ultrasound has a pro-inflammatory, not an anti-inflammatory action. Increased local blood flow is sometimes claimed as a result of therapeutic ultrasound. However, Rubin *et al.* (1990) noted that the acute effect of ultrasound is to vasoconstrict the small arterioles to a point that local decreases in blood flow occur.

Proliferative (granulation) stage

This begins approximately 3 days after injury and is the stage at which the connective tissue framework is laid down by fibroblasts for the new blood vessels. During repair, fibroblasts may be stimulated to produce more collagen; it has been shown that ultrasound can promote collagen synthesis (Harvey *et al.*, 1975). This is thought to be due to increased cell membrane permeability, caused by ultrasound, allowing the entry of calcium ions which control cellular activity (Dyson, 1987). Not only is more collagen formed but it is also of greater tensile strength after ultrasound treatment.

Ultrasound is also believed to encourage the growth of new capillaries in chronic ischaemic tissue and the same could happen during repair of soft tissues after injury (Dyson, 1987). The enhanced release of growth factors from macrophages following exposure to therapeutic ultrasound has also been observed (Young, 1988). This may well account for the proliferation of fibroblasts that occurs due to therapeutic levels of ultrasound, since there appears to be no direct stimulatory effect on fibroblast cells.

In a review paper, Maxwell (1992) noted that ultrasound can generate free radicals which, if excessive, could be harmful. She concludes that ultrasound may potentiate or inhibit inflammation, and that the timing of therapy may be critical. In this context, Dyson (1989) suggests that ultrasound treatment given during the first 2 weeks after injury accelerates bony union, but, if given to an unstable fracture during the phase of cartilage formation, it may result in the proliferation of the cartilage and consequently delay bony union.

Remodelling stage

This stage can last months or years until the new tissue is as near in structure as possible to the original tissue. Ultrasound is considered to improve the extensibility of mature collagen such as is found in scar tissue (Lehmann and deLateur, 1982). This is believed to occur by promoting the reorientation of the fibres (remodelling) which leads to greater elasticity without loss of strength. These beneficial changes appear to occur most evidently when treatment is started in the inflammatory stage.

There are several studies on animals that show that ultrasound at therapeutic intensities facilitates wound healing. While some studies are inconsistent and have not clarified the mode of action of ultrasound, one well-executed study on pigs (Byl *et al.*, 1992) found that ultrasound significantly increased the strength and rate of closure of the wound. Although the visual quality of the wounds was unaffected, there was higher degranulation of mast cells on the treated side. These results occurred in the first week of treatment and the collagenous changes were quantified, being around 25% greater than the controls.

Similarly, in a study on rates of wound contraction in rats, Hart and Dyson (1991) found that both 0.1 and 0.5 W/cm² 5-min applications of 3 MHz ultrasound given daily, caused significantly greater wound contraction than occurred in the sham-treated controls. The treatment was applied for 5 days, but wound measurements continued for 11 days.

For an authoritative account of the influence of ultrasound on tissue healing, particularly the '*in vitro*' effects, see Young (1996).

DISCUSSION OF THERAPEUTIC USES

Therapeutic ultrasound has been applied to an enormous range of conditions with claims of successful outcomes. These include acute and subacute traumatic and inflammatory conditions, chronic rheumatoid and arthritic conditions, scar and excessive fibrous tissue and for pain relief.

Reviews. The efficacy of these treatments is still a matter of uncertainty, even after 50 years of widespread clinical use and numerous reported trials. Several reviews of such trials reflect this uncertainty, are critical of the methodology of much of the published research and call for further studies. Of these, Holmes and Rudland (1991) considered 18 papers relating to acute soft tissue injury of which the only three they considered to be methodologically satisfactory reached different conclusions. Schlapbach (1991) reviewed nine trials involving musculoskeletal disorders noting that many questions remain to be answered. This latter review considered ultrasound to be effective for the treatment of lateral humoral epicondylitis based on a careful study by Binder *et al.* (1985). Holdsworth and Anderson (1993) also concluded that ultrasound does bring about a favourable response in the majority of patients with this condition – see also Lundeberg *et al.* (1988), Haber and Lundeberg (1991) and Pienimäki *et al.* (1996) for other views. Kitchen and Partridge (1990) likewise noted a lack of well controlled replicable clinical trials to test the effects of ultrasound in a wide-ranging review. Partridge (1987) reached similar conclusions and McDiarmid and Burns (1987) concluded that 'in seeking scientific evidence to verify the benefits of ultrasound or to decide on the optimum treatment parameters, physiotherapists are confronted with inadequate and often confusing evidence'.

Varicose ulcers. A number of controlled trials have demonstrated the effectiveness of ultrasound therapy to promote the healing of varicose ulcers (Dyson and Suckling, 1978; Roche and West, 1984; Callam *et al.*, 1987) and pressure sores (McDiarmid *et al.*, 1985).

Pain relief. There have also been favourable reports of pain relief for herpes zoster (Garrett and Garrett, 1982; Jones, 1984; Payne, 1984). Patrick (1978) suggested its use for low back pain and Nwuga (1983) for prolapsed intervertebral discs.

Acute tissue injury. Benefit has been found after dental surgery (El Hag *et al.*, 1985), in soft tissue and sports injuries (Dyson, 1989), in occupational injuries (Middlemast and Chatterjee, 1978) and post-natally (Ferguson, 1981; McLaren, 1984). However, subsequent larger controlled trials (Grant *et al.*, 1989; Everett *et al.*, 1992) on the value of ultrasound for perineal post-natal pain, were unable to demonstrate a clear, overall significant benefit beyond the placebo effect (see also Hay Smith and Reed, 1997). Everett *et al.* did, though, find the treated group had significantly greater improvement in certain of the pain/discomfort measurements.
Munting (1978) reported improvement for painful shoulders but Downing and Weinstein (1986) subsequently found little benefit.

Scar tissue. Improvements in the quality of scar and excessive fibrous tissue have been reported by Patrick (1978), in Dupuytren's contracture by Markham and Wood (1980), in painful, indurated episiotomy scars by Fieldhouse (1979) and in plantar fasciitis by Clarke and Stenner (1976).

Blood flow. In an investigation of the effect of continuous ultrasound on blood flow (Robinson and Buono, 1995), a dose of $1.5 \, \text{W/cm}^2$ for 5 min applied to the forearm did not alter the skeletal muscle blood flow.

Bone injury. Ultrasound therapy in the first 2 weeks after bony injury can increase bony union, but, given to an unstable fracture during the phase of cartilage proliferation, it may result in the proliferation of cartilage and therefore decrease bony union (Dyson, 1989).
Ultrasound has also been used in the early diagnosis of stress fractures. A moderate dose applied over the site of the fracture leads to immediate pain, whereas the same applied to the opposite side has no effect. Thus ultrasound can identify stress fractures but has no place in their treatment (Lowden 1986).

Trials. This paucity of controlled trials of ultrasound is a little surprising in view of the fact that it is relatively easy to arrange a double-blind trial, since the patient is unaware of any sensation at

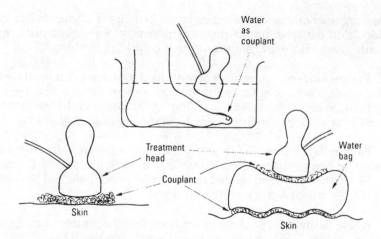

Fig. 6.7 Direct contact, immersion and water bag applications.

normal therapeutic intensities and the functioning of the machine can easily be concealed from the physiotherapist. An interesting point in this connection is that these and other studies assume that benefits due to sham treatment with an inactive treatment head are a placebo effect (e.g. Hashish *et al.*, 1986). It is possible that the local gentle massage due to the movement of the transducer over the skin has some direct beneficial effect, which is a point noted by Schlapbach (1991).

Summary

The principal therapeutic uses of ultrasound include promoting the:
- healing of chronic ulcers
- healing of acute soft tissue injuries
- relief of both neurogenic and chronic pain
- improvement of scar tissue.

Diagnostically it may be used to:
- identify stress fractures.

PRINCIPLES OF APPLICATION

Couplant.   Adequate transmission of ultrasonic energy to the tissues depends on having a couplant that provides a good match of acoustic impedance between the metal of the transducer head and the skin. There is virtually no transmission of ultrasound from the transducer to air; the energy being reflected causes heating of, and possibly damage to, the transducer itself. Water is a good couplant (see below) but has to be held in place between the treatment head and the tissues in some way. It is therefore made into a gel, held in a plastic or rubber bag or the whole body part is immersed in water with the treatment head (Figure 6.7). All three methods are in use but the first, called the direct contact method, is most commonly found.

Continuous movement of treatment head.   With all methods it is important to move the treatment head continuously relative to the tissues for the following reasons:

- the ultrasound beam is very irregular in the near zone
- the pattern of energy absorption in the tissues is very irregular due to reflection and refraction
- standing waves can be formed that might lead to temporary stasis of circulating blood cells and to endothelial damage
- at high intensities unstable cavitation or excess heating could occur causing tissue damage.

Steady movement of the treatment head will even out the dose delivered to the target tissues and will eliminate the risks of damage due to local high-intensity 'hot spots'. If the patient complains of any increased pain or discomfort during treatment, it should be terminated.

Direct contact application

Thixotropic substances are gels that become fluid on vibration and thus make ideal couplants for ultrasound. Various agents of high molecular weight may be added to water to form a suitable gel provided they are non-irritant to the tissues and not corrosive to the metal of the treatment head. While tests have shown differences in the ability of different gels to transmit ultrasound (Docker and Patrick, 1982), most of the commercial gels are acceptable. KY gel has the advantage of very high viscosity and is available in sterile form. Creams, which are emulsions of light oils in water, are also widely used. Requirements for the couplant are that it has:

- an acoustic impedance similar to the tissues
- high transmissivity for ultrasound
- high viscosity
- low suspectibility to bubble formation
- a chemically inactive nature
- a hypoallergenic character
- relative sterility.

Other desirable features are that it is cheap, can be hygienically and conveniently applied and is transparent. The couplant also serves the important purpose of acting as a lubricant to allow the treatment head to move smoothly over the skin.

Transmission of ultrasound is sometimes expressed as a percentage relative to that of water, which is taken to be 100% (see Table 6.6). Tap water has been shown to be a satisfactory couplant for ultrasound, being significantly better than mineral oil or glycerin (Griffin, 1980). Although all studies do not agree on the superiority of water (Reid and Cummings, 1977) the differences are small and it is safe, cheap and convenient. However, Ward and Robertson (1996) found that large corrections to the intensity output are required to compensate when using ultrasound in water at different applicator to skin distances. They suggest for a 1 cm distance increase by 30%, for 2 cm 55% and for 3 cm 80%.

Technique

Preparation of patient.

Explanation: The nature of the treatment, need for a couplant and stability of the area are all explained to the patient. The duration of the treatment as well as any particular co-operation required is indicated.

Examination and testing. The skin surface to be treated should be inspected; inflammatory skin conditions should be avoided.

Preparation and testing of apparatus. Prior to any treatment it is sensible to check that there is an output from the machine. This can be done by placing the treatment head just below the water surface in a suitable container and observing the disturbance which appears in the water. This, and similar methods, only indicate the presence of an output but to quantify it a radiation balance should be used regularly. Many surveys of ultrasound equipment over the years have shown that between 60 and 90% do not meet the appropriate national standard for output power (see earlier). Assessing the output by measuring the temperature rise in a standard volume of water has also been suggested, and shown to be a simple and reliable method (Pye *et al.*, 1994).

Preparation of part to be treated. The couplant should be applied to the skin surface.

Setting up. The physiotherapist should be comfortably seated with arm supported as skill is needed to apply efficient ultrasound, ensuring close contact, appropriate movement and correct angle of the transducer at all times.

The treatment head is placed on the skin before the output is turned on. This is to avoid damage to the transducer which can occur if the energy is reflected back into the transducer at its interface with air. Some machines have a monitoring system. If the ultrasound energy reaching the tissues becomes much less than the set intensity, the output is greatly reduced, the timer stops, and the operator is alerted in some way.

Instructions and warnings. The patient is asked to keep the part to be treated still and relaxed and to report any increase of pain or other sensations immediately.

Application. The treatment head is moved continuously over the surface while even pressure is maintained in order to iron out the irregularities in the sonic field. The emitting surface must be

---

Practical point
It is helpful if the position of the patient can be arranged so that the treatment head is applied downwards and moved horizontally as the weight of the treatment head contributes to the pressure, making it easier for the physiotherapist to control it. Furthermore, the couplant is more easily kept in place as it does not tend to move downwards away from the area.

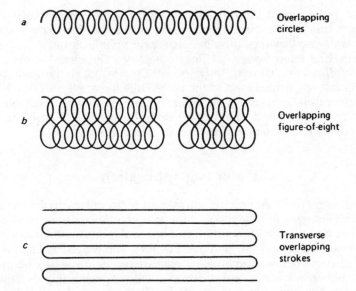

a   Overlapping
circles

b   Overlapping
figure-of-eight

c   Transverse
overlapping
strokes

Fig. 6.8 Patterns of movement of the ultrasonic transducer on the skin surface.

kept parallel to the skin surface to reduce reflection and pressed sufficiently firmly to exclude any air. The rate of movement must be slow enough to allow the tissues to deform and thus remain in complete contact with the rigid treatment head but fast enough to prevent 'hot spots' developing when using a higher-intensity treatment. The pattern of movement can be a series of overlapping parallel strokes, circles or figures-of-eight (see Fig. 6.8).

Termination.   The intensity is returned to zero, either manually or automatically, before the transducer is removed from the water bath or tissue contact. The skin is cleaned of couplant or dried. The transducer should also be cleaned after each use with a non-corrosive, non-abrasive antiseptic solution.

Recording.   The following should be recorded: machine used, SATA or SATP intensity, frequency, pulse mode, insonation time, couplant, region and area of insonation and response to treatment.

Water bath application

When direct contact is not possible because of the irregular shape of the part, or because of tenderness, a water bath may be used. As the part to be treated is immersed in water this can only reasonably be applied to the hand, forearm, foot and ankle. Testing the output of the machine and inspection of the part to be treated precede treatment, as above. The patient is seated and the part is put in water of a comfortable temperature, in such a position that it is suitably supported. The treatment head is placed in the water and moved parallel to the surface of the part which is being treated and as close to the skin as possible. The treatment head and skin will need to be wiped periodically to remove air bubbles which will reflect much ultrasound. If degassed water, produced by boiling the water and then cooling it, is used, no bubbles form.

The Chartered Society of Physiotherapy's *Guidelines for the Safe Use of Ultrasound Therapy Equipment* (1990) state that, 'If the operator's hand has to be immersed in the bath while the applicator is active, care should be taken to minimize exposure to any reflected or scattered ultrasound; this can be done by wearing a dry knitted glove inside a waterproof rubber or plastic glove'.

Water bag application

Another method of applying ultrasound to irregular surfaces which cannot conveniently be placed in a water bath is to use a plastic or rubber bag filled with water, forming a water cushion between the treatment head and the skin (see Fig. 6.7). The water bag can be an ordinary rubber balloon but condoms are more satisfactory because the rubber is thinner and of better quality. Special devices which perform the same function are made. The bag should be filled with warm water, degassed if possible. All visible air bubbles should be squeezed out before knotting the neck of the bag to seal it. Couplant is smeared onto the surface of the bag, skin and treatment head. The bag is then held in place over the irregular surface to be treated; this takes a separate pair of hands, which can be the patient's in some circumstances. The treatment head is then pressed firmly onto the bag so that a layer of water about 1 cm thick separates it from the surface. Inevitably some bubbles will form and it is important to ensure that these are in the sides of the bag and not in the region transmitting the ultrasound. The treatment head is then moved mainly by deforming the bag although it can also be moved over the surface of the bag. It is likely that there will be increased energy losses at the many interfaces but as there seems to be no information on their magnitude it is suggested that the output intensity should be increased by perhaps 50% over what would be appropriate for a direct contact treatment.

Solid sterile gel as couplant

Ultrasound treatment cannot conveniently be given over open wounds or injured skin because there is a risk of transmitting infection and the moving treatment head may cause further damage. To solve these problems a polyacrylamide agar gel in a 3.3 mm sheet can be used as a couplant. In a hydrated form this material is sold in sterile packs and is used for wound dressings and over skin grafts. It is 96% water but impermeable to bacteria, and is conveniently transparent.

The flexible sheet, cut to an appropriate size, is placed over the open wound with a little sterile saline to ensure that there are no air bubbles between the gel sheet and the raw surface. The slightly wetted outside surface of the gel sheet will allow the treatment

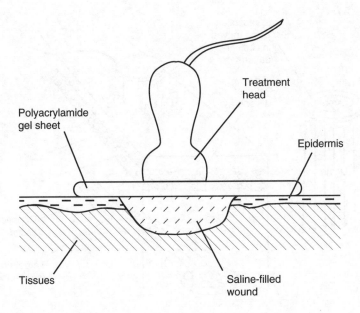

Polyacrylamide
gel sheet

Treatment
head

Epidermis

Tissues

Saline-filled
wound

Fig. 6.9 The application of ultrasound to
an open wound by means of a gel sheet.

head to move smoothly over it. The gel has been found to transmit
95% of the applied ultrasound energy (Brueton and Campbell, 1987)
(see Fig. 6.9).

Polyurethane film dressings are used in the same way. These and
similar wound dressings available have high ultrasound transmissiveness compared to water (Pringle, 1995).

Summary

Therapeutic ultrasound may be applied to the tissues:

- by direct contact using coupling gel
- in a water bath
- through a water bag
- via a solid gel sheet.

DOSAGE

Three factors determine the ultrasound dosage (see Fig. 6.10):

- size of area to be treated
- depth of lesion from surface
- nature of lesion.

The parameters of ultrasound include:

- mode
- frequency

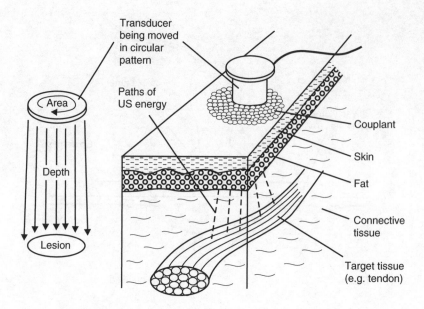

Fig. 6.10 The three determinants of ultrasound dosage: area, depth and nature of lesion.

- intensity
- duration of treatment.

As there is no certain way of knowing how much energy is absorbed in any particular tissue, decisions about dosage become a matter of judgement to some extent. This judgement must be based on the known factors governing ultrasound absorption. Any reference to dose should make clear whether the dosage is that applied at the surface or the estimated dose at the target tissue. These are not the same.

Mode – continuous or pulsed output

Continuous mode will produce some heat in the tissues if the intensity is great enough, whereas pulsed ultrasound at the same instantaneous intensity would have a much lower time-averaged intensity, and hence negligible heating (e.g. $0.5\,\mathrm{W/cm^2}$ pulsed at 1:4 will deliver the same energy as $0.1\,\mathrm{W/cm^2}$ on continuous mode). The difference lies between continuous small taps at a nail or a few stronger blows.

Continuous mode has been recommended for musculoskeletal disorders such as muscle spasm, joint stiffness or pain (Lehmann and de Lateur, 1982), whereas pulsed mode is preferred for soft tissue repair (Young, 1996).

Frequency

As attenuation increases with rising frequency effectively the lower frequencies penetrate further (Table 6.3). Thus much of the energy

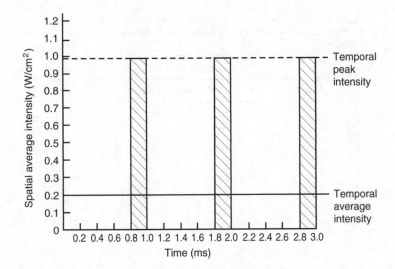

Fig. 6.11 The relationship between temporal peak and temporal averaged intensity for ultrasound SATP output of 1 W/cm², pulsed 2 ms on and 8 ms off. Thus, mark : space ratio 1 : 4 and duty cycle 20%.

carried in 3 MHz utrasound is absorbed in the superficial tissues whereas 0.75 MHz ultrasound will penetrate deeply through the tissue; that is it has a large half-value depth. While it makes sense to use higher-frequency ultrasound, such as 3 MHz, to treat superficial tissue it must be remembered that significant amounts of energy from lower-frequency therapeutic ultrasound are also absorbed by the superficial layers.

Intensity

Power, that is the total energy per second supplied by the machine, is measured in watts. Since this is spread over the whole face of the transducer, and transducers are of different sizes, it is more useful to give the intensity in W/cm². Most therapeutic sources emit up to a spatial average maximum of 2–3 W/cm².

It has already been explained that the ultrasound beam is very irregular so a useful measure is the average intensity of the peaks and troughs of the sonic field over a specific area, usually the transducer face; this is the space-averaged intensity. A pressure balance measures total power output from the transducer. A hydrophone scanning technique measures the beam profiles. From the total power output and the beam profile, the effective radiating area and the beam non-uniformity ratio (BNR) can be calculated. The lower the BNR, the less likely are high intensity peaks.

Time-averaged intensity is an important value in pulsed treatments. The intensity shown on the meter is usually the space-averaged temporal peak (SATP) intensity. During pulsed treatments the SATA intensity is obviously much lower; this may be indicated by the meter (see Fig. 6.11 and Table 6.5). It is worth noting that a SATP intensity of 2 W/cm² at a 1:4 pulse ratio is equivalent to a

Table 6.5 Examples of SATA outputs from an ultrasound source with a temporal peak display meter and maximum output of 3W/cm²

SATA intensity (W/cm²) at transducer face	Intensity shown on meter (W/cm²)		
	Continuous	Pulsed 1:1	Pulsed 1:4
0.1	0.1	0.2	0.5
0.2	0.2	0.4	1.0
0.3	0.3	0.6	1.5
0.4	0.4	0.8	2.0
0.5	0.5	1.0	2.5
0.75	0.75	1.5	—
1.0	1.0	2.0	—
1.5	1.5	3.0	—
3.0	3.0	—	—

SATA intensity (continuous mode) of 0.4 W/cm². Conversely, a SATA intensity of 0.1 W/cm² is equivalent to a SATP intensity at 1:4 pulse ratio of 0.5 W/cm².

It is reasonable to increase the intensity to compensate for losses due to absorption and scattering when treating more deeply placed targets. By estimating the depth of the target tissue from the surface and knowing the half-value depth, an appropriate intensity can be selected. For example, the intensity required to treat a lesion situated at the half-value depth of the ultrasound would be twice that needed for a similar surface lesion.

Any record of dosage should always make clear whether it is the surface intensity, as indicated by the meter or the intended estimated dose at the target. It is also essential to specify whether SATA or SATP intensity is being described and the duty cycle if pulsed.

When treating 'thin' areas, such as the hand, it may be necessary to reduce the surface intensity to allow for possible reflection of the ultrasound beam from the further skin–air interface.

The intensity applied should be in accordance with the nature of the lesion. For acute and immediately post-traumatic lesions surface intensities in the range of 0.1 to 0.25 W/cm² SATA, modulated to take account of depth of structure, may be appropriate. For chronic lesions and scar tissue, surface intensities in the region of 0.25 W/cm² up to 1 W/cm² SATA may be necessary. It must also be remembered that different tissues absorb ultrasound to different degrees according to their protein content (see p. 181), so that somewhat lower intensities may be used for densely collagenous targets.

Dyson (1987) states that intensities towards the upper end of the range available on most ultrasound machines are potentially damaging. The lowest intensity required to produce the desired therapeutic effect should therefore be used.

Duration of treatment

The amount of energy applied to the tissues and hence the effects will depend not only on the intensity but also on the length of time for which it has been applied. Quite short treatment times of a few minutes are usually considered to be sufficient. As the treatment head is moved continuously over the treated area the size of this area must be the most important determinant of the treatment time. There are differing opinions but a convenient guide is to give 1–2 min of treatment for every 10 cm^2 of surface covered (many transducer heads have an area of 5 cm^2 and the palm of a small hand is about 50 cm^2). Minimum treatment times are considered to be 1–2 min, maximum 10–15 min and an average would be in the region of 5 min. It is also suggested that chronic lesions benefit from longer treatment times.

The surface dosage chosen is inevitably a compromise. Some factors determine an increase, while others dictate a decrease in the parameters discussed above. Herein lies some of the skill in the successful application of ultrasound. In general, the smallest effective dose should be used.

Progression and timing

Recent injuries and acute conditions should be treated as soon as possible after the occurrence and thereafter once or twice daily. Chronic conditions may be treated on alternate days.

Progression is based on the outcome of previous treatment. If there is subjective and objective improvement the treatment should be continued at the same dose. If the symptoms are unpredictably worse the treatment should be reduced or discontinued. If there is no change when one would be expected the dose should be increased one parameter at a time until some change is apparent or until a number of applications have been tried without result, in which case the ultrasound should be discontinued.

Summary

Dosage parameters:

- mode – pulsing gives less power than continuous output
- frequency – lower frequency gives greater depth of penetration
- intensity – measured in W/cm^2 and usually as the SATP intensity
- time – duration of each treatment, in minutes, related to the size of area being treated
- treatment repetition – once or twice per day for acute lesions, less frequently for chronic.

POSSIBLE DANGERS

Apart from an instance of extreme abuse with self-administered treatment (Levenson and Weissberg, 1983) there seems to be no reported evidence of damage due directly to therapeutic ultrasound but it is reasonable to suppose that injury could occur under some conditions.

- burns could occur if the heat generated exceeded the physiological ability to dissipate it
- tissue destruction would result from transient cavitation
- blood cell stasis and endothelial damage may occur if there is standing wave formation.

These dangers would be more likely with high-intensity continuous output with a stationary head or over bony prominences. If the patient feels any pain, aching or prickling during the application the intensity should be reduced or the treatment terminated.

Extraneous radiation from the transducer into the physiotherapist's hand (maximum permissible value $100\,\text{mW/cm}^2$; International Electrotechnical Commission, 1984) is minimized by good design, the use of a glove as noted above and by holding the treatment head at a point furthest away from its transmitting surface.

CONTRAINDICATIONS

Rapidly dividing tissue

Since ultrasound has been shown to affect tissue repair it is possible that it could affect abnormal tissue activity so that it might encourage neoplastic growth and provoke metastases (Maxwell, 1995). Therefore, treatment over tumours or over tissue in precancerous states should be avoided.

Similarly, any risk to the rapidly dividing and differentiating cells of the embryo and fetus should be avoided by not applying treatment over the pregnant uterus. Diagnostic ultrasound is entirely safe and it is probable that low doses of therapeutic ultrasound would have no ill effects.

It may be wise to avoid the epiphyseal plates.

Spread of infection

It has been suggested that bacterial or viral infection could be spread by ultrasound, presumably by facilitating micro-organism movement across membranes and through the tissues. In spite of the lack of evidence this seems a reasonable supposition with respect to acute infections with marked inflammatory reactions, which should not be treated. The low-grade chronic infections of venous ulcers, or similar, would seem to be safe to treat.

Due to the possible risk of reactivating encapsulated lesions tuberculous regions should also not be treated.

Vascular problems

Circumstances in which haemorrhage might be provoked should not be treated – for example, where bleeding is still occurring or has only recently been controlled, such as an enlarging haemarthrosis or haematoma or uncontrollable haemophilia.

Severely ischaemic tissues should be avoided because of the poor heat transfer and possible greater risk of arterial thrombosis due to stasis and endothelial damage.

Treatment over recent venous thrombosis might extend the thrombus or disrupt its attachment to the vein wall forming an embolus. Areas of atherosclerosis are best avoided for the same reason.

Radiotherapy

Areas that have received radiotherapy in the last few months should not be treated because of the risk of encouraging pre-cancerous changes.

The nervous system

Normal doses of ultrasound have been applied for many years to the tissues around the spinal cord without any ill effects. In fact treatment of the spinal nerve roots and over the apophyseal joints is particularly common. Since the central nervous system is deeply buried beneath thick muscle and, more importantly, bone tissue it seems reasonable to suppose that only trivial amounts of energy could reach it. Where nerve tissue is exposed, e.g. over a spina bifida or after a laminectomy, ultrasound should be avoided. Statements are sometimes made to the effect that treatment over the cervical ganglia or vagus nerve might be dangerous in cardiac disease (Forster and Palastanga, 1985).

Specialized tissue

The fluid-filled eye offers exceptionally good ultrasound transmission and retinal damage could occur.

Treatment over the gonads is not recommended.

Implants

Although metal implants in the tissues would reflect the ultrasound at their interfaces and thus lead to more energy absorption in these areas, this does not lead to a large temperature rise in the region because the amount of heat generated is easily conducted by the metal to other cooler areas. Experiments with implanted metal in pigs showed no ill effects when ultrasound was applied (Lehmann and de Lateur, 1982). The effects might, however, be different with smaller and more superficial implants, like metal bone-fixing pins subcutaneously placed; as a precaution, low doses should be used in these circumstances.

Plastics used in replacement surgery, such as high-density polyethylene and acrylic, should also be avoided since their effect on ultrasound absorption is unknown (Lehmann and de Lateur, 1982).

Treatment over implanted cardiac pacemakers should not be given because the sonic vibration may interfere with the pacemaker's stimulating frequency. Additionally, the radio-frequency radiation emitted by an ultrasound therapy unit may disturb pacemakers.

Anaesthetic areas

There are some circumstances in which caution should be exercised. High doses should not be given over anaesthetic areas. It must be realized that the most common pain produced by high-intensity ultrasound is deep periosteal pain, probably due to the large amount of energy absorbed at the bone–tissue interface where there is not only reflection but shear waves may also occur, as explained earlier. Thus the cutaneous thermal sensation is of no consequence as regards protection, except where heating is occurring in or on the skin.

Summary of contraindications:

- malignant and precancerous tissue
- pregnant uterus
- gonads
- acute infections
- tissue at risk of haemorrhage
- severely ischaemic tissue
- recent venous thrombosis
- exposed nerve tissue
- the eye.

PHONOPHORESIS

Phonophoresis is the movement of drugs through skin into the subcutaneous tissues under the influence of ultrasound. Many drugs are absorbed through the skin only very slowly; high-frequency sonic vibration may accelerate this process. Such treatment has been in use since the early 1950s but not by many physiotherapists. It is also known as sonophoresis or ultrasonophoresis.

In Chapter 2 it was explained how iontophoresis achieved this same effect, that of driving drugs through the skin, by means of electrical forces. Phonophoresis relies on perturbation of the tissues causing more rapid particle movement and thus encouraging absorption of the drug. The effects of phonophoresis are those of the particular drug employed, combined with the effects of ultrasound. In studies on various musculoskeletal lesions it is difficult to separate these effects. For a review see Byl (1995).

Penetration of phonophoretically driven drugs

The depth to which drugs can be made to penetrate is a matter of particular uncertainty. As occurs with iontophoresis (see Chapter 2), once the drug has passed through the epidermis it is likely to be dispersed in the circulation to an extent which depends on the vascularity of the tissues concerned and the ease with which molecules of the drug can enter blood vessels. In any case dispersion will occur in the tissues. However, several studies quoted by Skauen and Zentner (1984) showed that cortisol could be driven into pig muscle and nerve by phonophoresis; further, the therapeutic effects reported by several studies, e.g. Kleinkort and Wood (1975, could only result if significant quantities of anti-inflammatory drug had penetrated to the affected tissue. In some of these studies ultrasonic frequencies rather lower than those customarily employed, 0.33 or 0.25 MHz, were found to be more effective. In fact, it has been concluded that lower frequencies lead to greater penetration (Skauen and Zentner, 1984).

It must be realized that deeper penetration does not necessarily infer greater effectiveness. If the therapeutic effects occur in the dermis and epidermis, such as the cutaneous anaesthetic effect of lignocaine, then it might be expected that higher frequencies would be a more effective delivery system since the ultrasound energy is largely absorbed in the superficial tissues. This has been shown to occur in that 1.5 and 3 MHz ultrasound appeared to be more effective in achieving absorption of local anaesthetic than 0.75 MHz (Benson *et al.*, 1988). Interestingly, this same study showed that pulsed was rather more effective than continuous ultrasound in achieving transfer of this particular cream. This provides evidence for a specific effect due to the pulsing of ultrasound.

Summary

In phonophoresis:

- ultrasound facilitates the passage of some drugs into and through the skin
- the effects are due both to absorption of the drug and to the ultrasound
- lower ultrasonic frequencies appear to lead to deeper drug penetration
- pulsing the ultrasound may lead to better drug penetration
- the quantity of drug entering the skin is proportional, in general, to the time and intensity of ultrasound application.

Drugs used in phonophoresis

The anti-inflammatory drug hydrocortisone has been widely used. High concentrations of the drug (Kleinkort and Wood, 1975, found 10% ointment more effective than 1%) can be driven through the skin with relatively high intensity ultrasound. Many inflammatory skin conditions have been treated with hydrocortisone. A pilot study comparing hydrocortisone phonophoresis with simple ultrasound (Holdsworth and Anderson, 1993) was unable to demonstrate a statistically significant difference between the treatments. In this study, all patients received ultrasonic treatment and the vast majority of acute lesions appear to have benefited. It is possible that ultrasound having a pro-inflammatory effect and steroids an anti-inflammatory effect are conflicting therapies.

Numerous other steroid-type drugs can be applied by phonophoresis as well as many non-steroidal anti-inflammatory drugs, mainly salicylates. An anti-inflammatory, analgesic cream (trolamine salicylate) has been recommended. A study to investigate the effectiveness of this agent on delayed onset muscle soreness in normal subjects (Ciccone *et al.*, 1991) found that ultrasound alone increased the symptoms, while ultrasound with trolamine salicylate had no such effect. It was concluded that the anti-inflammatory activity of this drug was able to offset the increased soreness due to the pro-inflammatory effect of ultrasound.

Phonophoresis of hydrocortisone has been used in the treatment of many skin conditions including psoriasis, scleroderma and pruritus. A lotion containing zinc oxide, tannic acid, urea and menthol has been applied by phonophoresis to treat herpes simplex virus type II in both oral and genital infections with good results (Fahim, 1980). Antibiotics such as penicillin have been given by phonophoresis for the treatment of skin infections.

Some suggested products appear not to be transmitted; e.g. Difflam Cream (benzydamine hydrochloride). This was tested in a double-blind controlled study (Benson *et al.*, 1989) in which the drug in a gel was recovered from the skin surface and measured; no significant difference was found between treatments with the ultrasound on and those with it off. As suggested above, if the base, cream or ointment in which the drug is dissolved is not a good ultrasonic transmitter then it seems unlikely that treatment would work effectively.

Cameron and Monroe (1992), while discussing the transmission of ultrasound through phonophoretic media, recommend a simple evaluation of transmission. Wide, sticky tape is fixed around the face of the transducer to produce a 1 cm well. The substance to be tested is placed on the transducer surface and the remainder of the well filled with water. If the medium transmits ultrasound, the water will be agitated at intensities of $1–2 \, W/cm^2$.

Application

The drug to be driven into the tissues is combined in a suitable gel or cream which forms the couplant. It is smeared onto the part,

Table 6.6 Transmission characteristics of various compounds

Product	Active ingredients	Transmission relative to water (%)		
		0.75 MHz	1.5 MHz	3 MHz
Steroids				
Cobadex cream	Hydrocortisone, dimethicone	55	67	75
Locoid lipocream	Hydrocortisone butyrate	38	61	71
Anti-inflammatory drugs				
Intralgin gel	Benzocaine salicylamide	87	11	120(sic)
Movelat cream	Corticosteroids, heparinoid, salicylic acid	33	48	69
Local anaesthetics				
Emla cream	Lignocaine, prilocaine	83	90	95
Xylocaine ointment	Lignocaine hydrochloride	2	2	0

From Benson and McElnay (1988).

using a spatula so that it is not applied to the physiotherapist's fingers. The treatment head is moved over the skin in the usual manner. Relatively high intensities of 1 and 1.5 W/cm^2 have been used. The depth of the target tissue determines the frequency used. The time of treatment depends on the area over which phonophoresis is to be applied; 1 min treatment for every 10 cm^2 area is reasonable, although Griffin *et al.* (1967) suggest 5 min for each 25 in^2, i.e. about 1 min for 30 cm^2. Most reported applications of phonophoresis have used continuous ultrasonic energy but Benson *et al.* (1988) used both continuous and pulsed energy to produce skin anaesthesia with Emla cream; the pulsed mode appeared to be more effective in these circumstances, as noted above.

When treatment is completed the remaining couplant, containing the drug, should be removed from both the patient's skin and the ultrasound transducer. It is essential to ensure complete removal from the treatment head since any drug remaining may be inadvertently and inappropriately applied to the next patient treated.

Since the cream or gel containing the drug is being used as the couplant it is important that it transmits ultrasound adequately. This has been considered by Benson and McElnay (1988; 1994), who investigated the transmission characteristics of a large number of different products and found wide variations. In general they found that gels were more efficient coupling agents than creams, particularly for higher (1.5 and 3 MHz) frequency ultrasound. Several were poor transmitters. Examples from these studies are given in Table 6.6, but for fuller information the original articles should be consulted.

Contraindications

The same considerations apply when giving phonophoresis as apply when giving ultrasound for its intrinsic effect (see p. 200). The effect of the drug must also be considered; for example, anti-inflammatory drugs may suppress necessary inflammatory reactions, such as local skin infections, allowing them to become more serious. If local skin-anaesthetizing drugs are being driven in by ultrasound it must be remembered that skin sensation under the treatment head will gradually be lost so that the patient may no longer detect excessive heat; high intensities should not therefore be used for these drugs.

LONGWAVE ULTRASOUND

This chapter has considered therapeutic ultrasound at megahertz frequencies, but there are machines with lower frequency outputs of 45 kHz. The wavelength of 3.3 cm is, therefore, some twenty times that of 1 MHz ultrasound, hence it is called 'longwave' ultrasound.

At this frequency the ultrasonic beam in the tissues would spread out very much more and be less rapidly attenuated than MHz frequency ultrasound. The consequence of this marked divergence and greater reflection from the irradiated surface is strong, superficial energy absorption and in spite of the greater penetration depth, consequent heating occurs in a few millimetres of tissue at the surface, like that due to infrared radiation or a hot pack (Robertson and Ward, 1997).

The particle displacement at 45 kHz is far greater than at 1 MHz at the same acoustic pressure and this is said to be one of the key issues in the effectiveness of longwave ultrasound (Dyson *et al.*, 1999).

Therapeutic benefit beyond that due to MHz ultrasound has been claimed for treatment with longwave ultrasound (Bradnock *et al.*, 1996), but the supporting study has been heavily criticized (Robertson and Ward, 1997).

ULTRASOUND IMAGING

Ultrasound is widely used in obstetrics to obtain foetal images. It is also used for tissue measurements, such as the cross-sectional area of the thigh musculature (Howe and Oldham, 1995). An important recent use is for the non-invasive investigation of changes in superficial wounds. This is a particularly elegant method of monitoring wound healing and holds the promise of valuable insights into tissue changes during healing. For further descriptions see Young (1996).

COMBINATION THERAPY

The application of two therapeutic modalities at the same time, and at the same site, is described as combination therapy. The most widely used combinations are those of ultrasound with some form of nerve and muscle stimulating current (e.g. ultrasound and interferential). This can be done because the ultrasonic transducer provides low-resistance electrical contact with the skin. It might be said that phonophoresis is a form of combination therapy, since it applies both ultrasound and drug therapy.

The production, application and therapeutic effects are those of the individual therapies as described in this text. The justification for the use of combination therapy is principally that the beneficial effects of both modalities may be achieved at the same time, thus making the therapy efficient, at least in terms of time committed by both therapist and patient. A second justification is that there may be an enhancing effect of one therapy upon the other, making the combination more effective than each therapy alone. While there is a paucity of evidence supporting the value of combination therapy, and indeed describing it, there have been several suggestions that different modalities of therapy, not necessarily applied at the same time, are more effective than a single therapy.

REFERENCES

Benson H. A. E., McElnay J. C. (1988). Transmission of ultrasound energy through pharmaceutical products. *Physiotherapy*, **74**, 587–9.

Benson H. A. E., McElnay J. C. (1994). Topical non-steroidal anti-inflammatory products as ultrasound couplants: their potential in phonophoresis. *Physiotherapy*, **80**, 74–6.

Benson H. A. E., McElnay J. C., Harland R. (1988). Phonophoresis of lignocaine and prilocaine from Emla cream. *Int. J. Pharm.*, **44**, 65–9.

Benson H. A. E., McElnay J. C., Harland D. R. (1989). Use of ultrasound to enhance percutaneous absorption of benzydamine. *Phys. Ther.*, **69**, 113–18.

Bierman W. (1954). Ultrasound in the treatment of scars. *Arch. Phys. Med. Rehabil.*, **35**, 209–13.

Binder A., Hodge G., Greenwood A. M. *et al.* (1985). Is therapeutic ultrasound effective in treating soft tissue lesions? *Br. Med J.*, **290**, 512–14.

Bradnock B., Law H. T., Roscoe K. (1996). A quantitative comparative assessment of the immediate response to high frequency ultrasound and low frequency ultrasound ('longwave therapy') in the treatment of acute ankle sprains. *Physiotherapy*, **81**, 78–84.

Brueton R. N., Campbell B. (1987). The use of Geliperm as a sterile coupling agent for therapeutic ultrasound. *Physiotherapy*, **73**, 653–4.

Byl N. N. (1995). The use of ultrasound as an enhancer for transcutaneous drug delivery: phonophoresis. *Phys. Ther.*, **75**, 539–53.

Byl N. N., McKenzie A. L., West J. M. *et al.* (1992). Low dose ultrasound effects on would healing: a controlled study with Yucatan pigs. *Arch. Phys. Med. Rehabil.*, **73**, 656–64.

Callam M. J., Harper D. R., Dale J. J. *et al.* (1987). A controlled trial of weekly ultrasound therapy in chronic leg ulceration. *Lancet*, **ii**, 204–6.

Cameron M. H., Monroe L. G. (1992). Relative transmission of ultrasound by media customarily used for phonophoresis. *Phys. Ther.*, **72**, 142–8.

Chartered Society of Physiotherapy. (1990). *Guidelines for the Safe Use of Ultrasound Therapy Equipment*. London: Chartered Society of Physiotherapy.

Ciccone C. D., Leggin B. G., Callamaro J. J. (1991). Effects of ultrasound and trolamine salicylate phonophoresis on delayed onset muscle soreness. *Phys. Ther.*, **71**, 666–75.

Clarke G. R., Stenner L. (1976). Use of therapeutic ultrasound. *Physiotherapy*, **62**, 185–90.

Docker M. F., Patrick M. K. (1982). Ultrasound couplants for physiotherapy. *Physiotherapy*, **68**, 124–5.

Downing D. S., Weinstein A. (1986). Ultrasound therapy of subacromial bursitis: a double-blind trial. *Phys. Ther.*, **66**, 194–9.

Dyson M. (1985). Therapeutic applications of ultrasound. In *Biological Effects of Ultrasound* (Nyborg W. L., Ziskin M. C., eds) London: Churchill Livingstone.

Dyson M. (1987). Mechanisms involved in therapeutic ultrasound. *Physiotherapy*, **73**, 116–20.

Dyson M. (1989). The use of ultrasound in sports physiotherapy. In *Sports Injuries (International Perspectives in Physiotherapy 4)* (Grisogono V., ed.) Edinburgh: Churchill Livingstone.

Dyson M., Pond J. B. (1970). The effect of pulsed ultrasound on tissue regeneration. *Physiotherapy*, **56**, 136–42.

Dyson M., Pond J. B. (1973). The effects of ultrasound on circulation. *Physiotherapy*, **59**, 284–7.

Dyson M., Pond J., Woodward B. *et al.* (1974). The production of blood cell stasis and endothelial cell damage in the blood vessels of chick embryos treated with ultrasound in a stationary wavefield. *Ultrasound Med. Biol.*, **1**, 133–48.

Dyson M., Preston R., Woledge R., Kitchen S. (1999). Longwave ultrasound. *Physiotherapy*, **85**, 40–49.

Dyson M., Suckling J. (1978). Stimulation of tissue repair by ultrasound: a survey of the mechanisms involved. *Physiotherapy*, **64**, 105–8.

El Hag M., Coghlan K., Christmas P. *et al.* (1985). The anti-inflammatory effects of dexamethasone and therapeutic ultrasound in oral surgery. *Br. J. Oral Maxillo. Surg.*, **23**, 17–23.

Evans P. (1980). The healing process at cellular level: a review. *Physiotherapy*, **66**, 256–9.

Everett T., McIntosh J., Grant A. (1992). Ultrasound therapy for persistent post-natal perineal pain and dyspareunia. *Physiotherapy*, **78**, 263–7.

Fahim M. (1980). New treatment for herpes simplex virus type 2. (Ultrasound and zinc, urea and tannic acid ointment.) Part II. Female patients. *J. Med.*, **11**, 143–67.

Ferguson H. N. (1981). Ultrasound in the treatment of surgical wounds. *Physiotherapy*, **67**, 12.

Fieldhouse C. (1979). Ultrasound for relief of painful episiotomy scars. *Physiotherapy*, **65**, 217.

Forster A., Palastanga N. (1985). *Clayton's Electrotherapy: Theory and Practice*. London: Baillière Tindall.

Frizzel L. A., Dunn F. (1982). Biophysics of ultrasound. In *Therapeutic Heat and Cold* (Lehmann J. F., ed.) Baltimore: Williams & Wilkins.

Fyfe M. C., Bullock M. I. (1985). Therapeutic ultrasound: some historical background and development in knowledge of its effects on healing. *Aust. J. Physiother.*, **31**, 220–4.

Fyfe M. C., Chahl I. A. (1982). Mast cell degradation: A possible mechanism of action of therapeutic ultrasound. *Ultrasound Med. Biol.* (Suppl. 1), 62.

Garrett A. S., Garrett M. (1982). Ultrasound for herpes zoster pain. *J. R. Coll. Gen. Pract.*, **32**, 709, 711.

Grant A., Sleep J., McIntosh J. *et al.* (1989). Ultrasound and pulsed electromagnetic energy treatment for perineal trauma. A randomized placebo-controlled trial. *Br. J. Obstet. Gynaecol.*, **96**, 434–9.

Griffin J. E. (1980). Transmissiveness of ultrasound through tap water, glycerin and mineral oil. *Phys. Ther.*, **60**, 1010–16.

Griffin J. E., Echternach J. L., Bowmaker K. L. (1970). Results of frequency differences in ultrasonic therapy. *Phys. Ther.*, **50**, 481–6.

Guirro R., Serrão F., Elias D., Bucalon A. J. (1997). Calibration of therapeutic ultrasound equipment. *Physiotherapy*, **83**, 419–32.

Haber E., Lundeberg T. (1991). Pulsed ultrasound treatment in lateral epicondylitis. *Scand. J. Rehab. Med.*, **23**, 115–18.

Hart J., Dyson M. (1991). The effect of therapeutic ultrasound on wound contraction. *WCPT 11th International Congress Proceedings, Book III*, London: World Confederation for Physical Therapy, p. 1391.

Harvey W., Dyson M., Pond J. B., Grahame R. (1975). The 'in vitro' stimulation of protein synthesis in human fibroblasts by therapeutic levels of ultrasound. *Proceedings of 2nd European Congress on Ultrasonics in Medicine*, pp. 10–21.

Hashish I., Harvey W., Harris M. (1986). Anti-inflammatory effects of ultrasound therapy: evidence for a major placebo effect. *Br. J. Rheumatol.*, **25**, 77–88.

Hay Smith E. J., Reed M. A. (1997). Physical agents for perineal pain following childbirth: a review of systematic reviews. *Phys. Ther. Rev.*, **2**, 115–21.

Holdsworth L. K., Anderson D. M. (1993). Effectiveness of ultrasound used with a hydrocortisone coupling medium or epicondylitis clasp to treat lateral epicondylitis: Pilot study. *Physiotherapy*, **79**, 19–24.

Holmes M. A. M., Rudland J. R. (1991). Clinical trials of ultrasound treatment in soft tissue injury: a review and critique. *Physiother. Theory Pract.*, **7**, 163–75.

Hoogland R. (1986). *Ultrasound Therapy*. Delft: Enraf Nonius.

Howe T. E., Oldham J. A. (1995). Reliability of measuring quadriceps cross-sectional area with compound B ultrasound scanning. Abstract from Physiotherapy Research Workshop at Manchester Royal Infirmary, Nov. 1994, *Physiotherapy*, **81**, 241.

International Electrotechnical Commission (1984). *Testing and Calibration of Ultrasound Therapeutic Equipment*. Geneva: Bureau Centrale de la Commission Electrotechnique Internationale.

Jones R. J. (1984). Treatment of acute herpes zoster using ultrasonic therapy. *Physiotherapy*, **70**, 94–6.

Kitchen S. S., Partridge C. J. (1990). A review of therapeutic ultrasound. *Physiotherapy*, **76**, 593–600.

Kleinkort J. R., Wood F. (1975). Phonophoresis with 1 per cent versus 10 per cent hydrocortisone. *Phys. Ther.*, **55**, 1320–4.

Kramer J. F. (1987). Sensory and motor nerve conduction velocities following therapeutic ultrasound. *Aust. J. Physiother.*, **64**, 1–9.

Lehmann J. F. (1965). Ultrasound therapy. In *Therapeutic Heat and Cold* (Licht S., ed.) pp. 321–86. Baltimore: Elizabeth Licht Publisher, Waverly Press Incorporated.

Lehmann J. F., de Lateur B. J. (1982). Therapeutic heat. In *Therapeutic Heat and Cold*, 3rd edn (Lehmann J. F., ed.) Baltimore: Williams & Wilkins.

Lehmann J. F., Guy A. W. (1972). Ultrasonic therapy in interaction of ultrasound and biological tissues. *Workshop Proceedings* (Reid J. M., Sikov M. R., eds). US Dept of Health Education and Welfare publication (FDA) 73, 73–8008, pp. 141–52.

Levenson J. L., Weissberg M. F. (1983). Ultrasound abuse: a case report. *Arch. Phys. Med. Rehabil.*, **64**, 90–91.

Lowden A. (1986). Application of ultrasound to assess stress fractures. *Physiotherapy*, **72**, 3, 160–1.

Lundeberg T., Abrahamsson P., Baker E. (1988). A comparative study of continuous ultrasound, placebo ultrasound and rest in epicondyalgia. *Scand. J. Rehabil. Med.*, **20**, 99–101.

Markham D. E., Wood M. R. (1980). Ultrasound for Dupuytren's contracture. *Physiotherapy*, **66**, 55–8.

Maxwell L. (1992). Therapeutic ultrasound: its effect on the cellular and molecular mechanisms of inflammation and repair. *Physiotherapy*, **78**, 421–6.

Maxwell L. (1995). Therapeutic ultrasound and tumour metastasis. *Physiotherapy*, **81**, 272–5.

McDiarmid T., Burns P. N. (1987). Clinical applications of therapeutic ultrasound. *Physiotherapy*, **73**, 155–62.

McDiarmid T., Burns P. N., Lewith G. T. *et al.* (1985). Ultrasound and the treatment of pressure sores. *Physiotherapy*, **71**, 66–70.

McLaren J. (1984). Randomised controlled trial of ultrasound therapy for the damaged perineum. *Clin. Phys. Physiol. Measure.*, **5**, 40.

Middlemast S. J., Chatterjee D. S. (1978). Comparison of ultrasound and thermography for soft tissue injuries. *Physiotherapy*, **64**, 331–2.

Mortimer A. J., Dyson M. (1988). The effect of therapeutic ultrasound on calcium uptake in fibrinoblasts. *Ultrasound Med. Biol.*, **14**, 499–506.

Munting E. (1978). Ultrasound therapy for painful shoulders. *Physiotherapy*, **64**, 180–1.

Nwuga V. C. O. (1983). Ultrasound in the treatment of back pain resulting from prolapsed intervertebral disc. *Arch. Phys. Med. Rehabil.*, **64**, 88–9.

Partridge C. J. (1987). Evaluation of the efficacy of ultrasound. *Physiotherapy*, **73**, 166–8.

Patrick M. K. (1978). Applications of therapeutic pulsed ultrasound. *Physiotherapy*, **64**, 103–4.

Payne C. (1984). Ultrasound for post-herpetic neuralgia. *Physiotherapy*, **70**, 96–7.

Pienimäki T. T., Tarvainen T. K., Siira P. T., Vanharanta H. (1996). Progressive strengthening and stretching exercises and ultrasound for chronic lateral epicondylitis. *Physiotherapy*, **82**, 527–30.

Pringle D. W. (1995). Therapeutic ultrasound: acoustic transmissiveness of wound dressings. Abstract from Physiotherapy Research Workshop at Manchester Royal Infirmary, Nov. 94. *Physiotherapy*, **81**, 240.

Pye S. (1996). Ultrasound therapy equipment – does it perform? *Physiotherapy*, **82**, 39–44.

Pye S., Hildersley K., Somer E. *et al.* (1994). A simple calorimeter for monitoring the output power of ultrasound therapy machines. *Physiotherapy*, **80**, 219–23.

Reid D. C., Cummings G. E. (1977). Efficiency of ultrasound coupling agents. *Physiotherapy*, **63**, 255–7.

Robertson V. J., Ward A. R. (1997). Longwave ultrasound reviewed and reconsidered. *Physiotherapy*, **83**, 123–30.

Robinson S. E., Buono M. J. (1995). Effect of continuous-wave ultrasound on blood flow in skeletal muscle. *Phys. Ther.*, **75**, 145–50.

Roche C., West J. (1984). A controlled trial investigating the effect of ultrasound on venous ulcers referred from general practitioners. *Physiotherapy*, **70**, 475–7.

Rubin D., Kuitert J. H. (1955). Use of ultrasonic vibration in the treatment of pain arising from phantom limbs, scars and neuromas: a preliminary report. *Arch. Phys. Med. Rehab.*, **36**, 445.

Rubin M. J., Etchison M. R., Condra K. A. *et al.* (1990). Acute effects of ultrasound on skeletal muscle oxygen tension, blood flow and capillary density. *Ultrasound Med. Biol.*, **16**, 271–7.

Schlapbach P. (1991). Ultrasound. In *Physiotherapy: Controlled Trials and Facts* (Schlapbach P., Gerber N. J., eds) Basel: Karger, pp. 163–70.

Skauen D. M., Zentner G. M. (1984). Phonophoresis. *Int. J. Pharm.*, **20**, 235–45.

Summer W., Patrick M. K. (1964). *Ultrasonic Therapy. A Textbook for Physiotherapists.* London: Elsevier.

ter Haar G. (1978). Basic physics of therapeutic ultrasound. *Physiotherapy*, **64**, 100–3.

ter Haar G. R. (1987). Basic physics of therapeutic ultrasound. *Physiotherapy*, **73**, 110–13.

ter Haar G. (1996). Electrophysical principles. In *Clayton's Electrotherapy*, 10th edn (Kitchen S., Bazin S., eds) Philadelphia: W. B. Saunders.

ter Haar G. R., Daniels S. (1981). Evidence for ultrasonically induced cavitation in vivo. *Physics Med. Biol.*, **26**, 1145–9.

Wadsworth H., Chanmugan A. P. P. (1980). *Electrophysical Agents in Physiotherapy.* Marrickville, NSW, Australia: Science Press.

Ward A. R. (1986). *Electricity Fields and Waves in Therapy.* Marrickville, NSW, Australia: Science Press.

Ward A. R., Robertson V. J. (1996). Dosage factors for the subaqueous application of 1 MHz ultrasound. *Arch. Phys. Med. Rehabil.*, **77**, 1167–72.

Williams R. (1987). Production and transmission of ultrasound. *Physiotherapy*, **73**, 113–16.

Young S. R. (1988). The effect of therapeutic ultrasound on the biological mechanisms involved in dermal regeneration. PhD Thesis, University of London.

Young S. (1996). Ultrasonic therapy. In *Clayton's Electrotherapy*, 10th edn (Kitchen S., Bazin S., eds) Philadelphia: W. B. Saunders, pp. 243–67.

Young S. R., Dyson M. (1990). Macrophage responsiveness to therapeutic ultrasound. *Ultrasound Med. Biol.*, **16**, 261–9.

7 Heat and cold

Heat and cold are probably the oldest of all physical therapies; hot and cold water seem to have been applied to the body for healing throughout recorded history.

This chapter deals with the underlying basic concepts, while therapeutic applications to the body surface are considered in the next two chapters and deep heating in other chapters.

Despite the fact that heat and cold are very familiar ideas, the fundamental nature of heat is often not well understood, so that a study of the basic science of heat is central to recognizing the way in which therapy works.

To this end the general principles, including the meaning of temperature, quantity of heat, heat transfer and energy conversions, are all considered at the beginning of the chapter.

The thermal regulatory mechanisms of the body are described and explained, with the physiological consequences of temperature changes at the body surface. This forms the bulk of the chapter.

Finally, the therapeutic effects of local tissue heating, but not cooling, are addressed.

GENERAL PRINCIPLES

To understand what happens when matter becomes hot it is necessary to consider the microstructure of matter.

Solids are formed of collections of atoms or molecules closely packed together in a regular pattern, so that each can only move a short distance. The atoms or molecules vibrate about their equilibrium positions and it is these movements – kinetic energy – which are recognized as heat. If more heat energy is added the amount of motion increases and usually (but not in all circumstances) the matter becomes hotter, i.e. the temperature increases.

In *liquids* the atoms or molecules have a rather greater amplitude of vibration and can partly overcome the interatomic forces of their immediate neighbours. The atoms have greater speeds because of their increased temperature and move randomly.

In *gases* the atoms are widely spaced and move randomly over much larger distances. Again adding heat causes more motion so that the average positions of the atoms become further apart so the matter has expanded. This is very evident in gases because of the large interatomic distances but less obvious in liquids and still less in solids. This property of expansion is utilized in engines to convert heat energy to mechanical energy and in the measurement of temperature.

The idea that heat is a form of energy and is conserved is asserted by the first law of thermodynamics.

Temperature

Temperature is a measure of the level of heat. Humans assess this level through special temperature receptors in the skin. The judgement made by the central nervous system is not absolute; rather it is a comparison of skin temperatures. If the right hand is immersed in hot and the left in cold water and both hands are then placed in tepid water it feels cold to the right hand and hot to the left. This illustrates a general feature of perception in the nervous system which tends to recognize contrasts.

Most simple thermometers utilize expansion to measure temperature, mercury in glass being the familiar form. Mercury expands much more than glass on being heated and if it is only allowed to expand along a very narrow tube quite a small temperature change will cause a large movement of mercury along the tube. To measure temperature two fixed points, the melting point of ice and the boiling point of water, are found and the region between them divided into 100 parts, called degrees. Such a scale, in which 0°C is the freezing point of water and 100°C is its boiling point, is known as the Celsius scale, abbreviated to C. The Fahrenheit scale was formerly used and may still be found.

As temperature is due to the kinetic energy of atoms and molecules there is no upper limit, but there is a definite lower limit where no motion occurs at all. This point is called absolute zero, and is -273.2°C. For much scientific work the more logical kelvin scale is used; this is the SI unit of temperature. This treats absolute zero as 0 K and uses the same degrees as the Celsius scale so that the freezing point of water becomes 273 K and its boiling point 373 K.

Quantity of heat

If a kettleful of boiling water is poured into a bath of tepid water the bath water may become perceptibly warmer but not nearly as hot as the water in the kettle. Clearly when a small quantity of water is added it carries a small quantity of heat which when spread throughout the larger volumes leads to little rise in temperature. To describe the quantity of heat a unit called the calorie was formerly used. This is the amount of heat needed to raise the temperature of 1 g of water 1°C; but since it is an energy measurement the appropriate SI units are now used, i.e. 4.18 kJ/kg/°C for water. In dietetics the kilocalorie is still widely used and is confusingly called the Calorie (with a capital C); this is therefore equal to 4.18 kJ. This amount of heat energy applied to a unit mass of a material to raise the temperature 1°C is known as the specific heat of the material.

Table 7.1 Specific heat

	Specific heat (kJ/kg/1°C)
Water	4.185
Air	1.01
Aluminium	0.904
Copper	0.402
Mercury	0.14
Glass	0.77
Paraffin wax	about 2.7
Rubber	2.01
Whole human body	3.56
Skin	3.77
Fat	2.3
Muscle	3.75
Bone	1.59
Whole blood	3.64

Data from Sekins and Emery (1982).

Water has a much greater specific heat than other common materials (Table 7.1) so that it takes a great deal of heat energy to raise the temperature of water and conversely hot water stores much heat per unit mass.

The specific heat of the human body is close to 3.5 kJ/kg/°C (Sekins and Emery, 1982) which is not surprising since it is 70% water. To raise the temperature of a 50 kg woman 2°C it takes 350 kJ of energy ($50 \times 3.5 \times 2$). Notice that this would be additional to the energy continuously being generated in the body. In fact, even at rest the basal metabolic rate leads to the emission of heat.

The addition of heat

When heat is added to matter it can cause expansion (an increase in volume or, if the volume is restricted, an increase in pressure) or it may change the physical state of the material, by melting or vaporizing it, or it may cause a temperature rise in the material, or any combination of these. When water boils a change of state occurs in which the liquid is changed into gas. The heat energy is used in separating molecules, disrupting the bonding forces and changing the state from liquid to gas, rather than increasing the kinetic energy; therefore there is no rise of temperature during the process. Exactly the same thing happens when the solid form, i.e. ice, is melted to water and when any other substance is vaporized or melted. As the energy used to make these physical changes does not appear as temperature rises the energy is stored in the microstructure of the material and can be returned as heat if the process is reversed. It is therefore known as latent heat. The quantity of heat per unit mass is characteristic for any material. For water it takes approximately 2260 kJ to change each kilogram into water vapour and about 333 kJ for the change from ice to water. Other substances have different latent heats.

In solids atoms are more strictly confined by neighbouring atoms so that the addition of heat leads to each atom oscillating more vigorously, increasing the average separation from other atoms, and hence expanding the whole material. When heat energy is added it not only goes to increasing the kinetic motion of the molecules, thus raising the temperature, but also to increasing the intramolecular and intra-atomic energies.

Liquids have rather more space between molecules than solids but much less than in gases. Almost all liquid states are therefore less dense than the solid states. Water is exceptional in that the molecules are more closely packed together at around 4°C than when the crystalline solid, ice, is formed; thus ice will float on water. The same thing happens when molten bismuth solidifies.

Clearly, increasing the energy of the microstructure of matter will lead to many other effects, notably the acceleration of chemical reactions (Van't Hoff's law) and the production of electromagnetic radiations, described in Chapter 11. The electron agitation can also lead to a potential difference between two dissimilar metals (the Seebeck effect) or electrons leaving the metal surface (thermionic emission). The viscosity of fluids is reduced, since the increased molecular motion diminishes the cohesive attraction.

Summary

Heating of matter may lead to:

- expansion
- a change of state; solids melting, liquids vaporizing
- an increased rate of chemical reaction
- production of electromagnetic radiations
- a p.d. between dissimilar metals
- thermionic emission
- reduced viscosity in fluids.

Energy conversions

Heat, the energy of the microstructure of matter, can be converted to other forms of energy, but not with 100% efficiency. Similarly, if one form of energy is converted to another, say chemical to mechanical, there is always some part converted to heat in the material so that such conversions can never be 100% efficient. Of course, the general law of conservation of energy – energy can neither be created nor destroyed – holds true for the total energy exchange. Since all energy ultimately ends as heat in the structure of matter it is sometimes described as the basic form of energy, but it is simply the tendency to randomization.

Heat transfer

Conduction.   One method of transferring heat from place to place is by the kinetic motion of atoms and molecules being passed from one to the next, dramatically described as 'atoms jostling one another'. This is called *conduction* and is easily demonstrated, especially in metals; if one end of a metal bar is heated the other end becomes hotter in time. (This concept is familiar to most of us as a consequence of leaving metal spoons and forks in the cooking pot!) Conduction is an inevitable consequence of molecular and atomic motion in the microstructure of any material and it would be expected that 'jostling' would be more effective in transmitting energy if the molecules are closer together, as happens in solids, and this is broadly the case.

Metals make good heat conductors while liquids and gases are much less effective. Notice that if two different materials are in contact heat can be transferred from one to the other in the same way, the molecules of the hotter material knocking into and so giving kinetic energy to those of the cooler. Heat flow through matter varies with the nature of the material and is called thermal conductivity.

Convection.   A second way of transferring heat energy is by bulk movement of the moving molecules themselves. When hotter atoms or molecules move from one place to another, as can easily occur with liquids and gases, the heat energy is said to be moved by *convection*. The fluid movement can be due to being pumped – the distribution of heat around the body is due to the heart circulating the warm blood – or it can be due to the fact that the heated liquid or gas, being less dense, tends to float upwards on the cooler fluid. This latter is called thermal convection and is familiar in many situations, from making marmalade to meteorology. The evaporation of gas molecules away from a surface, such as occurs in sweating, is a particular form of convection.

Radiation.   The third way in which heat energy can be transferred is by *radiation*. This is really the conversion of heat energy to an electromagnetic radiation. The most familiar radiations are infrared radiations, visible and microwave radiations which can all lead to heating when they are absorbed.

The amount of radiation produced depends on the temperature of the object; it is proportional to the fourth power of the kelvin temperature. The wavelength is also dependent on temperature so that emissions of shorter and shorter wavelength are given off with higher temperatures. Radiations travel through space so that heat is transferred without any intervening matter; hence the heat of the sun can be transmitted to the surface of the earth.

Although heat transmission is customarily described in terms of conduction, mainly in solids, convection in fluids and radiation, it must be recognized that in many real-life situations all three operate as complex chains of heat exchanges. For example, central heating radiators are warmed by hot water pumped through them (forced convection) and they warm air in contact with their surfaces (conduction) which rises (thermal convection) to warm the room. The radiator also emits infrared radiations which are absorbed by other objects and people in the room, which causes further heating. Obviously the contribution from both radiation and convection will increase with increasing temperature but whereas convection increases approximately linearly, radiation increases exponentially; thus at low temperatures energy is transferred predominantly by convection.

Summary

Heat may be transferred by:

- conduction
- convection – either forced or thermal
- radiation.

The concept of cold is due to human perception. It is the absence of heat and is recognized when heat energy is being transferred away from the body.

Thermometers

A thermometer is an instrument that measures temperature. It may utilize any physical change that correlates with heating and cooling. By far the most familiar is the mercury-in-glass thermometer. This device depends on the expansion of mercury which is much greater than that of glass when both are heated. The mercury-filled bulb is heated and the expansion is made visible because a thin line of mercury is forced along a narrow glass capillary tube. A typical clinical thermometer with a range of 30–45°C has a constriction in the capillary tube which breaks the mercury thread, preventing its return to the bulb as cooling occurs. This allows an accurate reading of the maximum temperature reached. The glass cylinder acts as a lens to enlarge the mercury thread. These thermometers can be extremely accurate: when new the vast majority are accurate to within 0.1°C (Cetas, 1982). Alcohol-in-glass thermometers work in the same way, are usually larger and can be made easier to read by colouring the alcohol. They are often used for checking room or waterbath temperatures.

Another widely used thermometer depends on the difference in expansion of two metals when they are heated. Such devices are sturdy but often inaccurate and are often used as a thermostat to open or close a switch at a pre-set temperature. This kind of system is found controlling the temperature of domestic water heaters, room temperature, electric blankets, electric heater pads and the paraffin wax baths used in physiotherapy departments, as well as many other situations.

Other thermometers use different effects. In the thermistor, which is a semiconductor, the electrical resistance decreases exponentially with rise in temperature. They can be manufactured to be very small – a tiny bead or disc on the end of two fine wires – and are relatively accurate. For these reasons they are used as thermal probes in hypodermic needles for testing temperature deep in the tissues. They are also found in little discs of epoxy resin of some digital readout skin thermometers.

Thermography

Thermography is the term used for the process of sensing the temperature of quite large areas of the body by photographing the surface using an infrared sensitive film. The film can be made to give a colour response to different temperatures, thus giving a colourful map of the temperature of the surface being investigated. This technique is used in the detection of underlying areas of inflammation or hot spots and for other purposes. Special video cameras can be used in a similar way.

Numerous other types of thermometers have been developed for special purposes. For clinical and general use electronic thermometers are no more accurate, and sometimes less reliable, than the mercury-in-glass type originally developed over 300 years ago (Cetas, 1982).

THERMAL REGULATORY MECHANISMS

Body temperature

It is well understood that humans are homeothermic in respect of their core temperature, that is the temperature of the deeply placed structures and organs. Skin and subcutaneous tissue temperatures are much more variable. Normally there is a circadian variation in the core temperature of about 1°C, being lower in the early morning and higher in the afternoon and evening (Hardy, 1982). Other variations also occur such as ovulatory cycles. Most people have core temperatures around 36.8°C but individuals vary and children tend to have slightly higher temperatures. Oral and rectal temperatures, which are conveniently measured, approximate to the real core temperature but are more variable. Vigorous exercise will temporarily raise the core temperature above these limits. It is largely through the skin that heat exchange with the environment takes place.

Table 7.2 Causes of heat gain and loss

Causes of heat gain	*Causes of heat loss*
Basal metabolism	Radiation to the environment
Metabolism of muscle contraction	Conduction to cooler objects
Metabolism of other tissues beyond basal, e.g. digestion	Conduction to air, continually removed by convection
Absorption of radiation from the environment	Evaporation of water from skin – 'insensible perspiration' – vapour carried away by convection
Conduction from hotter objects	Evaporation of sweat – water vapour carried away by convection
	Exhaled warm air – forced convection
	Excretion of urine, faeces and other fluids

Maintenance of homeothermy

The core temperature is dependent on a balance between heat loss and gain. The main features are identified in Table 7.2.

Although all the effects noted in Table 7.2 occur, the major heat gain is from metabolism, which is vastly increased during vigorous exercise: some 75% of the energy applied to muscle contraction appears as heat. At moderate environmental temperatures radiation accounts for some 60% of heat loss (Hubbard and Mechan, 1987).

As the outside temperature rises, approximating the body surface temperature, the effectiveness of radiation and conduction becomes less and less. If the outside temperature is above body temperature the body gains further heat by radiation from the surroundings. In these circumstances heat loss is entirely due to the evaporation of sweat from the skin. This is a very efficient method of heat loss as the evaporation of each gram of sweat at body temperature takes some 2.5 kJ of heat energy. Under suitable conditions a man can lose 1 kg of sweat per hour, thus achieving a cooling rate of nearly 700 W ($2500 J \times 1000 g/3600 s = 694.4 W$; Holwill and Silvester, 1973).

The difference between the core temperature and the normally lower body surface temperature is critical in controlling the heat loss from the body because the rate at which heat can be lost from the body surface depends on the temperature difference between that surface and the environment. A large temperature difference can be maintained between the core and the outer shell of the body because of the low thermal conductivity of tissue, especially fat tissue. The flow of heat from the deep tissue to the skin is largely due to the blood flow – forced convection. Heat is thus transmitted through the thermal barrier provided by the subcutaneous fat. This concept of a temperature gradient between the core and surface can be expressed schematically by the isothermal lines shown in Figure 7.1 and the tissue temperature gradients shown in Figure 8.1. There are variations of skin temperature on different areas of the body. The forehead skin is often at a higher temperature and there tends to be a progressive fall in temperature towards the periphery so that at toe-level skin temperature can be at room temperature.

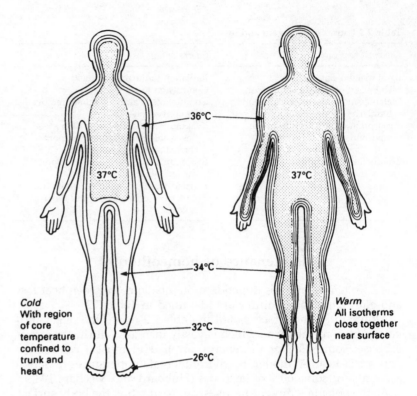

36°C

37°C

37°C

34°C

32°C

26°C

Cold
With region of core temperature confined to trunk and head

Warm
All isotherms close together near surface

Fig. 7.1 Body isotherms. Left: cold, with region of core temperature confined to trunk and head. Right: warm, with all isotherms close together near surface.

When the body is exposed to cold the loss of heat can be much reduced by vasoconstriction which greatly reduces the blood flow to the extremities and skin of the trunk so allowing skin and subcutaneous tissue temperature to fall. Conversely if the body retains too much heat vasodilation of skin vessels vastly increases the blood flow and hence the skin temperature. The isothermic lines are close to the surface, showing that there is now less difference between the surface and the core temperature (Fig. 7.1).

The thicker layer of subcutaneous fat in women gives them better thermal control than men. At low environmental temperatures their skin is colder but becomes warmer in hotter environments (Hardy, 1982) (see Fig. 7.2). However, it appears that sweating starts earlier and tends to be more extensive in men.

Counter-current heat exchange

Counter-current heat exchange is another aspect of thermal regulation in the body. Heat can be exchanged between the warm arterial blood moving from the body core to the periphery and the cooler venous blood returning from the extremities. If arteries and veins lie close together, as in the limbs, where the venae comitantes are situated on each side of a medium artery, heat can pass from the warmer artery to the cooler vein. Since arterial blood loses heat as it passes to the periphery and venous blood gains heat as it moves centrally, the heat gradient between them remains

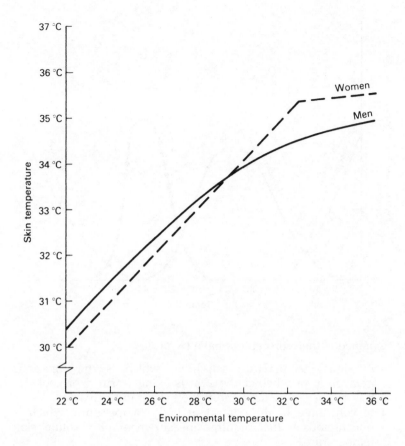

Fig. 7.2 Skin temperatures resulting from environmental temperatures. Modified from Hardy (1982).

much the same, thus heat exchange continues throughout the length of the vessels. The value of this arrangement is that body core heat in the arterial blood is conserved in the central parts by being used to heat the incoming venous blood instead of the extremities which are maintained at a lower temperature than the core.

While this counter-current mechanism is of great importance in some animals its effectiveness in humans is in question. Estimates of the heat savings vary from a negligible 5% to a significant 50% (Hardy, 1982).

Cutaneous thermoreceptors

Receptors in the skin signal temperature changes; some are heat receptors but many more (about eight times as many) are cold receptors. Many of those are identical to pain nerve endings (C fibres; group IV unmyelinated) and thermal perception seems to involve interpretation of the impulses from cold, warm and pain receptors by the central nervous system.

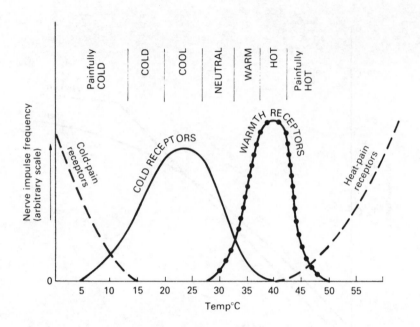

Fig. 7.3 Response of thermal receptors in skin.

Cutaneous thermoreceptors have two roles:

- to signal temperature sensation, which is the conscious perception of whether the skin is being warmed or cooled – this requires measurement of the temperature change
- to contribute to the control of body temperature, which is unconscious – this requires measurement of absolute skin temperature.

The perception of thermal sensation is also influenced by the size of the area stimulated and, importantly, by the rate of change of the stimulation.

Pain nerve endings discharge at the extremes of the temperature range – where the temperature stimulus becomes merged with pain – beyond 45°C for heating and 15°C for cooling. These endings are sometimes described as warmth-pain and cold-pain endings respectively. The more numerous cold receptors discharge over a wide range; different neurons have different ranges and different peak discharges, many around 25°C as shown in Figure 7.3. The warm receptors also vary greatly, many with peaks around 40°C (see Fig. 7.3).

The continuous discharge of receptors shown in Figure 7.3 depends on the absolute skin temperature as shown but if the skin is suddenly heated there is an abrupt decrease in cold receptor activity and a corresponding increased frequency of warm receptor discharge. Both frequencies slowly return to the frequency appropriate for the new absolute skin temperature. Thus information from these receptors is used to perceive skin temperature and temperature changes as well as to contribute to subconscious temperature regulation (Fischer and Solomon, 1965). The perception of temperature change on the skin is extraordinarily sensitive. At

Table 7.3 Temperature ranges*

Environmental temperature		Temperature (°C)	Skin surface temperatures	
			Subjective feeling	Effect
Behavioural regulation		60		Tissue damage
		55		
		50		
		45	Pain	
		40	Very hot	
		35	Hot	
Region of physiological temperature regulation	Region of thermal comfort	30	Warm neutral	
		25	Cool	
		20	Cold	
		15		
		10	Very cold	
		5	Pain	
Behavioural regulation		0		Tissue damage
		−5		
		−10		

* The range of body core temperature lies between 36.3°C and 37.3°C.

skin temperatures around 30°C changes of as little as 1°C can be recognized under some conditions. At colder or hotter skin temperatures, and if the change is slow, larger changes of 5 or 10°C are needed before temperature change is recognized.

The usual method of testing thermal sensitivity by applying warm and cold water-filled test tubes to the skin, being about 10°C above and below skin temperature respectively, should thus allow easy .recognition of the temperatures unless there is a significant sensory deficit.

The sensations associated with different surface temperatures are shown in Table 7.3 but it must be realized that this is a very subjective matter.

THERMAL REGULATION

There are two facets of human heat regulation:

- *physiological*, controlled by the hypothalamus, which is itself sensitive to blood temperature – this involves metabolic, vasomotor and hidrotic control
- *behavioural*, controlled in the higher centres.

Metabolic control

When much heat is being lost from the body some restoration can be made by increasing the metabolic activity. The most evident form this takes is shivering, in which irregular muscle contractions are provoked by stimulation of the sympathetic nervous system. Over short periods shivering can produce quite good heating but

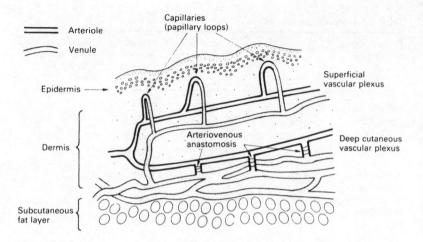

Fig. 7.4 Section through skin and subcutaneous tissue to illustrate vascular arrangements.

for several hours of cold exposure it can only double the resting metabolism on average (Hardy, 1982).

Brown adipose tissue is fatty tissue with more than the usual vascularity, hence making it look brown. It is found in a number of sites in the trunk close to the heart and kidney and between the scapulae. Fat metabolism can occur locally in this tissue in a way that releases energy entirely as heat. While important in newborn infants the value of this mechanism to adults is uncertain. It is stimulated by adrenaline release.

At rest most body heat (about 70%) is produced in the viscera of the trunk and in the brain. On activity most of the heat (about 90%) is produced by the muscles and skin, which moves the sites of major heat production nearer to the surface and to the extremities (Hardy, 1982). Of course, the increased blood flow needed to maintain oxygenation and nutrition to sustain continuous muscle contraction serves to dissipate heat from the working muscles to the rest of the body.

Vasomotor control

The blood flow in the skin not only serves the usual nutritional role but also acts as a heat transfer system. Arterioles feed capillary loops in the dermis forming papillae which drain via venules to a network of small veins. Slightly more deeply placed are rather larger venous plexuses: blood moving through these transfers heat to the overlying skin (see Fig. 7.4). Over most of the skin surface the blood flow is regulated by the lumen of the arteriole which is under the control of the sympathetic nervous system. In the skin of the hands, feet, ears, lips and some mucous membrane surfaces arteriovenous anastomoses are present between the arteriole and the large venous plexuses. These are regulated by vasoconstrictor impulses from the sympathetic nervous system so that when closed, in cold conditions, the flow of blood in the veins is reduced to almost nothing but the nutritive blood flow through the papillae is maintained. On dilation they allow a large flow of venous blood through plexuses causing a marked rise in skin temperature and thus loss of heat from the surface.

At rest the skin contains some 20 times as much blood as is needed for nutrition alone. Under cold conditions the blood flow to each 100 g of skin can be reduced to as little as 1 ml/min whereas in hot conditions this can rise to 150 ml/min (Hubbard and Mechan, 1987).

Sweating

As noted earlier, water evaporation from the skin surface is a very efficient way of losing heat; in fact it is the only way when the environmental temperature is the same as or even greater than the skin temperature. It is not difficult to see why so much energy (2.5 kJ/g) is used since the energy leads to increased movement of the water molecules, giving them a range of kinetic energies. The ones with the highest kinetic energy will be 'thrown off' the water surface to form vapour which moves away from the skin surface by convection. At all times under all circumstances the body is losing heat by evaporation (about 500 g/day for a 1.5 m² surface area, e.g. the 50 kg woman considered previously). About half of this is the water vapour of expired air while the remainder is due to the steady transpiration of water through the skin, the so-called insensible perspiration. This is more or less constant at environmental temperatures below about 30°C but at higher temperatures, or when metabolic heat is produced by vigorous exercise, active sweating occurs and the amount of sweat vaporized increases with temperature (see Fig. 7.2).

There are an enormous number of eccrine sweat glands in the skin under sympathetic nervous system control via cholinergic nerves (glands of the palms and soles may have additionally adrenergic fibres). Large amounts of sweat can be produced when needed, but vaporization – hence cooling – depends both on temperature and humidity. In dry conditions body cooling is therefore much more efficient.

Behavioural regulation

These are familiar responses which depend on sensations of heat and cold being interpreted as discomfort (Table 7.3). In temperate and cold climates the main method of behavioural regulation is wearing clothes, which provide thermal insulation by trapping a layer of air close to the skin surface. In other words, clothes prevent heat loss due to thermal and forced convection of air warmed by the skin. The effectiveness of air as an insulator is noticed when clothes become wet and immediately feel much colder. This occurs because the thermal conductivity of water is nearly 25 times that of air. Similarly, restricting the movement of cold air close to the body by maintaining a draught-free environment or wrapping the body in blankets acts in the same way. Using a material that reflects infrared radiations (survival sleeping bags) cuts down the heat loss further by blocking radiation emission from the body. Vigorous voluntary muscular activity is also used to increase metabolic heat.

Opposite behaviours encourage heat loss in a hot environment. Thus air-trapping by thick clothing is reduced; light loose-fitting clothing reduces absorption of radiation while allowing air convection currents close to the skin. Applying a steady draught of air by a fan or other means assists cooling. Avoiding radiation by remaining in the shade and limiting activity in hot environments also helps to control body temperature.

Summary

Thermal regulation is brought about by:

- Inputs from
  ○ temperature of blood perfusing hypothalamus
  ○ peripheral cutaneous receptors.
- Control via
  ○ hypothalamus
  ○ higher centres, i.e. behavioural
  ○ hormonal (adrenaline) response.
- Output, regulation
  ○ Involuntary (physiological)
    – metabolic control: shivering; metabolism of brown adipose tissue in babies
    – vasomotor control: blood flow in skin is varied
    – sweating: evaporation from skin varied.
  ○ Voluntary
    – insulation of body surface varied: clothes; shelter
    – voluntary increase/avoidance of metabolic activity: muscle contraction or inactivity
    – seeking or avoiding environmental heat.

Temperature regulation

The temperature-regulating centre is largely in the hypothalamus. It is effectively a thermostat responding to lowered blood temperatures by initiating heat-generating and conserving mechanisms and acting in the opposite way to raised blood temperatures. Heat-sensitive neurons in the anterior hypothalamus, affected by blood temperature, are integrated in the posterior hypothalamus with signals from peripheral receptors, thus providing overall control (Guyton, 1982). Adrenaline release is an important endocrine response to cooling. From what has been noted above there is also involvement of the higher centres.

Bacterial or viral infections of sufficient virulence lead to the release of substances which in some ill-understood way re-set the thermostat of the temperature-regulating centre. Thus the patient shivers and feels cold and the heat-conserving mechanisms come into play; cutaneous vasoconstriction makes the patient look pale.

Consequently the core temperature rises to a new, higher level for a time. When the infection has been overcome, aided by the higher metabolic rate and consequent increased activity of the immune system, the patient feels hot and cutaneous vasodilation occurs with sweating to bring the body temperature down as the thermostat is re-set back to the normal level.

Body temperature regulation is helped by the high specific heat (3.5 kJ/kg/°C) which means that it takes a large quantity of heat to raise, or heat loss to lower, the body temperature. Furthermore small temporary changes of core temperature, such as occur with exercise, are physiologically normal.

Since the principal source of heat is metabolism, which depends on tissue mass, and the principal source of heat loss is from the whole of the skin, which depends on the surface area, it is evident that body size will have an important effect. Babies have a larger surface area in proportion to their mass than adults, so that it might be expected that they would be at more risk from excessive heat loss. They appear to compensate by maintaining a higher metabolic rate and perhaps by means of the brown adipose tissue referred to above.

Even in healthy subjects the heat-regulating mechanisms can become overwhelmed by extremes of heat or cold. Feeling faint due to lowered cerebral blood pressure following prolonged standing or abrupt postural changes in the heat is familiar to most people. It can be called heat syncope and is caused by venous pooling; recovery is rapid once the subject lies down. A much more dangerous syndrome is heat stroke, when heat regulation fails, the person stops sweating and body temperature starts to rise. Urgent treatment to cool the patient and maintain body fluids is life-saving.

During hard work at high outside temperatures, body temperature is controlled by sweating and if water and salt are not replaced muscle cramps and fatigue result. Under extremely cold conditions the core temperature starts to fall, unconsciousness follows and unless rewarming can be effected thermal regulation is completely lost; this condition is fatal.

Stress due to extremes of temperature is a far more serious problem for those who have some deficiency in their normal response, either due to disease or old age. It has been noted that mortality rates go up during heatwaves or very cold spells, particularly amongst the elderly and those with chronic cardiovascular disease. As might be anticipated hypothermia is much the more significant problem in the UK, particularly among elderly people living alone. They may be unable to maintain their home at a suitable temperature so that body temperature falls leading to confusion and inertia, exacerbating the problem. It has been found (Fox *et al.*, 1973) that many of these elderly people have some failure of their temperature-regulating system – falling body temperatures do not provoke the normal shivering and vasoconstriction responses as quickly as usual.

There are a number of conditions in which exposure to extremes of heat or cold may lead to particular difficulties. For example, cystic fibrosis is associated with inefficient production of sweat and hence inadequate control in extreme heat.

THE PHYSIOLOGICAL EFFECTS OF TEMPERATURE CHANGE ON THE BODY TISSUES

Any form of local body tissue heating will lead to a complicated set of physiological changes which interact to produce still further complex responses. These merge with the systemic changes needed to maintain thermal homeostasis that have just been considered.

The various therapeutic modalities that produce tissue heating differ from one another in their effects due to the site of tissue heating rather than any difference in its nature. Thus the effects of local tissue heating will be considered as a whole in this chapter. The specific sites or other particular features of the modality are described in the chapters discussing: ultrasound (Chapter 6); conduction heating (Chapter 8); cooling (Chapter 9); shortwave diathermy (Chapter 10); microwave diathermy (Chapter 12); infrared therapy (Chapter 13).

It has already been noted that the terms 'heating' and 'cooling' are based on human perceptions, so that a skin temperature raised to 35°C would be considered warming, whereas lowering the deep tissue temperature to the same level is cooling. Cooling the tissues has effects which are not the simple reverse of those due to heating. The effects of tissue cooling are therefore considered separately in Chapter 9.

Living tissue appears to be affected by temperature changes in two fundamental ways, from which further changes emanate. These are:

- temperature dependent physical and chemical changes, as in metabolic rate, viscosity and collagen tissue extensibility
- changes related to physiological regulation, developed to protect the body from damage, such as occur in the vascular and nervous systems.

Metabolic activity

The rate of any chemical action that can be affected is increased by a temperature rise (Van't Hoff's law). Metabolism, being a series of chemical reactions, will increase with a rise and decrease with a fall of temperature. The actual change is about one-eighth (13%) for each 1°C so increasing the tissue temperature by, say, 4°C would increase the metabolic rate by some 60%. In the living organism increasing temperature tends to denature proteins and thus interfere with the enzyme (protein)-controlled metabolic processes. Thus after some increased activity an optimum temperature is reached at which metabolic activity is maximally stimulated by the heat and yet not sufficiently hot to destroy the necessary enzymes. This temperature point will differ for different reactions. At temperatures above 45°C so much protein damage occurs that there is destruction of cells and tissues. At low temperatures metabolism is progressively reduced and tissue destruction occurs if the intra- or extracellular fluid becomes frozen.

From a therapeutic point of view the local temperature changes that can, or should, be achieved are limited in the deeper tissues to about 5 or 6°C above or below core temperature; for skin and subcutaneous tissue much lower temperatures can be achieved. With an appropriate rise in temperature, all cell activity increases, including cell motility and the synthesis and release of chemical mediators. Furthermore, the rate of cellular interactions, such as phagocytosis or growth, is accelerated.

Viscosity

The resistance to flow in a blood vessel depends directly on the viscosity of the fluid and inversely on the fourth power of the radius of the vessel. This striking dependence of blood flow on the diameter of the blood vessel is the reason why the autonomic control of the arteriole diameter regulates the tissue blood flow so effectively.

Less dramatic, but still of consequence is the effect of viscosity. This property of moving fluids is sometimes described as friction between the moving particles. It is temperature dependent, so raising the temperature in liquids, but not gases, lowers the viscosity. Viscosity changes affect not only the fluids in narrow vessels (blood and lymph), but also fluid movement within and throughout the tissue spaces. Thus, although the effect is quite small, it is widespread.

Collagenous tissue changes

The changes that occur in collagen due to heating are well known in the cooking of meat. This renders the collagenous parts jelly-like, thus making the meat more tender. It has been shown that collagen melts at temperatures above 50°C (Mason and Rigby, 1963). At temperatures within a therapeutically applicable range (40–45°C), the extensibility of collagen tissue has been shown to increase (Lehmann *et al.*, 1970). This only occurs if the tissue is simultaneously stretched and requires temperatures near the therapeutic limit, but it is an important therapeutic effect. Kitchen and Partridge (1991), however, sound a note of caution in extrapolating the effects from *in vitro* experiments to therapy. Joint stiffness has been found to be reduced by heating (Wright and Johns, 1961); on cooling, joint stiffness is increased.

Nerve stimulation

Plainly heat and cold stimulate the sensory receptors of the skin since these sensations can be recognized (see earlier). Furthermore these receptors pass information to the heat-regulating centres, contributing to the control of body temperature. Afferent nerves stimulated by heat may have an analgesic effect by acting on the gate control mechanism in the same way as the mechanoreceptors (see Chapter 3); in the past, this effect was called a counter-irritant mechanism (Gammon and Starr, 1941). There is some evidence that stimulating heat receptors inhibits nociceptive impulses in rats (Kanui, 1985). This could account for the analgesic effects of local heating. There is evidence that cutaneous sensations are altered by local heating of the skin. Hyperalgesia occurs in the area of the heated region, which appears to be due to mechanisms in the central nervous system at subcortical level (Cervero *et al.*, 1993). This remains only for a few minutes after the cessation of heating.

It has been suggested that heating the secondary afferent muscle spindle nerve endings and Golgi tendon endings could be the way in which muscle spasm is reduced by heating (Lehmann and de Lateur, 1982).

Cooling has marked effects on peripheral nerves. Initially cold receptors are stimulated, adding to the overall sensory input, but at lower temperatures conduction rates are depressed. This occurs at first in the small myelinated fibres and later in large myelinated fibres. With sufficient cooling some nerve conduction is abolished so that numbness occurs. The therapeutic implications are considered in Chapter 9.

Blood vessel changes

Heat and cold applied to the skin have obvious effects. With heating the skin surface reddens, i.e. an erythema is produced, and with cooling it becomes pale due to vasoconstriction, although subsequent vasodilation due to cold may occur (see Chapter 9). The striking cutaneous hyperaemia due to heat leads to the idea that similar effects occur in other tissues but this is not the case. As noted already, the skin is specially adapted for heat regulation and what is being seen is a heat-blocking response.

Vasodilation occurs not only to distribute the additional heat around the body, allowing compensatory heat loss from other regions, but also to protect the heated skin. This is important because the skin surface is naturally heated from the outside and heat conduction is not effective through the subcutaneous fat; in fact the two mechanisms may be somewhat separate in that it has been found that directly heating the skin causes capillary dilation but the arteriovenous anastomoses are opened by reduced sympathetic tone for total body temperature regulation.

Vasodilation due to heat is caused by several mechanisms:

- there is thought to be a direct effect on capillaries, arterioles and venules, causing them all to dilate (Lehmann and de Lateur, 1982); the nature of this mechanism is not understood
- an axon reflex triggered by stimulation of polymodal receptors is an important cause of the vasodilation; in this mechanism only the peripheral branches of the afferent nerve fibres are involved

- increased metabolism will lead to further release of carbon dioxide and lactic acid, leading to greater acidity of the heated tissues, which tends to provoke dilation
- further heating can damage proteins; this may initiate an inflammatory reaction due to the release of histamine-like substances and bradykinins which evoke vasodilation (Lehmann and de Lateur, 1982).

It must also be recognized that the reduced viscosity of blood would contribute to the increase of blood flow. The foregoing accounts for the area being heated; other skin areas may well show cutaneous vasodilation to lose heat in response to impulses from the heat-regulating centre.

Cold induced vasodilation is somewhat different and the mechanisms are discussed in Chapter 9.

Increased blood flow in tissues other than skin has been shown to occur as a consequence of heating (Millard, 1961) but is much less marked and in some cases uncertain.

Blood and tissue fluid

As a consequence of the increased metabolic activity, decreased fluid viscosity and arteriole and capillary dilation (leading to a rise in capillary blood pressure and flow), there is an inevitable increase in fluid exchange across capillary walls and cell membranes. The acidity of the blood rises (pH falls) and both carbon dioxide and oxygen tensions increase. There is an increase in lymph formation and a higher blood leucocyte count.

Summary of the physiological effects of temperature change

Physical changes:
- metabolic rate raised by heating (about 13% per 1°C) and lowered by cooling (Van't Hoff's law)
- proteins denatured by sufficient heat, generally irreversible damage if maintained over 45°C
- freezing of fluids leads to tissue destruction
- blood and tissue fluid viscosity lowered by heating and raised by cooling
- softening of collagen due to heating.

Physiological changes:
- stimulation of sensory nerves by both heat and cold
- lowered nerve conduction due to sufficient cooling
- immediate skin arteriole vasodilation due to heating and vasoconstriction due to cooling
- subsequent skin vasodilation in some areas due to cooling (see Chapter 9)
- increased blood flow and tissue fluid exchange due to heating.

THERAPEUTIC EFFECTS OF LOCAL TISSUE HEATING

Encouragement of healing

From what has been considered above, it will be evident that any condition in which increased metabolic rate, cell activity and local blood flow were beneficial could be appropriately treated by mild heating. Thus heat has been found to encourage healing.

There seems to be general agreement that the application of heat to inflammatory injuries in the early stages is not beneficial, although it has been suggested that very mild inflammation may benefit from small temperature rises of between 2 and 5°C by increasing phagocytosis (Wadsworth and Chanmugan, 1980). Chronic inflammatory states and the stages of repair and regeneration are all appropriately treated with mild heating. All forms of therapeutic heating are applied to a wide range of chronic and post-traumatic conditions including the arthroses, soft tissue lesions and post-surgical healing.

Control of infection

The role of heat in the therapeutic control of infection by micro-organisms is not clearly defined. In so far as the defence mechanisms are enhanced by heat there is obvious benefit but, at the same time, heating may promote bacterial or viral growth and replication (Van't Hoff's law) thus negating any advantage. Historically, homely heat treatments, such as poultices, have been widely used. Some physiotherapeutic applications of heat to the surrounding healthy tissues of infected wounds have been used in the past. The availability of effective antibiotics has made this a largely otiose therapy over the past 40 years. However, all methods of enhancing the natural defence mechanisms, including heat, may be needed in the future.

Dry surface heating, achieved by infrared radiations or hot air, may have a particular role in the control of surface infections, such as chronic paronychia, a fungal (candida) infection, or other infections. Surface drying will diminish bacterial colonization.

Relief of pain

Therapeutic heat is widely used for the relief of pain. Several surveys of patients with persistent pain have found that some form of heat ranks highly, after analgesia, amongst the measures used by patients to control pain. For example, Barbour *et al.* (1986) found that heat was the most effective non-analgesic method of pain control being used in 68% of the cancer outpatients in their sample.

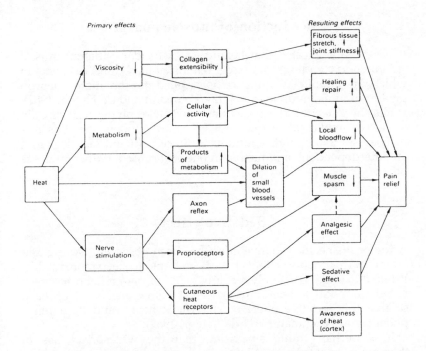

Primary effects

Resulting effects

Fig. 7.5 A simplified diagrammatic illustration of the pathways by which local tissue heating may alleviate pain. Heating the circulating blood will lead to cutaneous vasodilation in order to regulate body temperature. This is mediated via the hypothalamus and influenced by cutaneous thermoreceptors. This is in addition to the changes shown here.

Much therapeutic heating is of the skin. It is therefore reasonable to assume that the major pain relieving effects are mainly reflex as far as subcutaneous structures are concerned. Thus the stimulation of sensory heat receptors may activate the pain gate mechanism. The development of hyperalgesia as a consequence of mild heating (Cervero *et al.*, 1993) suggests that skin mechanoreceptor pathways are influenced which, in turn, may contribute to pain modulation, as discussed in Chapter 3.

A study investigating the sympathetic skin response to pain (Yagiz On *et al.*, 1997) found that therapeutic heat (hot packs giving skin temperatures near 45°C) significantly diminished the sympathetic palmar sweating response to painful electrical stimulation of a distant region. The authors suggest that this clear analgesic effect of heating may be due to suppression of cortical pain as a consequence of increased levels of endorphins and might also be due to local inhibition of both afferent and efferent C fibres.

Vascular changes could also reduce local pain. The increased blood flow that has been observed (Lehmann and de Lateur, 1982) could 'wash out' some of the pain provoking metabolites resulting from tissue injury (Wadsworth and Chanmugan, 1980). These include prostaglandins and bradykinin.

Other mechanisms that have been proposed to account for pain relief include the reduction of muscle spasm and the sedative effect (both considered below), as well as a decrease in sympathetic nervous system activity which is said to promote vasodilation in deeper blood vessels (Michlovitz, 1986).

The pathways by which local tissue heating may alleviate pain are illustrated in simplified form in Figure 7.5.

Reduction of muscle spasm

It has been suggested that heating the secondary afferent muscle spindle nerve endings and Golgi tendon organs could be a way in which an inhibitory influence is applied to the motor neuron pool to diminish muscle excitation (Lehmann and de Lateur, 1982). While this effect has been demonstrated by applying heat directly to nerves in the cat, it does not necessarily follow that this is a mechanism that operates in humans. Since pain and muscle spasm are interdependent, a reduction in one will cause a reduction in the other.

Sedative effect

A rather unspecific sedative effect has been observed. During and after heat treatments patients have been found to sleep more readily. While this might be simply a consequence of pain relief it has been noted that skin temperatures rise just before the onset of sleep so that this sedative effect of superficial heat could be a reflex phenomenon (Lehmann and de Lateur, 1982).

It is perhaps quite surprising that the widespread use of therapeutic heat for pain relief across many cultures and throughout recorded history is not yet afforded a satisfactory explanation. The use of heat is primarily based on empirical observation and the underlying mechanisms are unknown (Michlovitz, 1986). Despite the dearth of supportive clinical studies, there is still considerable acceptance of the use of heat for pain relief but its clinical use has declined over the last few decades.

It is well to remember the association of warmth with comfort and relaxation. This may lead to feelings of well-being when the body surface is warmed, which is a psychosomatic effect. Compare this with comments on cold in Chapter 9.

Increase of range of joint motion

There seem to be three mechanisms involved here:

- the analgesic effect of heat allows greater tolerance of stretching; a comparison of stretching the hamstrings with prior superficial heating gave a greater increase of hip flexion than stretching alone (Michlovitz, 1986)
- the viscosity of tissues will be reduced, which partly accounts for the reduction of joint stiffness that occurs with heating (Wright and Johns, 1961)
- increased collagen extensibility occurs at higher temperatures (Lehmann *et al.*, 1970).

Heat is therefore used prior to passive stretching and exercise to increase joint movement or lengthen scars or contractures, for example in the chronic stages of rheumatoid arthritis or any condition in which fibrosis is a marked feature. Similarly, scars in the skin or subcutaneous tissues would benefit by heat prior to stretching.

Apart from an increase in the range of joint motion, lowering the viscosity allows the joint, or other synovial tissue interfaces, to move more easily; the resistance to motion – stiffness – is reduced (Wright and Johns, 1961).

Prophylaxis of pressure sores

Heat applied to areas of skin subjected to prolonged pressure or friction has been suggested in order to promote a greater blood flow in the skin and thus decrease the risk of skin breakdown. Since the vasodilation effect is temporary – it lasts perhaps 30–60 min after the application – it would need to be repeated at intervals.

Oedema of the extremities

Heat has been recommended for the treatment of chronic oedema of the hand and foot (Wadsworth and Chanmugan, 1980). This must be given with the part in elevation since, as noted in Chapter 8, the application of superficial heating will tend to increase oedema if the part is dependent. Vessel dilation induced by heating will allow increased rates of fluid exchange and thus may help to increase the reabsorption of exudate. To be successful, the modality used would need to encompass the whole swollen region. Such heating arrangements coupled with active exercise are valuable in the treatment of hand injuries in general and those with an element of neurogenic pain, the reflex sympathetic dystrophies and in particular post-traumatic osteodystrophy.

Skin diseases

Fungal infections which are difficult to control and thrive in moist conditions, e.g. paronychia, are sometimes treated with regular infrared therapy, usually as a home treatment. The proper application may be taught to the patient by the physiotherapist. The thorough drying of the skin surface coupled with local vasodilation seem to be the effective factors.

Infrared radiation has also been used in the treatment of psoriasis on the grounds that moderate hyperthermia can affect cell replication and therefore could benefit a hyperproliferative disease like psoriasis. Note that psoriasis is commonly and effectively treated with ultraviolet (see Chapter 15). For studies involving the use of infrared radiations and other heat treatments for psoriasis see Westerhof *et al.* (1987) and Orenberg *et al.* (1980).

As a precursor of other treatment

Heat treatment is often used prior to other forms of treatment, e.g. muscle stretching, joint mobilization, massage or traction, in the belief that it will assist muscle relaxation and diminish pain. It is also used prior to exercise therapy for the pain-relieving effect and because it may contribute to muscle 'warm-up'.

Summary

The therapeutic effects of local tissue heating include:

- acceleration of healing
- control of infection
- pain relief and sedation
- reduction of muscle spasm
- facilitation of joint motion
- prevention of pressure sores
- reduction of oedema in elevated extremities
- resolution of some skin disease.

SITES OF TISSUE HEATING

Clearly the effects of local therapeutic heating will depend on the extent of heating – the volume of tissue heated and temperature reached – and on the particular tissues heated. The former is largely a matter of application and is determined by the extent and nature of the lesion to be treated. The latter is dependent on the modality used for heating. Thus modalities in which the energy is absorbed almost entirely at the surface, such as infrared radiation or conduction heating, will affect the skin and immediately underlying tissues, whereas the diathermies spread energy throughout deeper tissues. The important subject of energy distribution in the tissue is discussed with each modality in the appropriate chapter.

A further pertinent consideration is the spread of heat in the tissues. This occurs in two ways.

- conduction through the surrounding tissues (which is similar in most soft tissues to the conduction rate in water but notably less in fat and epidermis) is modest at the small temperature differences applied in therapy. The temperature of the epidermis has been shown to rise in an area only a few millimetres beyond the heated region (e.g. see Cervero *et al.*, 1993)
- dispersion of the heated blood accounts for most of the spread of energy in the tissues (i.e. thermal convection due to the blood flow). The increased blood flow in the dermis, as a consequence of heating the skin surface, is clearly evident as an erythema, and serves the protective function of dissipating heat from the skin to prevent a damaging skin temperature rise.

Ultimately, the raised systemic blood temperature and impulses from skin thermoreceptors will trigger reflex activity in the hypothalamus to stimulate the heat loss mechanisms of the body. This will cause vasodilation of other parts. This effect can be used therapeutically. If a proximal limb segment is heated the distal segment (and other parts) may show initial vasoconstriction followed by marked vasodilation. The initial brief constriction occurs to maintain normal blood pressure as the heated area of skin dilates. The subsequent vasodilation, to lose heat, increases the skin blood flow. Thus injuries involving the skin of the extremities can be treated without heating or even touching the affected tissues. Similarly, if skin ischaemia is present the blood flow can be increased without risk.

Such therapy is often called reflex heating and can be of considerable benefit in the treatment of injuries of the extremities, which should be elevated during treatment. It has also been used in the treatment of peripheral ischaemia due to arterial disease, but without evidence of any consistent long-term benefit.

Although temperature is the major factor controlling vasodilation, it must be recognized that other factors contribute and are superimposed upon the vascular reflex. The onset of vigorous exercise will lead to some cutaneous vasoconstriction, for example (Johnson and Park, 1982).

TISSUE DAMAGE DUE TO EXCESS LOCAL HEAT – BURNS

Burns are of considerable importance in medicine. Permanent skin damage or loss is a serious disability if anything more than a tiny area is involved.

It has been shown that skin temperatures over 45°C cause tissue damage but this depends on the length of exposure as well as the temperature. The sensation of heat gives way to one of pain at this same temperature; the pain increases in intensity with rising temperature. Both injury and the resulting pain are considered to be due to permanent damage to proteins in the basal skin cells.

It is important to understand the relationship between time, temperature and the resulting damage. Thus skin temperature around 45°C can be tolerated for, perhaps, an hour or so before damage occurs but with higher temperatures the period shortens so that 50°C can be tolerated for about 1 min or so and 65°C about 1 s or so (Hardy, 1982). This refers to skin temperature. Many much hotter objects can be touched for short periods without causing a burn but they do not necessarily lead to sufficient heat transfer to raise the skin to the same temperature. Most people have experience of touching a very hot object, say a saucepan of boiling water with a temperature about 100°C, yet because the hand is removed very quickly no damage occurs, except a transient erythema.

This has important implications in the immediate treatment of burns. The damaged area should be cooled as quickly as possible.

Table 7.4 Methods of heating and modes of heat transfer to the tissues

Method	Mode of transfer
Superficial heating	
Heat from outside transferred to skin by conduction, convection or radiation – does not pass the thermal barrier	Hot water bottle
	Hot pack
	Hydrocollator
	Hot water bath
	Hot muds
	Wax bath
	Electric heat pad
	Fluidotherapy
	Hot air/hairdrier
	Hydrotherapy
	Infrared radiation
Deep heating	
One form of energy converted to heat in the tissues – can pass the thermal barrier	Ultrasound
	Shortwave diathermy
	Microwave

Cold water should be applied at once; a scalded hand should be plunged immediately into cold water.

Testing thermal sensation

This is necessary in the safe application of heat treatments. The customary method is to apply two test-tubes of water at 40–45°C and 15–20°C randomly to the area, asking the patient to identify which is which with the eyes shut. The temperature difference between the tubes falls during the test so that patients are actually discriminating between only a few degrees Celsius. (Any other method that requires the patient to distinguish small temperature differences is perfectly satisfactory.) Temperatures over 45°C or much below 15°C should not be used because these may test pain rather than thermal sensations.

Summary

Therapeutic heating can thus be divided into:

- *Superficial heating* due to heat conduction or infrared radiation being produced by hot packs and similar means, as described in Chapter 8, and infrared lamps, as described in Chapter 13.
- *Deep heating*, also referred to as conversion or conversive heating, due to the conversion of energy passing through the tissues to heat, as with ultrasound (Chapter 6), shortwave (Chapter 10) and microwave diathermy (Chapter 12). (Strictly speaking, infrared radiation is also conversion heating.)

The distinction between these two groups is important; the skin and subcutaneous fat act as a thermal barrier to conduction and much radiation heating, thus limiting the heating of deeper tissues. There are, of course, indirect effects on deeper tissues mediated through the nervous system or due to the heated blood being carried to other parts. In contrast, the conversive methods, or diathermies, are able to generate heat in both superficial and deep tissues, as explained in Chapters 6, 10 and 13, much like metabolic heating (see Table 7.4).

REFERENCES

Barbour L. A., McGuire D. B., Kirchott K. T. (1986). Non-analgesic methods of pain control used by cancer outpatients. *Oncol. Nursing Forum*, **13**, 56–60.

Cervero F., Gilbert R., Hammond R. G. E. *et al.* (1993). Development of secondary hyperalgesia following non-painful thermal stimulation of the skin: a psychophysical study in man. *Pain*, **54**, 181–9.

Cetas T. C. (1982). Thermometry. In *Therapeutic Heat and Cold* (Lehmann J. F., ed.) Baltimore: Williams & Wilkins, pp. 35–69.

Fischer E., Solomon S. (1965). Physiological responses to heat and cold. In *Therapeutic Heat and Cold* (Licht S., ed.) Baltimore: Waverley Press, pp. 126–69.

Fox R. H., Woodward P. M., Exon-Smith A. N. *et al.* (1973). Body temperature in the elderly: a national study of physiological, social and environmental conditions. *Br. Med J.*, **1**, 200–6.

Gammon G. D., Starr I. (1941). Studies on the relief of pain by counterirritation. *J. Clin. Invest.*, **20**, 13–20.

Guyton A. C. (1982). *Human Physiology and Mechanisms of Disease*. Philadelphia: W. B. Saunders.

Hardy J. D. (1982). Temperature regulation, exposure to heat and cold and effects of hypothermia. In *Therapeutic Heat and Cold* (Lehmann J. F., ed.) Baltimore: Williams & Wilkins, pp. 172–98.

Holwill M. E., Silvester N. R. (1973). *Introduction to Biological Physics*. London: John Wiley.

Hubbard J. L., Mechan D. J. (1987). *Physiology for Health Care Students*. Edinburgh: Churchill Livingstone.

Johnson J. M., Park M. K. (1982). Effect of heat stress on cutaneous vascular responses to the initiation of exercise. *J. Appl. Physiol.*, **53**, 744–9.

Kanui T. I. (1985). Thermal inhibition of nociceptor-driven spinal cord nerves in rats. *Pain*, **21**, 231–40.

Kitchen S. S., Partridge C. J. (1991) Infra-red therapy. *Physiotherapy*, **77**, 249–54.

Lehmann J. F., de Lateur B. J. (1982). Therapeutic heat. In *Therapeutic Heat and Cold* (Lehmann J. F. ed.) Baltimore: Williams & Wilkins, pp. 404–562.

Lehmann J. F., Masock A. J., Warren C. G. *et al.* (1970). Effect of therapeutic temperatures on tendon extensibility. *Arch. Phys. Med. Rehabil.*, **51**, 481–7.

Mason T., Rigby B. J. (1963). Thermal transitions in collagen. *Biochim. Biophys. Acta*, **66**, 448–50.

Michlovitz S. L. (1986). Biophysical principles of heating and superficial heat agents. In *Thermal Agents in Rehabilitation* (Michlovitz S. L. ed.) Philadelphia: Davis, pp. 99–118.

Millard J. B. (1961). Effect of high frequency current and infra-red rays on the circulation of the lower limb in man. *Ann. Phys. Med.*, **6**, 45–60.

Orenberg E. K., Derau D. G., Farber E. M. (1980). Response of chronic psoriatic plaques to localized heating induced by ultrasound. *Arch. Dermatol.*, **116**, 893–7.

Sekins K. M., Emery A. F. (1982). Thermal science for physical medicine. In *Therapeutic Heat and Cold* (Lehmann J. F., ed.) Baltimore: Williams & Wilkins, pp. 70–132.

Wadsworth H., Chanmugan A. P. P. (1980). *Electrophysical Agents in Physiotherapy.* Marrickville, NSW, Australia: Science Press.

Westerhof W., Siddiqui A. H., Cormane R. H., Scholter A. (1987). Infrared hyperthermia and psoriasis. *Arch. Dermatol. Res.,* **279**, 209–10.

Wright W., Johns R. J. (1961). Quantitative and qualitative analysis of joint stiffness in normal subjects and in patients with connective tissue diseases. *Ann. Rheum. Dis.,* **20**, 36–46.

Yagiz On A., Colakoglu M. D., Hepguler M. D., Aksit R. (1997). Local heat effect on sympathetic skin responses after pain of electrical stimulus. *Arch. Phys. Med. Rehabil.,* **78**, 1196–9.

8 Therapeutic conduction heating

Body surface warming – a comforting warmth – is, perhaps, the most primitive panacea for pain. The therapeutic application of heated substances directly to the skin will be the subject of this chapter.

The transfer of heat to the body surface is largely by conduction, hence the title, but there is also some transfer by radiation since all heated bodies emit some infrared radiation. Although the effects are very similar, it seems sensible to describe pure infrared heating separately in Chapter 13.

First, some general points concerning tissue temperature changes as a consequence of local surface heating are discussed.

A list of superficial heating methods was given in Table 7.4 of the previous chapter. Some of those that involve conduction heating are then considered with their method of application; i.e. paraffin wax, hydrocollator packs, contrast and whirlpool baths, hot air treatment and fluidotherapy and finally electric heater pads.

The chapter concludes with some further consideration of the effects and therapeutic uses of conduction heating.

When local heating is applied to the body it does not normally cause a rise in core temperature. As already explained, the heat added in one place is dispersed throughout the body – by conduction and convection – to be lost at other surfaces. Thus local temperature rises will be a balance between heat input and dispersion. As noted above, if the temperature is high enough to cause tissue damage, that is above 45°C, the time in which this damage occurs becomes shorter as the temperature rises. In the therapeutic situation such high skin temperatures are not applied so that after a local rise in temperature the dispersion mechanism can keep pace with the heat input. This allows local heat to be applied indefinitely without producing tissue damage.

The rate of temperature rise at any given point in the tissues due to local heating depends on:

- the temperature applied
- the size of the area involved
- the thermal conductivity of the tissues.

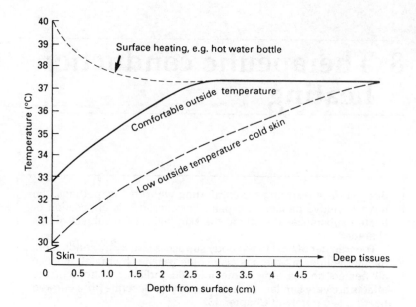

Fig. 8.1 Tissue temperature gradients.

Since epithelium and fat have lower conductivities than the watery tissues, heat will flow more readily in tissues deep to the skin and the superficial fat layer (Sekins and Emery, 1982). It follows that heat transfer by conduction within the tissues will be obstructed by the subcutaneous fat layer, and the temperature increase will tend to be confined to the area of skin heated. With a thicker subcutaneous fat layer the effect is more pronounced, which accounts for the slightly higher skin temperature found in women at environmental temperatures above 30°C, as illustrated in Figure 7.2.

The main way in which heat is moved through the tissues is by forced convection in the blood and lymph. Thus heat flow in the tissues is almost entirely due to blood flow. Consequently, cutaneous dilation will markedly increase heat transfer to the deeper tissues (see Fig. 7.4). As the specific heat of fat is only some 60% of that of blood, it takes more heat energy to raise the temperature of the subcutaneous tissue when it is highly vascularized. Thus, vasodilation inhibits rapid local temperature rise in both ways.

Local tissue heating is, of course, superimposed on the existing tissue temperature gradient which has been described in Chapter 7 in terms of temperature 'shells'. Application of heat to the surface will reverse this gradient locally (Fig. 8.1).

The rise in superficial tissue temperature does not occur instantly. As would be expected the skin temperature rises first, subcutaneous tissue temperature rises more slowly, and a very small change in superficial muscle temperature (of 1°C or so) takes as long as 20 or 25 min to occur. This is illustrated in Figure 8.2, which shows the temperature of various tissues against time: these data are based on studies by Lehmann *et al.* (1966) using the hydrocollator hot pack, and conform with others, e.g. Michlovitz (1986). The pattern

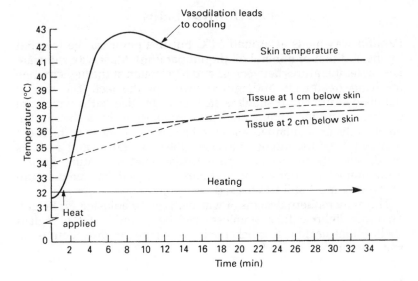

Fig. 8.2 Rise in temperature of tissues during heating.

would be similar whatever form of superficial heat were applied. Although the hot packs used cooled over the 30-min period, repeating the application every 10 min prolonged heating but made very little difference to the pattern (Lehmann *et al.*, 1966).

The marked rise in skin temperature of some 10°C contrasts with the trivial rise in deep-tissue (e.g. muscle) temperature of 1°C or so. Some experimental studies (on dogs) have demonstrated rather higher muscle temperatures of 4.7°C, when using hot packs on the skin (McMeeken and Bell, 1990). The skin temperature may actually decrease after some minutes, as shown, because the increased blood flow due to cutaneous vasodilation cools the skin. After some 25–30 min these vascular and tissue temperature changes have stabilized so that continued heating leads to no further change. This accounts for the customary practice of applying such treatments for 20–30 min. After the heat source is removed the tissue temperatures fall slowly back to normal, skin more rapidly than deeper tissues.

Summary

Local conduction heating of the skin surface leads to:

- a marked and rapid rise in skin temperature (sometimes followed by a slight fall) over some minutes – then a steady skin temperature is maintained
- marked cutaneous vasodilation evidenced by an erythema
- a slight rise in deep tissue temperature reaching a steady state in some 30 minutes or so
- dissipation to, and heat loss from, other parts to maintain heat balance.

Paraffin wax baths

Paraffin wax melts at around 54°C but this point can be lowered by the addition of mineral oil (liquid paraffin). Most wax baths are kept at temperatures between 42 and 52°C, often at the higher range for hand treatments and rather lower for the feet. The wax is maintained molten in stainless steel or enamelled baths which are electrically heated; temperature is kept constant by a thermostat. Some baths are contained within a heated outer water bath. There may be a fixed thermometer to check the temperature and a means of adjusting the thermostat setting to alter the temperature. Even if a thermometer is not an integral part of the bath the temperature of the wax must still be checked.

The more modern designs of wax bath can be adjusted for height. They are light, with a stainless steel bowl and outer fibreglass shell. Initial heating is quicker with this type because there is no waterjacket to be heated.

Method of application

The most widely used method of application is 'dip and wrap'. This can only be used for the extremities – hands, wrists, feet and ankles.

Preparation of the patient. The nature of wax treatment is explained and the area to be treated is inspected for contraindications.

Preparation of the apparatus. The temperature of the wax is checked.

Preparation of the part. The part is washed and thoroughly dried to prevent water being introduced into the wax bath. The patient is positioned to be able to dip the part in the wax in a convenient and comfortable way.

Application. The part is immersed for a second or so in the wax, withdrawn and allowed to cool for 2 or 3 s and then reimmersed. It is important to immerse the part briefly otherwise the outermost coating is melted off and the thickness of wax does not build. The procedure is repeated 6–12 times to produce a coating of wax 2 or 3 mm thick over the body part. The part is then put into a plastic bag or paper cover and wrapped in a blanket or towel to limit the rate of heat loss to the air. For any condition in which there is a proclivity for oedema the part should be elevated. Adequate elevation in which the part is kept above the level of the heart is of the utmost importance since otherwise the heating effect will tend to exacerbate swelling of the extremities.

Termination of treatment. The 'glove' of wax is normally left in place for some 15 min by which time the wax is completely solid although still malleable, so that it can be removed in one piece.

To achieve a higher skin temperature for longer periods the 'dip and leave in' method can be used. After a suitably thick layer of wax has been built up by a succession of dips the part is left in the wax bath for 15 or 20 min; this method can produce a much greater increase in tissue temperature (Abramson *et al.*, 1964), but it necessitates the hand or foot remaining dependent throughout the treatment, which is often deleterious.

If the part cannot be immersed in wax it is possible to coat the surface by either painting the wax on using a large brush, or ladling it over the part with a suitably large bowl placed beneath: the knees can be treated in this way. Alternatively, bandages of a suitable size and mesh can be soaked in the hot wax and then wrapped around the limb; additional wax can then be brushed over the bandage. These latter methods are infrequently used because of the inconvenience but are valuable if other methods are inappropriate. After use the wax is cleaned in a purifier and reused.

Mode of action of paraffin wax heating

Despite the fact that skin temperatures above 45°C can lead to damage it is possible to put the hand comfortably in a bath of wax at some 50°C. Water at the same temperature would be uncomfortably hot and ultimately cause damage. This is because the specific heat of paraffin wax is about 2.72 kJ/kg/°C, or less with added mineral oil, and therefore much lower than that of water at 4.2 kJ/kg/°C. Thus the amount of energy released by wax cooling 1°C is less than that of water. Perhaps more importantly, when the part is immersed in wax the cooler skin causes a thin layer of wax to solidify on the surface. Due to the relatively low thermal conductivity of wax this static layer acts to insulate the skin from the hotter surrounding wax: some air may be trapped between this solidified layer and the skin, adding to the insulating effect (Griffin and Karselis, 1988).

The wax transmits heat energy to the tissues by giving up energy as it solidifies – the latent heat of fusion – without any temperature change. This amount of energy is quite small: about 35 kJ/kg (Sekins and Emery, 1982). Although the temperature of the thin layer of wax on the tissues falls quite quickly on its outside surface the low thermal conductivity prevents much heat loss from the skin surface. It also prevents any evaporation of water from the skin thus further improving the insulating qualities. The net effect is to provide remarkably effective low-temperature heating of the part.

When it is considered that the hand and foot have a relatively large ratio of surface area to volume and that the wax is applied evenly over all this surface, as well as the fact that there is relatively little subcutaneous tissue separating the small joints of the fingers and toes from the skin, it can be understood why such mild heating appears to be therapeutically effective. Certainly there is widespread approbation amongst patients who suffer with painful and stiff joints for this form of heat.

As a consequence of preventing water loss from the surface of the skin the wax treatment tends to leave the skin with more

Practical point

A way of achieving the benefits of prolonged higher temperatures coupled with elevation is to place the wax-covered part in a loose-fitting plastic bag which is secured with a bandage around the wrist or ankle. The part is then elevated into a warm-air cabinet (simple heat cradle or infrared lamp will work); air temperature is about 70°C. This method can be combined with active exercise of the part while the limb is in elevation. The wax may fall away as it cools but a thin layer usually remains even as the fingers are moved. This method has been described for the treatment of post-traumatic osteodystrophy.

moisture hence feeling soft and pliable. This may be therapeutically valuable if the skin is dry. It is also claimed to soften adhesions and scars in the skin (Wadsworth and Chanmugan, 1980).

Contraindications and dangers

- Wax is, of course, sterile as no organisms can live in pure oil. Wax should not, however, be allowed to enter an open wound since it will set in the tissues acting as an inert foreign body and delay healing.
- Large pieces of dirt in the wax bath may harbour organisms but it is extremely unlikely that these could ever lead to infection.
- Patients with skin infections of the part are not usually treated as heat may increase the inflammatory activity.
- Some individuals may become allergic to the wax with extended and prolonged treatments but this is rare.
- Acute dermatitis may be made worse by wax, or indeed any form of heat on the skin.
- Circumstances in which there is defective thermal sensation coupled with deficient cutaneous circulation, as occurs with recently healed skin grafts, should not be treated.

Wax is highly inflammable if it becomes overheated so it is a sensible precaution to have a fire blanket and suitable carbon dioxide or foam extinguisher available. Pouring water on blazing wax is ineffective and dangerous because the wax floats on the water surface. Wax also renders the floor very slippery if spilt, so any spillage must be promptly dealt with.

Hydrocollator packs

These consist of a silicate gel, such as bentonite, enclosed in a cotton fabric container. This gel will absorb large quantities of water which, if it is hot, provides a considerable store of heat energy. The gel is contained in a set of separated fabric pockets, like a duvet, so that the whole pack is flexible and the gel confined. The packs are made in various sizes to fit different body areas. They are heated by being placed in a special tank of water warmed to 75–80°C by an electric heater controlled by a thermostat. The packs, supported on racks in the tank, take about 2 h to become fully heated from cold but rather less when being reheated.

The method of application follows the usual format, as described above, of explanation, preparation of patient and apparatus and the necessary checking for contraindications. This latter should include thermal sensitivity because, unlike wax treatment, the application is at a temperature that could cause tissue damage if the insulation is not adequate.

The hot packs are wrapped in towelling before being applied to the part so that some four to eight layers, depending on towel thickness, intervene between the pack and the skin. This provides thermal insulation, largely because of the air in the towelling, so that although the pack is at about 75°C the skin temperature does not rise above 42°C or so. It takes some time (about 8 min: Lehmann *et al.*, 1966) for the skin temperature to reach its maximum. During this time the pack temperature is falling but the towelling and pack prevent the skin surface from losing heat so that the skin and superficial tissue temperature rises, as indicated in Figure 8.2. The towelling can be separated from the wet pack by a plastic sheet which prevents wetting of the towel and thus enhances the insulating effect; in this case less towelling may be used. If lower temperature packs (e.g. 65°C) are used less thickness of towelling is needed.

The packs are left in place for 20–30 min.

Other packs

There are various forms of hot moist packs which have been used therapeutically. A piece of absorbant lint or woollen material soaked in almost boiling water and then wrung out (using gloves) can be applied to the skin when the temperature has fallen to about 60°C. After about 5 min the pack will have fallen to skin temperature, at which point it is replaced. Such packs, often called Kenny packs, have been widely used in the past as a means of reducing the muscle soreness and tightness associated with poliomyelitis.

Mud packs (peloids), notably kaolin and peat, have been used as hot moist packs because it was considered that their chemical composition gave them specific therapeutic properties. This is no longer believed; in fact some peat may cause skin irritation, so it is now usual to apply cleaner and more convenient moist packs such as the hydrocollator type, described above.

Contrast baths

Contrast baths involve alternate immersion in hot and cold water producing marked hyperaemia of the skin. Such treatment will cause considerable sensory stimulation as the cutaneous hot and cold receptors are alternately activated. This stimulation is relatively vigorous because each time neural accommodation starts to occur the temperature stimulation is reversed. This strong sensory stimulation may act to suppress pain by means of the gate mechanism (see Chapter 3) and account for the subjective relief of pain that occurs in many patients receiving this treatment. It is also considered by many that contrast baths will help to reduce local oedema by promoting alternate vasodilation and vasoconstriction.

Method of application

An explanation and examination are given in the usual way already noted. In this case, testing skin sensitivity is appropriate, not to obviate any risk but because the treatment is intended to provoke sensory stimulation.

Practical point
If a fresh hot pack is used every 10 min the heating may be prolonged but there is no difference in the temperature reached in the subcutaneous tissues (Lehmann *et al.*, 1966). This is due to the control of heating exerted by the insulating effect of the fat layer and the heat removed by convection in the blood due to vasodilation, as already explained.

Two suitably sized baths are filled, the hot at 40–45°C and the cold at 15–20°C (water from the cold tap is usually in this range). It is usual to start and finish with immersion in the hot water. The period of immersion in the hot water is longer – 3 or 4 min – while immersion in the cold water is kept to 1 min. This cycle is repeated three or four times so that the whole treatment lasts anything from 15 to 25 min. An initial hot immersion of 10 min has been recommended to achieve hyperaemia (Lehmann and de Lateur, 1982).

During the treatment the hot water will cool and the cold will be warmed, partly due to the transfer of the warm/cold wet limb from one bath to the other. It is therefore usually necessary to top up both baths during treatment. This is not a problem that arises with large volumes of water. A thermometer should be available to check the water temperature.

Hydrotherapy

Warm water has been used for therapeutic purposes since ancient times particularly where the presence of natural warm water has provided an opportunity for the development of spas. In thermal areas in some parts of the world such as Iceland or New Zealand, the water appears as geysers or bubbles up in hot mud. Such sources often contain sulphur and other minerals. Ground water is forced to the surface after permeating deeply placed, and hence hotter, rock formations. Also in some limestone areas, e.g. the Mendips, water is carried deeply in porous rock to become heated; it emerges at Bath at about 46°C.

Swimming and exercising in warm water have beneficial effects which were often ascribed to the minerals dissolved in the water. As the whole body is immersed and the major therapeutic effect is considered to be due to the exercise rather than the water temperature, hydrotherapy is outside the scope of this book and other texts such as *Hydrotherapy, Principles and Practice* by Reid Campion (1996) or *Duffield's Exercise in Water* by Skinner and Thomson (1983) should be consulted.

Whirlpool baths

Whirlpool baths are stainless-steel tanks or baths of various sizes. The smaller ones are made to accommodate one limb, while larger ones allow the patient to sit. The 'whirlpool' refers to turbulence produced by an electric pump, or compressed air, which mixes air and water into a jetstream. This water agitation can be varied in force by controls on the pump (or turbine) and air pressure. The direction of the stream can be altered by changing the position of the output nozzle. A mixing tap allows any desired water temperature; temperatures between 36 and 41°C are usually employed.

The agitation of the water, the whirlpool effect, serves to stimulate the skin surface mechanically. This stimulation of large-diameter mechanoreceptors and thermoreceptors may account for the analgesic effects (Walsh, 1986), being due to the gate mechanism discussed in Chapter 3. The mechanical effect is further used in the cleaning of open wounds – gentle debridement of dirt and necrotic tissue. Vigorous action can also destroy the delicate granulation. In circumstances where healing is slow, such as varicose ulcers, the mechanical effect is considered to provoke granulation tissue formation by increasing the local blood flow; this gives a gentle massaging effect. Although the water in these baths is changed for each patient it is often advisable to add an antibacterial agent to the water. Sodium hypochlorite (bleach) in 1 to 120 dilution is recommended (Walsh, 1986).

There is evidence that the temperature of the subcutaneous tissues rises with whirlpool bath treatment, like any other form of conduction heating (Borrell *et al.*, 1980), and thus there is a consequential increase in blood flow. There is also evidence that treatment in the whirlpool increases oedema; an increased tissue volume was found both in patients and in healthy subjects (Magness *et al.*, 1970). This is unsurprising since the extremities must be dependent during immersion in the warm water. If oedema is a likely problem it would be reasonable to modify the treatment so that it is followed by a period of warmth and/or exercise with the limb in elevation.

Treatment is usually given for a period of 20 min since longer treatments appear to give no greater benefit, at least in so far as tissue-heating is concerned. Prolonged immersion in hot water leads to temporary wrinkling of the skin which in healthy skin recovers rapidly on drying. However, repeated soaking tends to increase the risk of skin infection and exacerbate any infection already present; atrophic skin is particularly at risk.

Contraindications to treatment with hot water

There is very little chance of damage with these treatments since mild heat and simple, familiar materials are used:

- Local burns are only possible if very hot water is allowed to contact the skin; this could happen with the careless application of a hydrocollator pack or hot compress. With these treatments it is as well to be sure the patient has normal thermal sensitivity.
- Since local thermal regulation depends on the ability to increase cutaneous blood flow it is important to be aware of any ischaemic disease that might prevent an adequate vasodilatory response. This would apply to conditions in which the peripheral arteries were structurally damaged, such as arteriosclerosis or Buerger's disease, but not necessarily those due to vasospasm.
- If the whole body, or large segments, are immersed the heat loss mechanism of the body is affected because if the water temperature is above core temperature there is no way of losing heat from the areas under the water. Patients who have any deficiency of the cardiovascular or heat-regulating mechanism may be at risk in these circumstances.

- Apart from the risks associated with excess heat there are some infections that are encouraged by wetness of the skin, notably certain fungal infections, the best known being tinea pedis (athlete's foot) and paronychia, which thrive in warm moist conditions. The presence of such conditions indicates that some form of dry heat would be more suitable or the part should be enclosed in a thin plastic bag, achieving the thermal effects without wetting the skin.
- Acute dermatitis or eczema may be exacerbated by immersion in hot or warm water or, for that matter, by any other form of heat. Similar considerations apply to inflammation of the skin due to radiotherapy or chemical irritants of any kind; in these circumstances the application of heat should be avoided.
- The effects of heat and limb dependence have already been noted. Thus the presence of oedema can be seen as a contraindication in some circumstances.

Heated air treatment

Both simple hot, dry air and a mixture of air and water vapour are described as hot air baths. Small hot air cabinets – a metal box fitted with an electric fan or element heater, both thermostatically controlled – have already been mentioned in connection with wax treatment of the hand. They are useful for hand injuries with oedema and open wounds as the hand can be exercised in elevation and nothing but warm air comes in contact with the tissues. Temperature in the metal cabinet should be about 70°C, but because of the low thermal conductivity of air, the skin temperature is kept much lower.

Small fan heaters, such as hairdriers, are occasionally used to dry and give mild heating to open wounds such as bedsores. Hot or hot moist air has been applied by enclosing the whole body in special cabinets. This can produce a small rise in body core temperature and needs strict control and adequate body fluid replacement.

Fluidotherapy

Warmed air, thermostatically controlled, is blown through a mass of tiny cellulose particles (a powder) which become suspended in the moving air in a large metal cabinet. The effect is to produce a fluid-like mixture into which the distal part of the limb can be immersed through a hole in the box. The viscosity of the system is relatively low so that exercise can be performed in the moving particles – not unlike moving in warm water without the wetness.

The air temperature can be regulated; treatment is usually given at anything between 38 and 45°C although somewhat higher temperatures can also be used. The amount of particle agitation can be varied and this determines the amount of skin stimulation. This treatment differs from hydrotherapy in that sweating can still act effectively as a heat loss mechanism.

Treatment is usually given for 20 min and is considered useful because it provides mechanical as well as thermal stimulation.

To sterilize the powder and thus obviate any risk of cross-infection between patients an additional heater is used. Any open wound must be covered during this treatment to prevent the powder entering the tissues.

Electric heating pads

These vary from small pads about 30×30 cm to electric blankets. Electric resistance wire is contained in a suitable fabric and a set of resistances provided in a control unit so that the pad can operate at various temperatures. The resistance wire is heated and warms the fabric which when placed against the skin gives conduction heating. Such pads are often used as a convenient way of achieving muscle relaxation or relaxing muscle spasm prior to other treatments such as exercise or mobilization.

Heating and cooling apparatus

A device has been developed which can heat or cool the skin surface by means of varying the temperature of a circulating fluid. A flexible applicator, in which fluid circulates, is held in contact with the tissue surface. This 'cyclotherm' system is able to apply a temperature up to 40°C and down to 1°C, and vary it between these limits at a rate of approximately 13°C per minute. The device can be programmed to apply predetermined temperatures for pre-set times for thermotherapy, cryotherapy and, perhaps most usefully, thermal contrast therapy (see Contrast baths and Chapter 9).

Summary

Therapeutic thermal conduction methods:

- wax baths – heating and moistening skin
- hydrocollator packs – heating
- water and mud packs – heating
- contrast baths – heating and cooling
- whirlpool baths – heating and mechanical stimulation
- hot air – heating
- hot air and powder – heating and mechanical stimulation
- electrical heating pads – heating
- 'Cyclotherm' apparatus – heating and cooling.

THE EFFECTS OF SUPERFICIAL HEAT ON THE TISSUES

As has been explained, applying heat to the skin leads to reflex responses in order to dissipate the local heat. There is local skin vasodilation in the heated skin and subsequently vasodilation of skin vessels elsewhere to increase the body's heat loss. Thus when heat is applied to the skin surface, either as conduction heating or as radiation, little heating of the deeper tissues occurs because they are shielded by the thermal insulation provided by the subcutaneous fat and the fact that heat is removed in the increased skin blood flow.

However, some conduction to the local deep tissues does occur and it is this that justifies the use of superficial heat for the treatment of such structures; for example, applying hot packs to the knee for the treatment of chronic arthritis.

Weinberger *et al.* (1989) measured the intra-articular and skin temperatures of five patients with bilateral knee effusion. Hot packs at 42°C were placed on the right knee for 30 min and the temperature of both knees was recorded. Small but statistically significant rises in intra-articular temperature occurred in the treated knees a little later than the skin temperature rise. In the control knee there was no significant change in the intra-articular temperature but the skin temperature increased somewhat, although less than that of the heated knee. Other studies (e.g. Borrell *et al.*, 1980) have also found small temperature increases in joint structures due to superficial heating.

In an interesting study of the motor performance of normal hands, Kauranen and Vanharanta (1997) found that heat (hydrocollator hot packs) applied to the forearm and hand led to a small increase in finger tapping speed which persisted for at least 30 min. No effect on the speed of movement of the whole hand was found. In contrast, this study found quite marked changes due to cooling in several measures of motor activity (see Chapter 9). Hot packs also, rather curiously, were found to delay reaction time; an effect ascribed by the authors to diminished mental alertness as a consequence of greater relaxation induced by the warmth.

THE THERAPEUTIC USES OF SUPERFICIAL HEATING

The various forms of superficial heating are widely used for pain relief; the mechanisms have been discussed in Chapter 7. Since the effects are largely confined to the skin it is reasonable to propose that the major pain-relieving effects are largely reflex as far as subcutaneous structures are concerned. The other therapeutic effects due to heat, discussed in Chapter 7 and illustrated in Figure 7.5, are attributable to conduction heating.

Summary

Therapeutic uses of superficial heat:

- the relief of pain
- the relief of muscle spasm
- sedation
- acceleration of healing, especially of superficial injuries
- promotion of resolution of chronic inflammatory states
- increase of the range of joint motion or lengthening scar tissue
- facilitation of fine movements.

In spite of the fact that the main circulatory changes due to conduction heating occur in the skin, rather than in the underlying structures in which the painful lesion is often located, there is a widespread acceptance of the efficacy of mild superficial heating. This may be due to the excitation of cutaneous receptors, as discussed in Chapter 7. It has also been suggested that the very mild heating which occurs in the deeper tissues (see Figs 8.1 and 8.2) is particularly beneficial to promote resolution of mild inflammatory states and accelerate repair (Wadsworth and Chanmugan, 1980).

REFERENCES

Abramson D. L., Tuck S., Chu L. S. W. *et al.* (1964). Effect of paraffin bath and hot fomentations on local tissue temperature. *Arch. Phys. Med. Rehab.*, **45**, 87–94.

Borrell P. M., Parker R., Henley E. J. *et al.* (1980). Comparison of 'in vivo' temperatures produced by hydrotherapy, paraffin wax treatment and fluidotherapy. *Phys. Ther.*, **60**, 1273–6.

Griffin J. E., Karselis T. C. (1988). *Physical Agents for Physical Therapists*, 3rd edn. Springfield, Illinois, USA: Charles C. Thomas.

Kauranen K., Vanharanta H. (1997). Effects of hot and cold packs on motor performance of normal hands. *Physiotherapy*, **83**, 340–44.

Lehmann J. F., de Lateur B. J. (1982). Therapeutic heat. In *Therapeutic Heat and Cold* (Lehmann J. F., ed.) Baltimore: Williams & Wilkins, pp. 404–562.

Lehmann J. F., Silvermann D. R., Baum B. A. *et al.* (1966). Temperature distribution in the human thigh produced by infra-red, hot pack and microwave applications. *Arch. Phys. Med. Rehab.*, **47**, 291–9.

Lehmann J. F., Masock A. J., Warren C. G. *et al.* (1970). Effect of therapeutic temperatures on tendon extensibility. *Arch. Phys. Med. Rehab.*, **51**, 481–7.

Magness J., Garret T., Erickson D. (1970). Swelling of the upper extremity during whirlpool baths. *Arch. Phys. Med. Rehab.*, **51**, 297.

McMeeken J. M., Bell C. (1990). Effects of selective blood and tissue heating on blood flow in the dog hind limb. *Exp. Physiol.*, **75**, 355–66.

Michlovitz S. L. (1986). Biophysical principles of heating and superficial heat agents. In *Thermal Agents in Rehabilitation* (Michlovitz S. L., ed.) Philadelphia: F. A. Davis, pp. 99–118.

Reid Campion M. (1996). *Hydrotherapy, Principles and Practice*. Oxford: Butterworth-Heinemann.

Sekins K. M., Emery A. F. (1982). Thermal science for physical medicine. In *Therapeutic Heat and Cold* (Lehmann J. F., ed.) Baltimore: Williams & Wilkins, pp. 70–132.

Skinner A. I., Thomson A. M. (eds) (1983). *Duffield's Exercise in Water*, 3rd edn. London: Baillière Tindall.

Wadsworth H., Chanmugan A. P. P. (1980). *Electrophysical Agents in Physiotherapy*. Marrickville, NSW, Australia: Science Press.

Walsh M. (1986). Hydrotherapy: the use of water as a therapeutic agent. In *Thermal Agents in Rehabilitation* (Michlovitz S., ed.) Philadelphia: F. A. Davis, pp. 119–39.

Weinberger A., Fadilah R., Lev A. *et al.* (1989). Intra-articular temperature measurements after superficial heating. *Scand. J. Rehab. Med.*, **21**, 55–7.

Wright V., Johns R. J. (1961). Quantitative and qualitative analysis of joint stiffness in normal subjects and in patients with connective tissue diseases. *Ann. Rheum. Dis.*, **20**, 36–46.

9 Cold therapy

Cold therapy or cryotherapy refers to the use of local or general body cooling for therapeutic purposes. The latter is of importance for major cardiac surgery but it is the former – local cryotherapy – that is the subject of this chapter.

The effects of cooling the surface of the skin are dealt with first, followed by discussion of the therapeutic uses of cold therapy.

Major methods of applying cold are then described, including immersion, cold packs, ice towels, ice massage and evaporating sprays.

Finally, dangers and contraindications are noted.

Cooling the body surface is simply the transfer of energy away from the tissues. The result is to lower the local tissue temperature and provoke the thermoregulatory responses described in Chapter 7. Although cooling can be achieved in several ways, such as evaporating liquids or blowing cold air over the skin, the vast majority of cold treatments are given with crushed ice. Heat is thus transferred by conduction from the skin and the energy is used in changing solid ice to water. It takes a great deal of energy to melt ice ($333\,J/g$). In fact, more than twice as much energy is needed to melt 1 g of ice than is subsequently needed to raise the temperature of the resulting gram of water from 0°C to 37°C.

Temperature changes in the tissues will depend on both the rate and amount of heat energy removed. Thus for a constant source of cooling the temperature drop in the tissues will depend on:

- The temperature difference between the coolant and the tissues: the colder the application the greater the heat loss from the tissues.
- The thermal conductivity of the tissues. This differs from one area to another. In general, water-filled tissues, such as muscle, have a high thermal conductivity compared to fat or skin (see Chapter 7). Thus the cooling of deep tissue depends on the nature of the overlying tissue. The normal layer of subcutaneous fat serves as thermal insulation so that heat loss through the tissues – or cold penetrating the tissues, which is the same thing – is largely dependent on the blood flow.
- The length of time for which the cold is applied. The amount of energy loss is clearly dependent on time; temperature falls until energy lost at the surface is balanced by heat energy

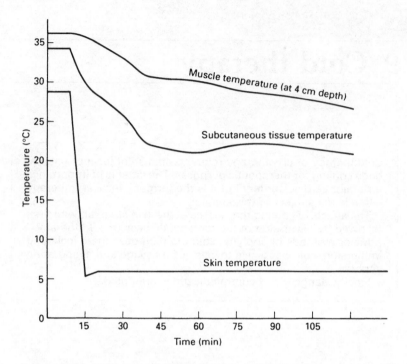

Fig. 9.1 Example of temperature changes in tissues of the calf on application of ice bags. Modified from Bierman and Friedlander (1940).

supplied from the rest of the body, at which point the temperature becomes constant.

• The size of the area that is being cooled. The larger the area, the more heat energy is lost.

While the skin temperature can be changed abruptly and markedly with the application of cold the deeper tissues are cooled much less and much more slowly. This has been demonstrated by several investigators. Figure 9.1 illustrates this point. In this example it takes some 30 min to lower the muscle temperature at a depth of 4 cm by 3.5°C or so. Muscle tissue at 2.5 cm can take up to 20 min or longer to drop 5°C (Palastanga, 1988).

Oosterveld *et al.* (1992) found that the intra-articular temperature of the knee joint fell by an average of 9.4°C due to the application of a 3 kg bag of ice chips applied for 30 min to the front of the knee. This remarkably low intra-articular temperature was associated with a fall of 16.4°C in the knee skin temperature of these normal subjects. The paucity of subcutaneous fat over the knee joint may account for the lower than expected intra-articular temperatures.

PHYSIOLOGICAL CHANGES DUE TO COOLING THE SKIN

Putting ice on the skin surface leads to local changes at the cooled site and general systemic changes as the heat-regulating mechanism of the body is activated (see Chapter 7).

The local effects

On cutaneous blood vessels

There is immediate vasoconstriction of cutaneous blood vessels, shown by the blanching that occurs. This restricts the blood flow in the skin so that heat loss is minimized. The speed with which this vasoconstriction occurs indicates that it is a reflex in the autonomic nervous system, which is triggered by stimulation of the thermal receptors in the skin. There is also considered to be a direct effect of cold on the smooth muscle of the arterioles. In addition the precapillary sphincters, which are influenced by local hormones (e.g. serotonin and bradykinin), may be involved in local thermoregulation (Lee and Warren, 1978). This vasoconstriction leads to a dramatic decrease in blood flow through the skin, and hence limits the conduction of heat to the body surface. The increased blood viscosity, due to cooling, will also contribute to the slowed blood flow.

After some minutes the vasoconstriction may give way to a marked vasodilation which itself may last some 15 min before being replaced by another episode of vasoconstriction. This alternation of constriction and dilation is called the Lewis 'hunting reaction' (Lewis, 1930), in the sense that the vessel 'hunts' or oscillates about its mean position. This cold-induced vasodilation occurs most easily when the rest of the body is relatively warm and is largely confined to certain body areas. It occurs most readily and most rapidly in the face, especially the nose and ears, but also in the hands, feet, patella region, olecranon, buttocks and some parts of the chest wall (Fox and Wyatt, 1962).

The explanation for this curious response to cold seems to be that it serves to protect the tissues from damage due to prolonged cooling and relative ischaemia. This idea is supported by the fact that it occurs most vigorously in areas that are exposed and in those regions on which pressure occurs – buttocks, anterior surface of knees and particularly the feet. Fox and Wyatt (1962) noted that cold-induced vasodilation was more readily induced in the lateral (weight-bearing) part of the sole of the foot than in the medial area. This response is variable from person to person. It tends to occur about 10 min after cold application and rather more rapidly, about 5 min, in the face. It will be noted that the peripheral areas that exhibit strong cold-induced vasodilation are well endowed with arteriovenous anastomoses in the skin (see Fig. 7.4), suggesting that these play a predominant role; however, cold-induced vasodilation is variable and does not always show the clear-cut cycling effect.

The cause of this vasodilation is still not completely elucidated. Originally an axon reflex mechanism involving a histamine-like substance (substance H) to cause local vasodilation was suggested (Lewis, 1930). As the increased blood flow washes out this substance the vessels constrict again thus continuing the cycle. Later suggestions include the possibility that as the temperature falls so smooth muscle activity is diminished and constriction is no longer possible. The consequent vasodilation rewarms the part, the smooth muscle recovers and it constricts again.

On muscle blood flow

The foregoing account applies to the skin only, a region involved in thermal regulation. The response of muscle blood flow to cooling is less dramatic. It seems likely that cooling provokes vasoconstriction in all vascular smooth muscle and the increased viscosity certainly reduces the blood flow.

Cooling a localized area of one forearm for 15 min has been shown to lead to a temperature drop not only in the underlying muscle, which reached maximum cooling about 18 min after cooling, but also in the same muscle on the other forearm (Wolf, 1971). The cooling of the contralateral forearm took much longer (42 min) to reach the lowest temperature. It is suggested that this effect might be therapeutically useful since it would allow some beneficial effects of muscle cooling to be achieved in, say, a hemiplegic patient by local icing of the unaffected side.

One striking feature of studies investigating muscle cooling is the length of time it takes to reach maximum cooling and the even longer period needed for rewarming. After heating, muscle temperatures rapidly return to normal because the vasodilation and lowered viscosity allow a high blood flow thus removing excess heat rapidly; after cooling the blood flow is diminished for the opposite reasons, so that muscle rewarming takes a good deal longer. The muscle is also shielded from warming from the surface by the subcutaneous fat layer.

On metabolic rate

The principal effect of cooling living tissue will be to reduce its metabolic rate in accordance with Van't Hoff's predictions discussed in Chapter 7. This will affect the activity of all tissues. Most evident will be the reduced oxygen uptake; in fact the erythema due to cold-induced vasodilation is distinguished from that due to heating due to its 'pinkness' because it contains less reduced haemoglobin. Thus cooling does not benefit the healing process.

On the peripheral nervous system

Cold applied to the skin provides a strong sensory stimulus by stimulating the cold receptors. This may be used therapeutically in the suppression of pain and treatment of hypertonicity. If the cold is sufficiently intense it reduces the conduction velocity of peripheral nerves. Synaptic transmission can also be delayed. All nerve fibres are not equally affected by cooling. As might be expected the small-diameter non-myelinated slow-conducting group IV C fibres are least affected; similarly, the B fibres, also small but myelinated and mainly preganglionic autonomic, are also little affected. The A delta fibres are the most susceptible to cold. These are small and thinly myelinated and are pain and temperature carriers; they are closely

Table 9.1 Peripheral nerve fibres affected by cooling

Most affected by cold		Moderately affected by cold	Least affected by cold
$A\beta(II)$	Intrafusal muscle fibres Low-threshold mechanoreceptors	$A\alpha$ Extrafusal muscle fibres Cutaneous, joint and muscle receptors	*B* Preganglionic efferent autonomic
$A\gamma$	Intrafusal muscle fibres		*C* Postganglionic efferent autonomic
$A\delta(III)$	Fast pain High-threshold mechanoreceptors Thermoreceptors above 45°C		Slow pain, polymodal Nociceptors Thermoreceptors

followed by A beta and A gamma fibres (Table 9.1) (Douglas and Malcolm, 1955). This evidence was gained from studies on isolated animal tissues and it must be recognized that it may not apply to intact human tissues. Both motor and sensory nerve conduction velocities have been shown to be reduced (in the ulnar nerve) by cooling (Lee *et al.*, 1978). This study, in common with several others, showed that the effect of cooling lasted considerably longer than the application of ice.

Abramson *et al.* (1966) showed that cooling the forearm led to a marked fall in the motor nerve conduction velocity of the median and ulnar nerves and that these changes were strongly correlated with the tissue temperature fall. (Warming tended to raise the motor nerve conduction velocity to a peak at a temperature a little above core temperature and higher tissue temperatures had an inconsistent effect.)

On the motor system

Muscle strength is diminished by cooling the limb in water at 10–15°C, probably because of its effect on viscosity and metabolic rate, but there is evidence that the strength increases over the original value about an hour or so after cooling has ceased. Briefly applied cold, i.e. 5 min of ice massage, has also been found to increase isometric strength (Michlovitz, 1986; see discussion below).

Motor skills are diminished as a consequence of local cooling, again unsurprisingly since the loss of dexterity in cold hands is a common experience. This effect occurs at temperatures above those at which muscle strength is decreased. Kauranen and Vanharanta (1997) have shown that an ice pack applied for 15 min to the forearm causes a significant decrease in the velocity of movement and finger tapping speed. These effects could be due to diminished nerve conduction and/or a direct slowing effect on muscle contraction.

Summary

The local effects of cooling include:

- Immediate perception of cold and pain:
  - cold receptors are stimulated
  - pain receptors responding to cold may be stimulated.
- Immediate vasoconstriction of cutaneous vessels followed by cold-induced vasodilation in some areas, which may continue in a cyclical manner.
- Lowered metabolic rate; Van't Hoff's law:
  - reduced oxygen uptake
  - reduced production of metabolites
  - reduced cellular activity
  - slowed healing.
- Subsequent reduced blood flow in muscle and other deep tissue.
- Effects on peripheral nervous system due to reduced nerve conduction; reduction of:
  - pain
  - hypertonicity
  - dexterity and speed of fine movement.
- Variable effect on muscle strength.

General effects of cooling

Cooling applied to the skin immediately stimulates cold receptors which are more numerous than heat receptors in any given area of skin. Although some of these cold receptors will be firing at normal skin temperatures their activity increases greatly as cooling occurs, diminishing somewhat when cooling becomes steady, i.e. they show adaptation. Extreme cold is experienced as pain, involving pain receptors (see Chapter 7). Both pain and temperature neurons synapse in the posterior horn of the spinal cord; the subsequent neuron ascends in the spinothalamic tract of the opposite side. Apart from a synapse in the thalamus with a neuron to the sensory cortex, giving awareness of cold, there are many collateral paths, particularly to the hypothalamus.

As explained in Chapter 7, the hypothalamus acts as a thermostat to maintain core temperature. The posterior hypothalamus is concerned with the response to body cooling, being affected by nervous input from the skin and probably other receptors as well as the blood temperature. To conserve heat the response, via the vasomotor centre, is cutaneous vasoconstriction. The skin blood flow can be increased (see Fig. 7.4) by vasodilation much more than it can be diminished (Hubbard and Mechan, 1987), indicating that humans are better adapted to a hot environment; this is also evidenced by the efficiency of the human sweating response. The degree of general vasoconstriction that occurs is dependent on the extent of the cooling. Further, if the temperature drop is great enough shivering will occur. This increases metabolism, and hence heat production, by irregular muscle contractions. The resting metabolic rate can be doubled by shivering over periods of several hours and rather more over shorter periods (Hardy, 1982). However, it is expensive in physiological terms in that energy is being expended. As noted in Chapter 7, brown adipose tissue in neonates is able to produce heat by directly metabolizing but this does not seem to occur significantly in adults. Shivering in the muscles of mastication gives rise to the familiar teeth chattering with cold.

Awareness of cold leads to behavioural responses to maintain body temperature such as increased activity or putting on more clothes.

THERAPEUTIC USES OF COLD

Recent injuries

Cold is widely used in the treatment of recent injuries. When bleeding occurs on the skin surface cold serves to promote immediate vasoconstriction and makes the blood more viscid; both diminish the flow. Combined with pressure over the wound such treatment leads to haemostasis. However, the cooling must not be so intense or so prolonged as to delay blood coagulation – clotting time is lengthened by cooling. When bleeding occurs deep in the tissues, forming an intramuscular haematoma, for example, the same principle would apply but much longer periods of cold application would be needed to achieve cooling at this depth, as illustrated in Figure 9.1 and noted earlier.

The immediate treatment of cutaneous heat burns requires rapid cooling of the area, as described in Chapter 7. Prompt cooling lowers the tissue temperature and thus limits tissue damage.

Soft tissue injuries of all kinds are almost universally treated by cold in the early stages. During this time the inflammatory changes occur in a well recognized sequence: the severity depends on the injury (see Chapter 1). The amount of pain will be related to the rate at which this oedema and chemical irritation occurs. Cooling will diminish the rate of swelling and production of irritants and so alleviate the pain. Compression and elevation of the part will also limit oedema formation. Thus the initial treatment of traumatic injuries can be defined by the acronym PRICE, standing for protection, rest, ice, compression and elevation.

The effect of cooling on metabolism is important in limiting the extent of the injury. Cell necrosis occurs over a period of several hours, releasing lysins and provoking local oedema. This leads to secondary cell damage which extends the area and severity of tissue injury. Therefore cooling in the early stages of injury, during the initial 2 h, will minimize secondary cell necrosis by reducing the metabolic rate (McLean, 1989). There is histological evidence that cooling can lessen the inflammatory reaction: experiments on pigs investigating the effects of ice on injured ligaments showed less inflammation when the ligaments were cooled compared to controls

(Farry *et al.*, 1980). This study also showed that some swelling occurred in the subcutaneous tissues after removal of the ice in both injured and uninjured joints; the significance of this finding and whether it occurs in humans is not known.

Pain

Pain can be alleviated by the application of cold in several ways. The reduction of oedema and decreased release of pain-inducing irritants, mentioned above, is one. A direct effect on the conduction of pain receptors and neurons, reducing the velocity and number of impulses, is another. It is evident that this latter effect would only occur in the skin and then only if the temperature is much reduced. It is unlikely that the unmyelinated C fibres would be affected since they have been shown to continue to conduct at very low temperatures (see Table 9.1). The thinly myelinated A delta fibres which carry well-delineated 'fast' skin pain would be more susceptible. However, the pain due to tissue injury would be carried by C fibres and this is the pain that is usually being treated.

The immediacy of the effect of cold on pain suggests that it may act like other sensory stimuli on the pain gate mechanism (see Chapter 3) and since cold stimuli are quite intense they may lead to the release of endorphins and encephalins by the same mechanism (Palastanga, 1988). The fact that cold will effectively relieve pain, at least temporarily, has been supported by many studies, e.g. Benson and Copp (1974).

Ernst and Fialka (1994), in their review paper, also concluded that ice may be useful for a variety of musculoskeletal pains, yet the evidence for its efficacy should be established more convincingly. Hay-Smith and Reed (1997) similarly found that while ice is commonly applied for perineal pain and that there is some evidence that it has a short-lived analgesic effect, there was a complete absence of trials comparing ice/cold with a control or no treatment group.

Muscle spasm

Muscle spasm is linked to pain in that the pain of an injury appears to provoke muscle spasm as a protective measure. It has been suggested that the consequence of muscle spasm in causing tissue ischaemia may provoke further pain leading to a self-perpetuating cycle (Lee and Warren, 1978). There is therefore a reasonable expectation that the application of cold would reduce muscle spasm and so allow an increased range of movement.

Spasticity

Cooling has been used clinically for many years to reduce muscle spasticity. There is good objective evidence to support this, for example cold producing a marked decrease in ankle clonus, described by Peterjan and Watts in 1962. The mechanisms by which the reduced spasticity may be brought about have been studied extensively (see reviews in Lee and Warren, 1978 and Lehmann and de Lateur, 1982) without being fully elucidated. It is apparently not only the hyper-reflexia which can be affected but skilled activity of the upper limb has been shown to improve in hemiplegic patients after cooling in a 12°C bath (Hedenberg, 1970). Thus cryotherapy can lead to an improvement of neuromuscular function.

There would appear to be more than one mechanism by which cooling can affect spasticity, operating at two different sites, one in the skin and the other in the muscle itself. The immediate effect of stimulating cold receptors in the skin is to provide stimulation to the central nervous system. This is used therapeutically to facilitate muscle contraction – briefly stroking with ice over the appropriate dermatome, for example. Ice cube stroking over the biceps for 1–2 min has been shown to enhance the motor unit activity of subjects who had learned to activate a single motor unit with the aid of electromyogram biofeedback (Clendenin and Szumski, 1971).

Cutaneous stimulation also appears to have reflex effects, diminishing gamma motor neuron activity or at least in some way diminishing the muscle spindle discharge, and so reducing spasticity. However, it is not known how much of the effect is due to cold and how much to mechanical stimulation. It is also possible that sympathetic stimulation may contribute. Such effects would occur almost immediately as the skin temperature fell; a drop in muscle temperature would take longer, as already noted, but would also last much longer (Peterjan and Watts, 1962).

It has been suggested that muscle cooling might lead to reduced muscle spasticity by reason of the differential effect of cooling on the small myelinated fusimotor efferents and secondary afferents on the one hand, and the large thickly myelinated motor nerves to the extrafusal fibres on the other. It will be recalled that conduction in the former is more easily affected by cooling than in the latter (Table 9.1). The muscle spindle activity is diminished, lessening the stretch reflex, while the extrafusal muscle fibres, supplied by the less susceptible A alpha nerves, are unaffected. Changes in the viscostatic properties of muscle tissue may also play a part since cooling makes the muscle – both intrafusal and extrafusal fibres – more viscid thus allowing less rapid stretching.

It must be recognized that there is a range of different responses to cooling; the responses of neurologically damaged patients are notably inconsistent (Urbscheit *et al.*, 1971). In order to ascertain the effectiveness of cooling as a means of reducing spasticity for any particular patient it would seem advisable to apply sufficient cold at least to reduce muscle temperature, i.e. for 25–30 min (Lehmann and de Lateur, 1982).

Muscle strengthening

There is evidence that cooling the skin surface can lead to greater strength of the underlying muscles, although there are also conflicting reports of a strength decrease following cryotherapy. Most investigators have concerned themselves with isometric strength. For example, Rajadhyaksha *et al.* (1982) found an increase of around 17% in the strength of the quadriceps after 30 min of ice applied to the anterior aspect of the thigh compared with a control group. Interestingly this was to some extent retained 24 h later.

The muscle strength increase has been ascribed to a facilitatory effect on the alpha motor neuron pool, at least in the short term. Sympathetic system stimulation has also been suggested as the mechanism for greater immediate muscle strength; cold stress has a potent effect on the sympathetic system and catecholamine release. On the other hand if the muscle is cooled it will be more viscid and thus use more energy on contraction, resulting in weakness. This, it has been suggested, would account for the finding of lowered muscle strength on cooling. These contradictory findings may thus be reflecting a difference in the degree of cooling in different investigations, the shorter applications stimulating the nervous system, while prolonged intensive cooling affects muscle metabolism leading to weakness.

Chronic inflammatory conditions

The value of cold therapy for acute inflammatory conditions is both rational and supported by clinical experience but this is not entirely the case with chronic inflammatory conditions. Many degenerative and chronic joint diseases have been treated successfully with cold therapy, including osteoarthrosis and chronic rheumatoid arthritis. Cold may well be beneficial in these conditions by virtue of its pain-relieving effect or because it may help to control such minor acute or subacute inflammatory changes as occur from time to time with degenerative joint conditions. Alternating hot and cold packs, or contrast baths, may be effective (Wadsworth and Chanmugan, 1980).

Chronic oedema and joint effusions

That cold treatment reduces chronic oedema is widely recognized. A study by Moon and Gragnani (1989) has attempted to quantify this effect in nine hemiplegic patients whose swollen hands were intermittently immersed in water at around 10°C for 30 min. Although hand volumes are variable, both between subjects and at different times in the same subject, there was a reduction in hand volume in all patients; it was statistically significant in eight of them. During both treatment and measurement these hands were dependent; combining treatment with elevation may lead to even better results.

As well as interstitial oedema, inflammatory joint effusions are benefited by cooling. The application of ice and a compression bandage for an acute joint effusion are almost universally recognized treatments. The application of cold for obstructive oedema, such as that due to deep vein thrombosis, has a less rational basis and is not usually recommended.

Other therapeutic effects

Ice massage has been used in treatment of pressure sores, as have ice packs, although the former is considered more effective (Lee and Warren, 1974). The beneficial effects are said to be due to the fact that cooling reduces vascular stasis.

The effectiveness of cryotherapy is widely asserted, particularly for acute lesions. A number of studies comparing cold with other therapies have supported the superiority of cryotherapy. However, as noted by Fahrer (1991) the results are not completely convincing and demonstrate what is described as 'a strong trend for effectiveness'.

Summary of the therapeutic uses of cold

- *Applied to recent injuries*:
  - limits bleeding by vasoconstriction and increased blood viscosity
  - limits pain by reducing the rate of oedema formation and production of pain nerve irritants
  - reduces the metabolic rate and hence secondary cell necrosis
  - reduces joint effusion/oedema.
- *Alleviation of pain*:
  - acts as above
  - reduces the conduction of some pain nerves in skin
  - provides sensory stimulation, acting on the pain gate
  - gives a strong cold sensation leading to endorphin release.
- *Reduces muscle spasm*:
  - is linked to the effect on pain above.
- *Reduces muscle spasticity*:
  - provides stimulation of cutaneous receptors and reflex inhibition of muscle activity
  - affects the muscle spindle directly by more prolonged cooling
  - increases viscosity which may diminish rapid stretch reflexes.
- *Facilitates muscle contraction and may affect muscle strength*:
  - provides brief stimulation of skin receptors – ice massage.
- *Others* include reduction of chronic inflammation and joint effusion.

METHODS OF APPLYING COLD THERAPY

Cooling of the body surface may be achieved by

- the application of a substance at a lower temperature, thus conducting heat energy away from the surface
- evaporating a chemical of low boiling point from the tissue surface.

The former is by far the most widely used and the majority of cold treatments are given with melting ice. To achieve cooling over any but the smallest body region it is convenient and efficient to use flaked (or crushed) ice since this provides a large surface area of ice from which melting can occur. Ice blocks have the disadvantage of exerting local pressure which can impede circulation. Flaked ice is conveniently made in ice-making machines which produce a continuous supply of consistently sized flakes and store them in a large container. These machines work on the same principle as an ordinary domestic electric refrigerator and are usually plumbed in to the water supply.

Technique of application of cold therapy

For all the different methods considered below the general features of the technique of application follows the format set out in Chapter 1.

Preparation of patient.   The reasons for, and nature of, the cold treatment are explained to the patient. This is perhaps particularly pertinent with ice treatment for the psychological reasons noted below. Examination of the area to be treated is carried out to ascertain the absence of any contraindications.

Preparation of apparatus.   The means of applying cold is checked, including the correct temperature of the water bath.

Preparation of part.   A suitable position and support for the part is arranged, depending on whether it is to be immersed or have a pack applied. The need for elevation and relaxation of the part are considered. Oil is applied to the skin if appropriate.

Instructions for the patient.   The patient is instructed what to do and warned to indicate any increased pain or discomfort.

Application.   During treatment it is appropriate to check the application every few minutes and inspect the skin at the same time. The onset of both vasoconstriction and vasodilation should be noted.

Termination.   The cold application is removed and the skin is dried and inspected once more.

Local immersion

This is the simplest method of all. It involves placing the part in a container of iced water – a mixture of water from the cold tap and flaked ice. The temperature can be controlled by varying the amount of ice used. At temperatures around 16–18°C continuous immersion can usually be tolerated for 15–20 min (Lee and Warren, 1978). At lower temperatures, such as around 10°C, continuous immersion is uncomfortable, so that intermittent application is usually given. This is done by leaving the part in the water for only 1 min or so at a time.

Clearly such treatment can only be conveniently applied to the extremities – hand, forearm, foot and leg – which can be placed in a water bath. When the limb remains still in the water bath for relatively long periods it is necessary to agitate the water occasionally because the layer of water in contact with the skin tends to warm up; also the water temperature should be checked from time to time as it will gradually become warm and more ice may need to be added.

Cold packs

Ice packs

Flaked ice is folded into damp terry-towelling or put into bags made of the same material and applied directly to the skin. They may be held in place by a plastic sheet wrapped around the part and the pack. Placing the pack beneath the part is not advisable because the weight of the tissues, causing local ischaemia, may allow excessive cooling, leading to an ice burn. A further towel or blanket is occasionally wrapped outside the plastic to decrease heat gain to the ice pack from the outside air.

Cooling of the skin is quite rapid at first as the ice-cold water seeps through the towelling but after a minute or so the layer of water in contact with the skin tends to warm up somewhat so that these packs are quite tolerable for some 20 min. If the pack is removed after a few minutes and immediately reapplied with a fresh cold surface in contact with the skin, greater and more rapid cooling is achieved. However, rapid cooling can sometimes lead to skin damage (see below) so it is sometimes recommended that a thin layer of oil is smeared over the skin and separated from the towelling with paper. The aim is to provide some insulation to reduce the rate of cooling and to cause a rapid run-off of water from the skin. In all ice pack treatments in which the pack remains stationary, a thin layer of water on the skin surface tends to be held at a higher temperature than that of the ice pack. This means that the skin temperature is usually above the 0°C of melting ice, often around 5–10°C.

Flaked ice may also be put in a suitably sized polythene bag; the top of the bag is tied to prevent water leaking out. This ice-filled bag can be moulded to fit the region to which it is being applied and a damp towel is used to separate the bag from the skin, with the skin oiled if there is thought to be any danger of cold injury to the surface. As the water from the melting ice is confined within the bag this is a clean and convenient method of application.

Comparisons between these two methods, in which a wet towel is placed between the ice and the skin, and the use of ice in a dry plastic bag, have been made (De Domenico *et al.*, 1991). No significant differences were found between the cooling efficiencies of the three methods when the ice was removed, and it is suggested that the methods are interchangeable.

In all treatments with ice packs the bag should be removed after a few minutes to inspect the underlying skin to determine the response, and if it is considered abnormal the pack is not replaced.

Commercial cold packs

These are basically plastic, often vinyl, bags filled with a mixture of water and some substance that prevents the water freezing solid; thus the pack will remain flexible and can be moulded to the part. Silica gels are the most common.

Commercial cold packs are of various sizes but normally small enough to store in the freezer compartment of a domestic refrigerator. The pack will therefore be stored at a temperature below 0°C, often −5°C or even −12°C. It is important to be aware that initially these packs are at a lower temperature than ordinary ice packs and therefore have the potential to cool the skin very rapidly. However, their temperature rises rapidly on application and most of the cooling is due to melting ice which is at 0°C.

Depending on their size such packs may provide adequate cooling for about 20 min. As a precaution these packs can be applied over a wet towel to prevent ice burns (Harrison, 1978). As long as the towel remains wet as opposed to frozen it ensures that the surface in contact with the skin is not below 0°C.

Patients are sometimes advised to use bags of frozen peas as an ice pack for home treatment. Again the wet towel should be placed between the skin and the pack to avoid excessive cooling.

A totally different kind of cooling pack consists of chemicals which are mixed by breaking a container within the main pack; the resulting endothermic reaction causes strong cooling of the pack. These are, of course, one-use-only packs and are thus more appropriate for first-aid applications. If such a pack should accidentally be ruptured the contents should not be allowed to remain on the patient's skin since some are strongly alkaline and can cause irritation.

The only advantage of commercial packs seems to be convenience since it has been found that ice packs lower subcutaneous temperatures better than the chemical packs (McMaster *et al.*, 1978).

Ice towels

If a terry-towel is put into a mixture of flaked ice and water and then wrung out, much of the chipped ice will be found to adhere to the cloth. This can be placed over quite a large area to give immediate surface cooling. The ice towel will need to be replaced by another one after 2 or 3 min (or after 1 min in the case of the first towel) to give adequate cooling; say 20 min in total. It is a particularly useful technique for the treatment of muscle and allows movement and/or exercise to be performed while cold therapy is being applied.

Ice massage

This is given with a solid piece of ice, either as an ice cube wrapped in paper or cloth or an ice 'lollipop' on a wooden stick. This latter can be made quite simply by putting a wooden tongue depressor (spatula) upright in a small plastic cup of water in the freezer. Being larger, the lollipop lasts longer and is easier to handle than the usual size of ice cube.

There are two distinct purposes for ice massage:

- For the relief of pain, the ice block is moved over the part using a slow circular motion for some 5–10 min. During this time the patient will feel cold, burning and then aching sensations before the part finally becomes numb.
- For neurological facilitation the ice should be applied only briefly, either dabbing for about 4 s at a time or short strokes. The application should be over the dermatome supplied by the same nerve roots as those of the muscle that is to be stimulated.

Cold-compression units

Cold therapy combined with intermittent compression devices to a limb segment are available. Cold water is circulated in a sleeve which is put over the limb and part of it is inflated at intervals. Cooling can also be achieved in a similar way with the 'cyclotherm' system, as described in Chapter 8.

Evaporating sprays

Spraying a rapidly evaporating liquid on the skin has the effect of using heat energy and hence cooling the surface. Ethyl chloride was originally used but it is highly inflammable and thus posed some risk. Other sprays, e.g. fluorimethane, are non-flammable. The liquid is sprayed on to the area to be cooled in a series of short strokes of about 5 s each with a few seconds' interval between each. The nozzle of the spray is held about 45 cm from the skin surface and close to a right angle. Cooling from such sprays can be very rapid but does not last very long. If spraying near the face care should be taken to avoid the eyes and prevent the vapour from being inhaled.

Summary of methods of application of cold therapy

- *Conduction cooling*:
  - immersion
  - cold packs
    - standard ice packs
    - commercially made cold packs, either reusable or single use
  - ice towels
  - ice massage
    - slow and prolonged (10–15 min) for pain relief
    - brief (few seconds) for muscle facilitation
  - cold-compression and cold fluid units.
- *Evaporative cooling*:
  - evaporating spray.

CONTRASTING HEAT AND COLD TREATMENTS

In the sense that heating the tissues adds energy whereas cooling extracts energy these are obviously opposite treatments. However, many conditions appear to benefit from either thermotherapy or cryotherapy. This is not a contradiction, for some of the effects are indirect and the total effect on the tissues is complex. The apparent paradox has spawned several studies of superficial heat and cold applied to the same condition for comparison. For example, a cross-over comparative trial on chronic rheumatoid arthritic knees (Kirk and Kersley, 1968) showed little objective difference but cold was associated with somewhat more pain relief. Pain thresholds in the shoulders of healthy subjects (Benson and Copp, 1974) were found to be raised by both heat and cold but significantly more so by the latter.

In summary:

- both heat and cold appear to be useful in relieving pain and muscle spasm
- spasticity is reduced by cooling
- recent trauma benefits from immediate cooling, reducing bleeding, rate of oedema formation and pain
- later, the same injury will benefit from mild heating to increase metabolism and gently increase the healing processes; cold has been shown to slow down healing
- the tendency to oedema is encouraged by heating but decreased by cooling
- skilled movements are impaired by cooling
- muscle activity can be facilitated by brief local cooling
- joint stiffness is decreased by heating and increased by cooling.

DANGERS AND CONTRAINDICATIONS

There are two ways in which tissue injury might occur.

- Excessive local cold causing damage to normal tissues.
- Normal local cooling causing damage due to some predisposing pathological condition.

Damage in either circumstance is rare.

Excessive local cold on normal tissue

The mildest form consists of the appearance of erythema and tenderness of the skin a few hours after the application of ice, subsiding in a day or two; this is called an ice burn. A more severe form, an ice burn with fatty necrosis, shows bruising as well as more tenderness and can last up to 3 weeks (Lee and Warren, 1978). Such injuries are rare and are said to occur in areas which are underlain by thick subcutaneous fat and which have been cooled rapidly. Inadequately crushed ice can lead to a large piece being held against the skin for a long time, which increases the possibility of an ice burn. There have also been some reports of peripheral nerve damage due to locally applied cold (Covington and Bassett, 1993). These have occurred in situations where the nerve is superficial.

With extreme cold freezing of the tissues can occur but this is extremely unlikely ever to occur with the treatment methods described above. What happens depends on the rate of cooling; if it is rapid ice crystals can form in the cells which may lead to cell death, whereas slower cooling tends to cause freezing of the extracellular fluid and withdrawal of water from the cells. This is referred to as 'frostbite' and only occurs if the body suffers extreme exposure; similar prolonged exposure to low temperatures without freezing the tissues, 'immersion foot' for example, can also produce severe tissue damage.

Certain pathological conditions

Cold sensitivity

Vasospasm. Raynaud's phenomenon is a condition often associated with connective tissue disorders in which excessive vasoconstriction, triggered by cold, occurs in the digital arteries. Obviously cold treatment should not be used to provoke vascular spasm. Some other vascular conditions may have an element of vasospasm as well as obstruction, such as thromboangiitis obliterans (Buerger's disease), and therefore should not be treated with cold. With vascular disorders which are primarily obstructive, such as arteriosclerosis, cold treatments are considered unsuitable by some, but the reasons are unclear. Since cold reduces the metabolic rate it is difficult to see what harm can occur as the tissues are already partly ischaemic; in fact cooling is temporarily beneficial in relieving pain.

Cryoglobinaemia.   An abnormal protein is present in the blood; it can form a precipitate at low temperatures blocking blood vessels and thus causing local ischaemia. Although not common, this condition can also be found in association with some of the connective tissue disorders such as systemic lupus erythematosus and rheumatoid arthritis.

Cold urticaria.   Cold causes the release of histamine from mast cells leading to a local weal and erythema and sometimes general (systemic) symptoms such as lowered blood pressure and raised pulse rate.

Cardiac disease

Coronary thrombosis and anginal pain have sometimes been provoked by cold, leading to the suggestion that locally applied ice may cause reflex vasoconstriction of the coronary arteries and should therefore not be given to patients who have coronary artery disease. Injunctions to avoid ice treatment, especially of the left shoulder, for such patients have frequently been repeated but with little supporting evidence. The matter has been studied by electro-cardiographically monitoring 25 patients who had known coronary artery disease while ice packs were applied to the left shoulder (Lorenze *et al.*, 1960). Only one of these patients showed changes in the electrocardiogram of any significance. It seems likely that any effect on the heart is due to greater demand due to increased blood pressure. Thus careful local cooling is reasonable for these patients but cooling large areas should be avoided (Lee and Warren, 1978).

Arterial blood pressure

Cooling larger areas, such as a limb segment, can lead to a transient rise in arterial blood pressure. This could well be dangerous for hypertensive patients or those with especially labile blood pressure. Monitoring the blood pressure during and for a short time after treatment would be advisable if large areas are to be cooled and there is uncertainty regarding the blood pressure response.

Summary

Contraindications to cold therapy:
- vasospasm
- cryoglobinaemia
- cold urticaria
- special care with
  - cardiac disease
  - hypertension
  - areas underlain by thick subcutaneous fat
  - close to superficial nerves.

Sensory deficiency

It is sometimes asserted that ice should not be applied to areas with some sensory deficiency (e.g. Wadsworth and Chanmugan, 1980), but this seems illogical since cooling can lead to partial sensory loss anyway and it can be safely applied to an anaesthetic area (Lee and Warren, 1978). However, two points must be borne in mind. First, the neurological effects of cooling, such as facilitation of muscle contraction, require intact sensory nerves; secondly, the normal circulatory response is altered if the autonomic nerves are affected so that tissue cooling occurs more rapidly and more deeply than normally. Therefore caution is required if skin with defective innervation is to be treated. In connection with this point thermal sensation testing is recommended by some as a necessary precaution prior to cryotherapy but there would seem to be little point in this, since there is no awareness of tissue damage until after it has occurred. Observing that normal vasoconstriction has taken place early in treatment – the autonomic response – is a sensible precaution.

Emotional and psychological features

Some patients may have a strong aversion to cold in any form or to local cold applications in particular. This may be partly due to cultural factors since our language abounds with metaphors in which 'cold' has some unpleasant connotations, e.g. in cold blood, cold-hearted. There is an obviously physiological association with fear – cold feet and cold sweat. Both cold and fear stimulate the sympathetic system. There is also an emotional link:

Pale grew thy cheek and cold,
Colder thy kiss
Truly that hour foretold
Sorrow to this!

Byron: 'When we two parted'

Even the medical term 'frozen shoulder' implies the concept of ice locking movable joints. The connection of cold with death is also well recognized. Thus the patient may exhibit a strong emotional disapprobation of cold which would make it inappropriate to use cryotherapy. It has been claimed that this is more likely to occur in elderly patients; this may be due to the fact that a greater range of skin temperature occurs in the elderly compared with young adults (Howell, 1982), presumably because the control mechanism is becoming less efficient in old age.

REFERENCES

Abramson D. I., Chu L. S. W., Tuck S. *et al.* (1966). Effect of tissue temperature and blood flow on motor nerve conduction velocity. *J.A.M.A.*, **198**, 156–62.
Benson T. B., Copp E. P. (1974). The effects of therapeutic forms of heat and ice on the pain threshold of the normal shoulder. *Rheumatol. Rehab.*, **13**, 101–4.

Bierman W., Friedlander M. (1940). The penetrative effects of cold. *Arch. Phys. Ther.*, **21**, 585–91.

Clendenin M. A., Szumski A. J. (1971). Influence of cutaneous ice application on single motor units in humans. *Phys. Ther.*, **51**, 166–75.

Covington D. B., Basselt F. H. (1993). When cryotherapy injures. *The Physician and Sports Med.* **21**(3), 78–93.

De Domenico G., Cotton S., Devereux D. *et al.* (1991). Skin temperature changes with different methods of cryotherapy. *WCPT 11th International Congress Proceedings Book II*. London: World Confederation for Physical Therapy, pp. 606–8.

Douglas W. W., Malcolm J. L. (1955). The effect of localised cooling on cat nerves. *J. Physiol.*, **130**, 53.

Ernst E., Fialka V. (1994). Ice freezes pain? A review of the clinical effectiveness of analgesic cold therapy. *J. Pain Symptom Manage.*, **9**, 56–9.

Fahrer H. (1991). *Therapeutic Cold (Cryotherapy) in Physiotherapy: Controlled Facts and Trials*. (Rheumatology, vol. 14) (Schlapbach P., Gerber N. J., eds) Basel: Karger, pp. 141–9.

Farry P. J., Prentice N. G., Hunter A. C., Wakelin C. A. (1980). Ice treatment of injured ligaments: an experimental model. *N.Z. Med. J.*, **91**, 14–16.

Fox R. H., Wyatt H. T. (1962). Cold induced vasodilation in various areas of the body surface in man. *J. Physiol.*, **162**, 289–97.

Hardy J. D. (1982). Temperature regulation, exposure to heat and cold and effects of hypothermia. In *Therapeutic Heat and Cold* (Lehmann J. F., ed.) Baltimore: Williams & Wilkins, pp. 172–96.

Harrison M. A. (1978). Effects of ice treatment. *Physiother. Sport*, October.

Hay-Smith E. J., Reed M. A. (1997). Physical agents for perineal pain following childbirth: a review of systematic reviews. *Phys. Ther. Rev.*, **2**, 115–21.

Hedenberg L. (1970). Functional improvement of the spastic hemiplegic arm after cooling. *Scand. J. Rehab. Med.*, **2**, 154.

Howell T. (1982). Skin temperature gradient in the lower extremities of old women. *Exp. Gerntol.*, **17**, 65–7.

Hubbard J. L., Mechan D. J. (1987). *Physiology for Health Care Students*. Edinburgh: Churchill Livingstone.

Kauranen K., Vanharanta H. (1997). Effects of hot and cold packs on motor performance of normal hands. *Physiotherapy*, **83**, 340–44.

Kirk J. A., Kersley G. D. (1968). Heat and cold in the physical treatment of rheumatoid arthritis of the knee. *Ann. Phys. Med.*, **IX**, 270–4.

Lee J. M., Warren M. P. (1974). *Cold Therapy in Rehabilitation*. London: Bell and Hyman.

Lee J. M., Warren M. P., Mason S. M. (1978). Effects of ice on nerve conduction velocity. *Physiotherapy*, **64**, 2–6.

Lehmann J. F., de Lateur B. J. (1982). Cryotherapy. In *Therapeutic Heat and Cold* (Lehmann J. F., ed.) Baltimore: Williams & Wilkins, pp. 563–602.

Lewis T. (1930). Observation upon the reactions of the vessels of the human skin to cold. *Heart*, **15**, 177–208.

Lorenze E. J., Carontonis G., DeRosa A. J. (1960). Effect on coronary circulation of cold packs to hemiplegic shoulders. *Arch. Phys. Med. Rehab.*, **41**, 394–9.

McLean D. A. (1989). The use of cold and superficial heat in the treatment of soft tissue injuries. *Br. J. Sports Med.*, **23**, 53–4.

McMaster W. C., Little S., Waugh T. R. (1978). Laboratory evaluation of various cold therapy modalities. *Am. J. Sports Med.*, **6**, 291–4.

Michlovitz S. L. (1986). Cryotherapy: the use of cold as a therapeutic agent. In *Thermal Agents in Rehabilitation* (Michlovitz S. L., ed.) Philadelphia: F. A. Davis, pp. 73–98.

Moon A. H., Gragnani J. A. (1989). Cold water immersion for the oedematous hand in stroke patients. *Clin. Rehab.*, **3**, 97–101.

Oosterveld F. G. J., Rasker J. J., Jacobs J. W. G., Overmars H. F. J. (1992). The effect of local heat and cold therapy on the intraarticular (sic) and skin surface temperature of the knee. *Arth. Rheum.*, **35**, 146–51.

Palastanga N. P. (1988). Heat and cold. In *Pain: Management and Control in Physiotherapy* (Wells P., Frampton V., Bowsher D., eds) London: Heinemann Medical Books, pp. 169–80.

Peterjan R. H., Watts N. (1962). Effects of cooling on the triceps surae reflex. *Am. J. Phys. Med.*, **41**, 240–51.

Rajadhyaksha V., Dastoor D. H., Shahani M. (1982). Influence of cooling of anterior aspect of thigh on maximal isometric tension of muscle quadriceps. In *Proceedings of the IXth International Congress of World Confederation for Physical Therapy*. Stockholm, pp. 494–8.

Urbscheit N., Johnston R., Bishop B. (1971). Effects of cooling on the ankle jerk and 'H' response in hemiplegic patients. *Phys. Ther.*, **51**, 983–8.

Wadsworth H., Chanmugan A. P. P. (1980). *Electrophysical Agents in Physiotherapy*. Marrickville, NSW, Australia: Science Press.

Wolf S. L. (1971). Contralateral upper extremity cooling from a specific cold stimulus. *Phys Ther.*, **51**, 158–65.

10 Electromagnetic fields: shortwave diathermy, pulsed electromagnetic energy and magnetic therapies

The subject of this chapter, as often occurs in electrotherapy, is plagued by a profusion and confusion of names.

The basic therapeutic mechanism being considered here is the passage of (relatively) high-frequency currents through the body to produce heating in both deep and superficial tissues. When little energy is applied due to the low intensity and/or the pulsing of the current, no heat may be evident. The consequences of such low-energy treatments are considered by some to be due to effects other than heating.

When detectable tissue heating occurs it is logically called 'diathermy' (a word, coined from the Greek, meaning 'through heating') – shortwave diathermy. Otherwise names such as pulsed electromagnetic energy (PEME) or pulsed shortwave abound. A description of these two entities form the bulk of this chapter.

First, the nature and production of such currents are briefly considered, followed by the way in which high-frequency currents are transmitted to the tissues. The principles of application are explored, including the important effects of varying the size, position and relationship of electrodes to the tissues on the heating pattern. The technique of application of continuous shortwave diathermy is next described with dosage and potential dangers.

Pulsed shortwave is then described, with comment on its application, dosage and contraindications.

The chapter concludes with some reference to low-power high-frequency energy, Indiba therapy and the use of magnetism in therapy. Finally, there is some comment on the current concern with the safety of all kinds of electromagnetic fields.

NATURE

Electromagnetic energy can be considered from three aspects:

- *Electrostatic* forces between stationary electric charges. There is an attraction between opposite charges and a repulsion of like charges. These forces act between any charges and their strength and direction can be described by drawing lines called lines of electric force. The area in which this force acts is called an electric field.

- When charges move it is referred to as an *electric current*. The effects on the tissues have been discussed in Chapters 2 and 3. An inevitable consequence of constantly moving charges is the formation of a magnetic force at right angles to the direction of the charge motion. The area in which the magnetic force is evident is called the magnetic field.

- If an electric charge is accelerated it causes the production of an *electromagnetic radiation*. This radiates away from the moving charge and once generated is independent of the charge.

If electric currents are made to oscillate, the rapid acceleration of charges causes the production of electromagnetic radiations whose wavelength and frequency are related to the frequency of oscillation, illustrated in the frontispiece. This is further described in Chapter 11. The radiations emitted by high-frequency oscillating currents are familiar as radio waves.

The electric field, i.e. electric force, is measured in volts and the rate of motion of the charges, i.e. electric current, is measured in amperes.

All electromagnetic radiations have the same velocity of 3×10^8 m/s and differ from one another in their wavelength and frequency. At frequencies of several hundred kHz the radio waves produced have wavelengths of about 1 km; at frequencies of 1 MHz they have wavelengths of 300 m and at 10 MHz the wavelengths would be 30 m. The bands of radio wave frequencies around these three regions are called long, medium and shortwave bands respectively. Modern radio receivers usually give the frequencies rather than wavelengths. All radio frequencies in the range of 10–100 MHz are called shortwave and because the device for producing therapeutic heating is in this range it is called 'shortwave diathermy'. The first part of the name is unfortunate since it suggests that 'shortwave radio waves' are the effective therapy, which is entirely untrue. The radiations are largely irrelevant to the therapy. It is the high-frequency oscillating currents generated in the tissues that cause the heating.

It may be wondered why heating should occur when high-frequency currents are passed through the tissues, since it was pointed out in Chapter 3 that therapeutic low-frequency currents produced negligible heating. The answer lies in the fact that much higher currents are being passed through the tissues with diathermy and the heating would depend on the square of the current (heating $= I^2Rt$ where $I =$ current intensity, $R =$ resistance, and $t =$ time) so that a greater current would lead to very much greater heating. The low-frequency currents of Chapter 3 were mostly of a few milliamperes – or even a few microamperes – whereas diathermy heating might involve total currents of 0.5–1 A, although it is the current density (current per unit area) that matters.

Table 10.1 Assigned frequencies and wavelengths

Frequency (MHz)	Wavelength (m)
13.56 ($\pm$6.25 kHz)	22.124
27.12 ($\pm$160 kHz)	11.062
40.68 ($\pm$20 kHz)	7.375

The reason why large currents can be passed through the tissues if they are oscillating rapidly enough – i.e. have a high enough frequency – is that there is not enough time at each oscillation for nerve or muscle tissue to be affected. It will be recalled that excitable tissue is affected by altering the ionic balance across the membrane, as explained in Chapter 3. Single pulses (phases) of voltage need to pass for about 0.1 ms to stimulate a nerve with minimal voltage. Shorter pulses would need higher voltages or a series of such pulses would be interrupted or modulated to provoke a nerve impulse. At the usual shortwave diathermy frequency of 27.12 MHz the voltage phases would be less than 1/50th of a microsecond so that no excitatory effect on muscle or nerve can occur.

PRODUCTION OF SHORTWAVE DIATHERMY

Since electromagnetic radiations are emitted in the radio and television bands certain specific frequencies have been allocated by international agreement for industrial, scientific and medical purposes to prevent interference with communications. These frequencies and their wavelengths are shown in Table 10.1. Of these the 27.12 MHz frequency is by far the most widely used because it has the widest frequency band; that is to say, the extent to which it is allowed to drift off the assigned frequency is much greater than the others.

High-frequency current is generated by an oscillator circuit consisting of a capacitance and an inductance whose dimensions are arranged to allow electron oscillation at a precise frequency, e.g. 27.12 MHz. The frequency (f) at which such a circuit will oscillate depends only on its electrical size, that is the product of capacity (C) and inductance (L):

$$f = \frac{1}{2\pi\sqrt{LC}}$$

In order to maintain the regular oscillation, electrical energy must be fed into the circuit in bursts at exactly the right moment in the cycle to make good the losses. This is achieved by means of an electronic switch – either a thermionic valve or a transistor – which is coupled to the circuit so that current is added in time with the oscillations. The circuit can be either:

- a power oscillator in which the electrical oscillations are generated at the required power and frequency using a valve and a cavity (pot) resonator

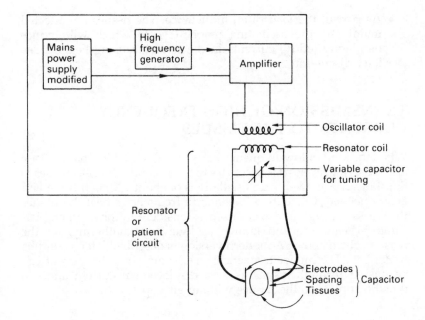

Fig. 10.1 Block diagram to show short-wave diathermy generation.

- a crystal-timed transistor controlled low power circuit, which is amplified to a level appropriate for therapy.

The part to be treated is included in the 'patient' or resonator circuit which is coupled inductively to the oscillator circuit (Fig. 10.1). This involves a coil in each circuit being placed close together, forming a transformer, so that the magnetic field generated by the oscillator circuit induces a current in the resonator coil. Energy will be effectively transferred if the two circuits are in tune, i.e. have the same frequency. Since the frequency of both circuits is proportional to $1/(2\pi\sqrt{LC})$ it is only necessary to arrange it so that the product of capacity and inductance in one circuit is the same as the product of capacity and inductance in the other.

The capacity of the resonator circuit will vary because the tissues contribute to the capacity so a variable capacitor must be adjusted to bring the circuits into resonance. This tuning can either be done manually, using the excursion of a meter or brightness of a light to indicate maximum resonance, or automatically. In this latter case a motor drives the tuning capacitor and is itself regulated by the output from the resonator circuit. This automatic mechanism, another example of negative feedback, keeps the machine tuned even if the patient moves a little.

Once tuned, the heating of the tissues is controlled by regulating the output of the machine. This is done in different ways in different machines.

The tissues may be coupled into the shortwave field in two ways:

- As part of the dielectric of a capacitor, as in Figure 10.1; this is called a capacitive method. The tissues are affected principally by the oscillating electric field.

- As part of the load of an inductance. The tissues are affected mainly by the oscillating magnetic field which will induce oscillating (eddy) currents in the tissues causing heating; see later discussion.

TRANSMISSION OF HIGH-FREQUENCY CURRENTS TO THE TISSUES

When the kind of low-frequency currents discussed in Chapter 3 are applied to the tissues it is necessary to apply conducting electrodes to the skin surface. Even with oscillations of about 1 MHz this method is still needed. Currents of megahertz frequencies heat the tissues they pass through and were used extensively by physiotherapists some 50 years ago and known as longwave diathermy, for the reasons given above. A modern version is described later as 'Indiba treatment'. For higher frequencies, i.e. shortwave, the current can be passed through insulators as a displacement current and can thus be applied to the tissues with an air gap.

Effects of high-frequency currents on the tissues

The major effect of passing currents of sufficient intensity at frequencies above 1 MHz is to cause heating. The nature of heat was considered in Chapter 7 and it will be recalled that heat is energy, basically the amount of random molecular and atomic motion in a material. Anything that increases the internal kinetic energy of matter causes heating, usually accompanied by a temperature rise in the material.

Vibration of ions

The tissues contain large numbers of ions, which are the charge carriers when a current flows in the tissues (convection current; see Chapters 2 and 3). If an electric field is applied first in one direction and then in the other the ions will be accelerated first one way then the opposite, colliding with adjacent molecules to give up some energy to them and so increasing the total random motion, that is heating. At the most commonly used therapeutic frequency of 27.12 MHz the movement is more of an oscillation about a mean position but the rapid acceleration affects nearby particles leading to significant heating (Fig. 10.2(a)).

Dipole rotation

The tissues are, of course, largely water. Water molecules behave rather differently because, although electrically neutral as a total molecule, they are polar, that is the ends of the molecule carry small opposite charges. Because of this they are sometimes called dipoles. When rapidly reversing charges are applied to polar molecules they

(a)

Ionic
motion

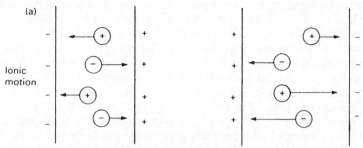

Positive and negative ions move to and fro under the
influence of an oscillating electric field.

(b)

Dipole
rotation

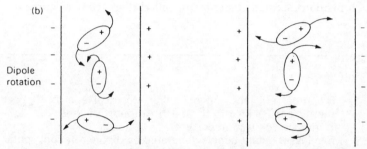

Polar molecules rotate to and fro as the electric field oscillates.

(c)

Electron
'cloud'
motion

'Molecular
distortion'

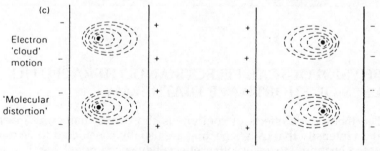

The paths of orbiting electrons are distorted first in one
direction then in the other as the electric field oscillates.

Fig. 10.2 The effects of oscillating high-
frequency electric fields on the molecules
and ions of the tissues.

will rotate to and fro (Fig. 10.2(b)). This rotational energy disrupts
the motion of adjacent molecules causing more total random motion
and hence heat.

Molecular distortion

Atoms and molecules which are not charged can also be affected
by the rapidly oscillating electric field in that the paths of their
orbiting electrons are distorted (i.e. they will polarize). As the electric
field changes direction one side becomes more positive and the

other more negative so the average position of the electron 'cloud' shifts, being attracted to the positive and repelled from the negative side (Fig. 10.2(c)). This does not cause motion of the molecule but the interaction with other neighbouring molecules leads to more random motion and therefore some heating. However, it must be appreciated that very little energy is converted to heat by this latter mechanism. As far as tissue heating is concerned it is the least important. Ionic movement is the most consequential as it is a very efficient converter of electrical energy to heat (Ward, 1986).

It follows from what has just been said that if high-frequency currents are applied through non-polar materials there will be little energy lost as heat. This explains why the plastic covers of the shortwave electrodes do not become hot; neither does the insulation of the wires, nor for that matter the air spacing between electrode and patient. The oscillating electrical force will readily pass through such insulators. Such currents are called displacement currents.

Summary

- The most efficient conversion of electrical energy to heat energy occurs by the to and fro motion of ions – a high-frequency convection current.
- To a lesser extent heat is generated by dipole rotation – polar molecules rotating back and forth.
- The least efficient conversion is by electron cloud movement – molecular distortion.

PHYSIOLOGICAL EFFECTS AND THERAPEUTIC USES OF SHORTWAVE DIATHERMY

The therapeutic effects of continuous shortwave diathermy given at an intensity that causes heating are usually considered to be due to the heating. However, other effects have been noted, e.g. Bansal *et al.* (1990).

The application of shortwave diathermy by several of the methods described below has been shown to cause rises in both skin and intramuscular temperature (Hansen and Kristensen, 1973; Verrier *et al.*, 1977; Verrier *et al.*, 1978). The actual temperature rises vary widely, but skin temperatures of 3–6.6°C, and muscle temperatures a degree or so lower, were achieved. Intra-articular heating has also been demonstrated (Whyte and Reader, 1952; Oosterveld *et al.*, 1992).

The effects of heating and the therapeutic uses have already been considered in Chapter 7. The only difference to be considered when using shortwave diathermy is the site and pattern of heating in the tissues.

PRINCIPLES OF APPLICATION

The methods of applying shortwave therapy are:

A. *Inductive method*:

- Using a small flat metal coil enclosed in a plastic drum (with a capacitor in parallel). This is sometimes called a monode.
- Using a long tubular flexible conductor covered in thick rubber called a cable or coil. This may be wrapped round the part to be treated in a spiral manner or made into a flat spiral. The cable forms an inductance and is separated from the skin by towel spacing.

B. *Capacitive method*:

- Using rigid metal plates enclosed in plastic. These are called rigid or plate electrodes or space plates and are positioned by means of supporting arms.
- Using flexible or malleable electrodes encased in thick rubber which can be positioned under the part to be treated with spacing provided by suitable material.

While there is a distinction between the capacitive and the inductive methods, it must be recognized that the application of any form of inductive coil will produce heating due to both the magnetically induced eddy currents and currents due to the electrostatic (capacitive) field (see later discussion and Fig. 10.7). It should be noted here and in the subsequent discussion that 'heat' and 'heating' refer to the physical effect in the tissues and may, or may not, be detected by the patient.

Heating pattern in the tissues – capacitor field method

Understanding and as far as possible controlling the distribution of the electric field of shortwave diathermy and hence the heating in the tissues is the central skill in this type of application. The electric field pattern, and hence the heating pattern, with various sizes, shapes and positions of electrodes relative to the tissues can be approximately predicted for homogeneous tissue. The tissues are, of course, far from homogeneous so that the field pattern is markedly altered by the nature and orientation of the tissue through which it passes.

The passage of the high-frequency current in the tissues depends on both conduction and the degree of polarization. This latter correlates with the dielectric constant or relative permittivity. The dielectric constant of air and other gases is close to one, but substances that polarize strongly have high dielectric constants, e.g. pure water at 81. It is low in most familiar insulators such as polythene (2.2) and glass (approx 9).

If an electric field is applied across homogeneous material it will be uniform but if there is a boundary between materials with different dielectric constants and/or different conductivities the electric field is refracted at the boundary. This is much the same as the refraction that occurs when visible radiation (or any wave motion) passes from one medium to another. In general, those tissues that have a high dielectric constant are good conductors, e.g. water and tissues with a high water content. The reverse is also evident; fat tissues have a low dielectric constant and low conductivity. Thus the electric field in the tissues tends to be refracted at various interfaces both at the surface and between various tissue layers. The overall effect is to spread the field within the tissues. For a fuller description and explanation of these factors see Ward (1986) and Guy (1982).

Some simplified illustrations of the effects of different sizes and orientations of electrodes are shown in Figure 10.3. The shape of the tissues will also have an effect.

To provide sufficient energy for heating in the tissues it is necessary to concentrate the field in the particular area to be treated. Equally it is important not to allow the field to be so concentrated as to produce excessive heating and hence damage. The following points should be considered in conjunction with Figure 10.3. The aim is to achieve a uniform field in the tissues.

Spacing of electrodes

- 2–4 cm skin–electrode distance.
- Wide spacing gives the most uniform field in the tissues.
- More heat per unit area is generated in the skin than in the deeper tissues. This ensures the safety of shortwave diathermy since the skin is highly sensitive to temperature changes (see Fig. 10.4).
- Closer spacing of one electrode leads to concentration of the field on that side.

Size of electrodes

- A little larger than the part to achieve a uniform electric field through the tissues.
- Unevenly sized electrodes may concentrate the field under the smaller electrode.

Positioning of electrodes relative to the tissues

- Electrodes parallel to the skin surface so that skin–electrode distance is as constant as possible.
- The field takes the shortest pathway and will preferentially pass through the material of least impedance.
- The distance between the electrodes must be greater than the combined skin–electrode distance of the two electrodes or the field will pass through the air between the electrodes rather than through the tissues.
- Uneven spacing leads to concentration of field at closest point.

285

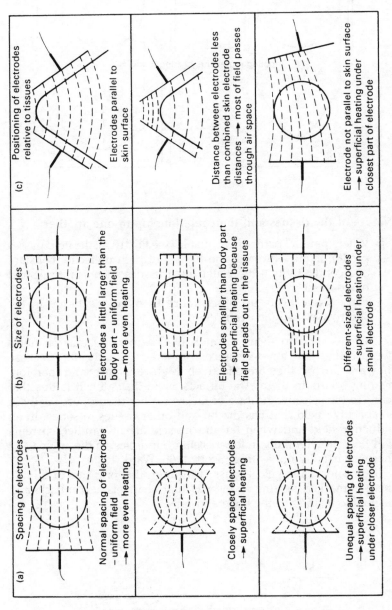

Fig. 10.3 The effect of positioning electrodes on the electric field through tissues using a contraplanar technique.

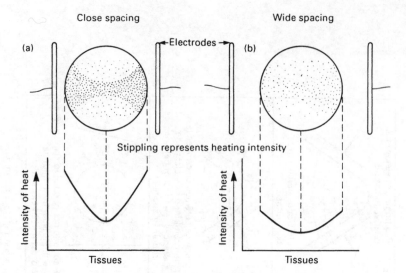

Fig. 10.4 Heating intensity (stippled area) in tissues with (a) close and (b) wide spacing.

Nature of the tissues and their relationship to one another

- Where parallel paths are available (see Fig. 10.5), the field passes predominantly through the tissues of high dielectric constant and conductivity – the water-filled tissues such as muscle and blood vessels.
- Fatty tissue heats up much more than muscle tissue in the shortwave field (Schwan, 1965).

Currents tend to focus through the narrow vascular channels because they are low-resistance compared with the fat. Because they are narrow, they are effectively high-resistance, and therefore heating occurs in them. The fat acts as an insulator. It is this that leads to the selective heating of fat over other tissues, especially in a capacitive field that has the fat and other tissues in series. In an inductive field and when fat and muscle are in parallel, currents will flow preferentially in low resistance muscles. In the air spacing there is virtually no heating (Scott, 1965; Ward, 1986).

If the shortwave field is passed through the long axis of a limb, there is marked heating in the vascular channels and muscle and negligible heating in the bone and fat.

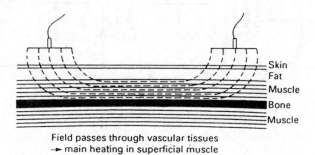

Fig. 10.5 Coplanar technique. The electric field passes through vascular tissues, therefore the main heating is in the superficial muscle.

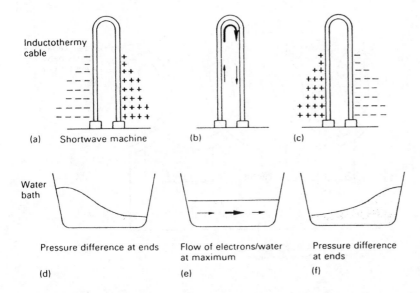

Inductothermy cable

(a) Shortwave machine

(b)

(c)

Water bath

Pressure difference at ends

(d)

Flow of electrons/water at maximum

(e)

Pressure difference at ends

(f)

Fig. 10.6 To illustrate the motion of electrons and water in half-wavelength 'containers'.

Heating pattern in the tissues – inductothermy

Heating by inductothermy is due to eddy currents. The difference between inductothermy and the capacitor field method lies in the way energy is introduced into the tissues leading to a different pattern of heating. The magnetic field is a result of electron movement (i.e. current), so it appears where there is maximum electron flow. The inductothermy cable or coil, whatever its configuration, is a part of the resonator circuit and is a conductor of high-frequency current, which behaves as an electromagnetic wave. To understand what happens, consider a cable of half the wavelength (i.e. 5.503 m) in which the high-frequency current is oscillating with a wavelength of 11.06 m, as shown in Figure 10.6(a). At some point in the cycle there will be a maximum potential difference between the two terminals of the machine and hence between the ends of the cable. At this instant there would be no current. As the cycle proceeds, electrons flow from the negative to the positive end. This current rises to a peak and then subsides as the difference of potential again develops between the terminals, this time in the opposite direction (see Fig. 10.6(c)). The process then reverses, the electrons moving back to the position shown in Figure 10.6(a) to complete the cycle. At a time half way between that shown in Figure 10.6(a) and Figure 10.6(c) there will be no difference of potential between the terminals or any part of the cable, but the current will be maximum, the greatest current intensity being half way between the terminals, as shown in Figure 10.6(b).

The mechanism is illustrated by analogy with a container of water. While soaking in the bath, some abrupt body movements can cause the water to swill from end to end. A wall of water at the tap end sweeps over the recumbent bather to be reflected from the other end, passing up and down the bath. This occurs in many situations and on different scales, from liquid slopping to and fro

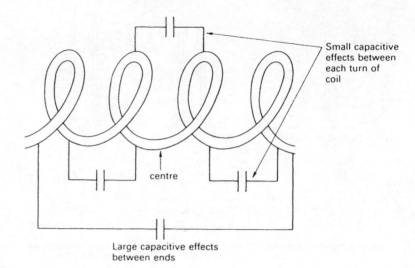

Small capacitive effects between each turn of coil

centre

Fig. 10.7 To illustrate capacitive effects between the ends and between each turn of the cable. There is a similar effect if the cable is wound as a flat spiral.

Large capacitive effects between ends

in a disturbed cup to tides that occur in large lakes. The important common feature is that the motion has a constant frequency. When the water is piled up at one end, there is a large difference of pressure between the two ends of the container. This is like the large difference of electrical potential and, in both cases, for an instant, there is no flow. As the water sweeps back in the bath there comes a moment when the two ends are at the same level (no difference of pressure), but there is maximum flow of water or electrons, as illustrated in Figure 10.6(b) and (e). Thus, the very middle of the cable (and the bath) experiences only a flow and the two ends only a pressure difference between them, with the result that the middle of the cable produces a strong electromagnetic field and hence has strong inductive effects, whereas the ends provide the strongest capacitive effects.

While this description has been based on a cable of exactly half the wavelength, and the inductothermy cable of many shortwave machines will be found to conform approximately, the same effect can be achieved by replacing part of the cable with a suitable capacitor. This is often what is used to provide a 'drum'-type electrode, with the centre of the cable formed into a flat spiral.

From Figure 10.7 and what has been described, it will be evident that energy will be introduced into the tissues due to both capacitive and inductive effects. The former will be strongest between the two ends of the cable but will also occur between other parts of the cable. Thus, as will be seen in Figure 10.7 there are capacitive fields between each turn of the cable, as well as inductive effects.

The inductive effects are due to the oscillating magnetic field generated by the large current at the centre of the cable. Since the tissues are virtually transparent to magnetic fields, the energy

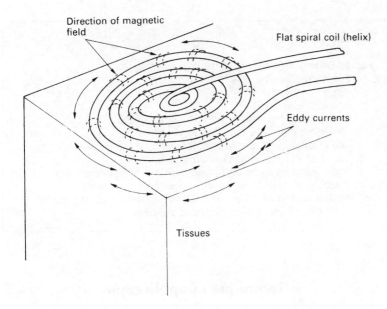

Direction of magnetic field

Flat spiral coil (helix)

Eddy currents

Tissues

Fig. 10.8 To show the directions of the magnetic fields and eddy currents due to a flat spiral coil.

spreads out in the tissues, interacting with the electric and magnetic fields of the atoms and molecules. The result is the electromagnetic induction of electric currents at right angles to the direction of the magnetic field. A typical flat spiral coil is illustrated in Figure 10.8. With such a coil, most of the heating would occur in the superficial tissues, but not predominantly in fatty tissues, as occurs in capacitive applications. This results in proportionally more energy being absorbed in the superficial muscle that underlies the fat and skin, and hence more heating in this region (Guy, 1982).

If an electrostatic screen (a wire mesh often called a faradic screen) is placed between the coil and the tissues, it will eliminate the electric field and leave only the magnetic field. When this is done experimentally, heating diminishes dramatically (Ward, 1986), showing that capacitive heating accounts for much of the heating due to the coil. Some drum-type electrodes have such a screen built in, so that only the magnetic field is applied.

If the cable is used it must be kept at a distance of 2–3 cm from the skin surface to give a sufficient spread of field. This is achieved partly by the rubber insulation of the cable and partly by applying the cable over a minimum of 1 cm thickness of towelling or other suitable material. It is also important that adjacent turns of the coil are evenly separated from each other by insulating material to avoid overheating of the cable and spread the field. Wooden or perspex spacers are provided for this purpose.

The plastic casing of the drum electrode ensures suitable spacing but an additional air gap is also needed to achieve adequate-depth heating (Lehmann and de Lateur, 1982); 1–2 cm is an appropriate distance.

Summary

Factors affecting heating pattern in the tissues:
- The capacitive field is influenced by:
  - spacing of electrodes
  - size of electrodes
  - relationship of electrodes to skin surface.
- The inductive field is influenced by:
  - relationship of coil to the tissues
  - part of the coil that predominates.
- Both capacitive and inductive fields are influenced by:
  - nature of tissues involved – dielectric constant
  - relationship of different tissues – in series or in parallel
  - boundaries between different tissues.

Technique of application

Preparation of patient.

Explanation: The nature of the treatment is described and whether heating of the part will be experienced.

Examination: The part is examined for possible dangers and contraindications.

For this, the area to be treated should be adequately exposed. Passing the field through clothing may cause several problems aside from obscuring the area. The clothing may:

- be made of inappropriate synthetic material
- contain metal fastenings
- be damp or conceal dampness on the skin
- constrict circulation to the part.

Thermal sensation must be tested and recorded.

Preparation of the apparatus.   The machine and apparatus are assembled and if deemed necessary tested with an output indicator.

Preparation of the part.   The part to be treated, and indeed the whole patient, must be supported in a position that is safe, convenient and comfortable. Metal objects, synthetic materials and any droplets of moisture should be removed from the area of the field. If the skin is moist it must be dried. Any skin surfaces that are in contact with each other must be separated by some absorbant material. Adequate support is particularly important if a manually tuned machine is used since any movement of the part disturbs the circuit tuning.

Setting up.   An appropriate method of treatment for the required effect is selected – capacitor field or inductothermy. The capacitor field method may be applied in different ways:

A. CAPACITOR FIELD

(a) *Contraplanar*

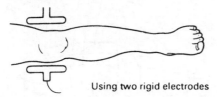

Using two rigid electrodes

(b) *Coplanar*

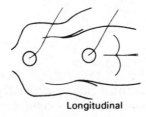

Longitudinal

B. INDUCTOTHERMY

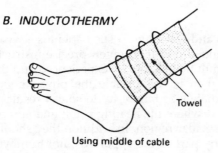

Towel

Using middle of cable

Fig. 10.9 Some techniques of application of shortwave diathermy.

- *Contraplanar*: electrodes are placed on opposite sides of the part, to treat deeply placed structures, e.g. joints (Fig. 10.9).
- *Coplanar* (Fig. 10.5 and 10.9): electrodes are placed on the same side of the part to treat more superficial structures, e.g. the spinal musculature.
- *Cross-fire* (Fig. 10.10): half the treatment is given with the electrodes in one contraplanar position and for the second half the electrodes are repositioned at right angles. This technique may be used to achieve more uniform heating of the tissues and particularly for the walls of air-filled cavities, e.g. paranasal sinuses.

Appropriate type and size of electrodes are chosen.
The inductothermy cable may be applied as:

- a monode or drum-type electrode (Fig. 10.11)
- a coil wound as a flat spiral (Fig. 10.8)
- a coil, wound round the circumference of a limb (Fig. 10.9B).

The electrodes are positioned relative to the tissues with appropriate spacing. Other parts of the body must be protected from the field set up from all aspects of the electrode and from the

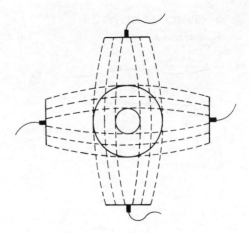

Fig. 10.10 The cross-fire technique and the passage of an electric field in tissues around an air-filled cavity.

connecting leads. The leads must not be closer together than the terminals of the machine nor close to any conductor in which they could induce heating.

Instructions and warnings. The patient is advised whether any heating is intended and if so given precise instructions about the degree of warmth that should be experienced and the warning that if it is hotter than is comfortable the physiotherapist should be notified immediately as failure to do so can result in a burn. They must also report where the heating is felt and any concentration of heat in one particular region. In addition they should be instructed not to touch any part of the apparatus, not to move or fall asleep. The patient is the only source of knowledge of what heating is occurring so it is essential for the patient to understand and co-operate fully in order to regulate the heating.

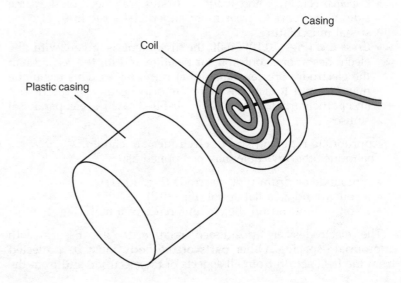

Fig. 10.11 A drum-type applicator (capacitor not shown).

(a) *Continuous shortwave*

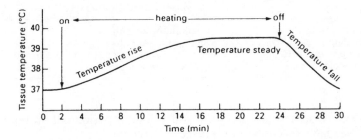

(b) *Pulsed shortwave*

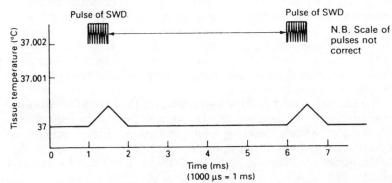

Fig. 10.12 (a) Continuous shortwave: as heat is added the local tissue temperature rises but at the same time the body's thermoregulatory system reacts, removing heat until a steady state is reached at a new higher temperature. (b) Pulsed shortwave: the small (negligible) temperature rise due to each impulse is dissipated during the pulse interval. *Note*: the different time and temperature scales of (a) and (b); pulse lengths and intervals are not to scale; the temperature changes shown in these figures are not based on actual measurements.

Application. The apparatus is then switched on, tuned, manually, if necessary, and the heating adjusted to the appropriate intensity as indicated by the patient. As vasodilation takes place, heat is dissipated and the intensity may have to be increased. It is equally important not to turn the intensity too high before this has occurred. If any pain or discomfort occurs during treatment the machine should be switched off at once.

Termination. At the end of treatment, which can last up to 30 min, the heating can be assessed to some extent by the presence and intensity of erythema on the skin and by palpating the skin and judging the increased surface temperature.

DOSAGE

If energy is added to the tissues faster than it is being dissipated the temperature must rise, which causes vasodilation to increase heat removal until the heat gain and loss are once more in balance at a new, higher local temperature (see Chapter 7 and Fig. 10.12(a)). It usually takes some 15–20 min for these vascular adjustments to occur and thus reach a steady state but it can be longer. This is the reason for applying such treatments for 20–30 min. Very low intensity applications, in which no vascular response would be

> **Practical point**
> Pain could be due directly to the treatment, overheating or causing increased local oedema for example. It could also be due to the position of the patient. If the patient is left in the same position for a few minutes after the heat has been turned off, the pain will diminish or disappear only if heating is the cause.

Table 10.2 Dosages of shortwave diathermy

Dosage	Description of heat to patient
Moderate heating	Comfortable warmth
Mild heating	Mild gentle warmth
Minimal perceptible heating	So that you can only just feel the warmth
Imperceptible heating	No feeling of warmth at all

evident, are sometimes given for much longer periods of an hour or so; see later discussion on pulsed shortwave.

As any heating due to shortwave treatments can only be known from descriptions given by the patient, it is important to be able to communicate the amount of heating. Since the shortwave field is strongest at the surface, any heat is detected by thermoreceptors in the skin. Dosage can be described as shown in Table 10.2.

The term 'subthermal' or 'athermal' for imperceptible heating is best avoided as these words suggest that no local heating occurs because it cannot be felt.

It must be stressed that the perceptions of the patient are the only safe guide to the heating in the tissues. Similar energy inputs can lead to widely differing heat perceptions due principally to differences in blood flow (Scott, 1957).

The minimum dose should be given that will achieve the required effect.

POTENTIAL DANGERS IN THE APPLICATION OF SHORTWAVE DIATHERMY

All the potential dangers inherent in any heat treatment must be taken into account (see Chapter 7).

In addition there are some specific considerations, as described below.

Burns

Burns can be due to:

- the patient being unaware of the heat because of defective thermal sensation or unconsciousness
- concentration of the shortwave field happening so quickly that a burn occurs before the patient has time to react.

Concentration of the electric field

- If there is a material of high dielectric constant/low impedance in the field, such as metal or moisture, this will concentrate the electric field and a burn can result. All metals are relatively low-resistance conductors and even if enclosed in plastic, as in the armpieces of spectacles, will provide a low-impedance pathway. Similarly many pieces of metal are to be found in

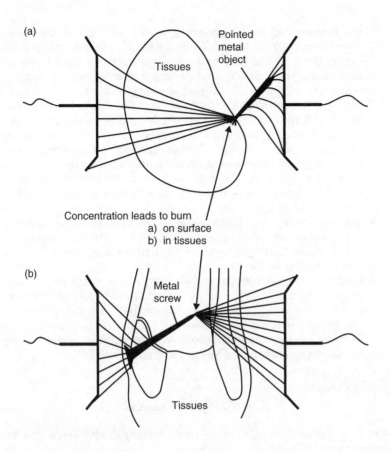

(a)

Tissues

Pointed
metal
object

Concentration leads to burn
a) on surface
b) in tissues

(b)

Metal
screw

Tissues

Fig. 10.13 The way in which (a) metal touching the skin surface and (b) metal implanted in the tissues may concentrate the current, leading to a burn.

clothing, e.g. zip fasteners, hooks-and-eyes, buckles, all of which can have the same effect.

Whether significant field concentration will occur or not depends on the size, shape and orientation of the metal with respect to the field. A long slender pointed piece of metal like a key or silver propelling pencil with its long axis parallel to the lines of force of the field and touching the skin at its point would provide a conductor concentrating the current at the point of contact with the skin (see Fig. 10.13). Notice that although the metal itself would become warmed by the passage of the current it is where the metal touches the high-resistance skin that maximum heating, and hence the burn, will occur.

Whether a burn occurs or not will depend on local field strength which is dependent on the output of the shortwave machine and to what extent the field is concentrated. Even something like an earring, although small, may cause burning because it has point contact with the tissues.

If a person in an electromagnetic field touches any conductor connected to earth, this may provide a route to ground for charge induced in the tissues (Martin *et al.*, 1991).

Metal implanted, such as fixation of fractures (see Fig. 10.13(b)) and metal arthroplasties, or accidently embedded in the tissues, can lead to burning at the junction of the metal with the tissues for the reasons explained above. In these cases the patient would not feel any heat because there are no thermoreceptors in the tissues and the evidence of damage would be deep pain. Small round pieces of metal such as tooth fillings have little or no effect but large wire dental splints may be a risk. Intrauterine contraceptive devices are usually regarded as a hazard during treatment of the pelvis or lower lumbar region. However, Nielson *et al.* (1979), who calculated the probable rise in temperature in the metal, consider them to be safe.

Water droplets on the skin, such as sweat or wet dressings, can also provide this low-resistance pathway and therefore carry the same risk.

- Inadequate spacing of electrodes or leads so that they come in contact with the part, or uneven spacing so that one section of the skin–electrode distance is less than the rest will also cause concentration of the field.
- Under some circumstances, and with the machine at high output, the field near the output cables could be so concentrated, due to being touched by the patient or therapist, that an electric arc breakdown of the insulation occurs. This would cause burning of the cable insulation, with consequent risk of injury to patient or therapist (Evaluation Report, 1987).

Cardiac pacemakers

Another possible danger is to those patients who have cardiac pacemakers. These can be affected by all kinds of electromagnetic fields, transformers, electric razors; a number of cases due to shortwave diathermy have been reported (Jones, 1976). Some demand-type (triggered) pacemakers can occasionally be affected but most modern pacemakers are relatively immune. Nevertheless it is important that patients with pacemakers that might be at risk be kept away from shortwave machines.

Although not as critical, electronic hearing aids can be affected by the shortwave diathermy field.

Synthetic materials

These may have the following disadvantages (personal communication (AR) with UK Dept of Health; Mann, 1989):

- they do not absorb moisture as readily as natural materials
- they ignite more easily than natural materials and can produce large volumes of toxic fumes – there have been a number of cases where shortwave electrodes or cables have overheated and caught fire
- the material itself or any coating applied (e.g. for fire resistance) may alter the field either by absorbing energy or by concentrating the field.

Distance from the shortwave machine

To restrict exposure, operators should remain 1 m from continuous wave therapeutic diathermy equipment, 0.5 m from pulsed treatment with capacitive electrodes, and 0.2 m from pulsed inductive applicators. Short excursions closer to the electrodes are permitted but only when necessary. Extra care should be exercised by pregnant operators. These precautions are recommended by The Chartered Society of Physiotherapy (1992), the Canadian Department of Health and Welfare (DHW 1983) and the Australian National Health and Medical Research Council. Martin *et al.* (1991) state that there is no reason to suspect any long-term health risk to physiotherapists working with diathermy equipment.

Obese patients

The subcutaneous fat layer is more readily heated than muscle, absorbing almost eight times that absorbed in muscle (Delpizzo and Joyner, 1987); see earlier discussion. Capacitive electrodes should be avoided with obese patients (those who weigh 20% or more than normal body weight); a magnetic field output, e.g. a drum-type electrode (coil), is more suitable to produce deep tissue heating (Kloth *et al.*, 1984).

The eye

Because of the poor dissipation of heat from the eye, it should have minimum exposure to shortwave diathermy. It may be wiser to remove contact lenses if the region of the eye is being treated as they may restrict heat loss.

Pregnancy

A study of birth outcomes among physiotherapists in Sweden found a very slightly higher than normal incidence of stillborn or malformed infants born to those operating shortwave diathermy units (Kallen, 1982). Taskinen *et al.* (1990) found a non-significant relationship between exposure to shortwave diathermy and spontaneous abortion, but a significant association with congenital malformations, though only in the low exposure category. They did not conclude that there was a causal relationship. Although no direct link has been found it is probably a wise precaution to avoid excessive exposure to shortwave diathermy during pregnancy and direct application to the area of the uterus.

Implanted slow-release hormone capsules

It is sensible to avoid treating the area where the capsule is implanted.

CONTRAINDICATIONS TO SHORTWAVE DIATHERMY

From the foregoing a list of conditions and circumstances in which the application of shortwave might be dangerous or damaging can be deduced:

- Implanted pacemakers.
- Metal in the tissues.
- Metal on the surface of the tissues that cannot be removed, such as forms of external skeletal fixation or dental splints.
- Impaired thermal sensation.
- Patients unable to control their movements or whose co-operation cannot be presumed, for example the very young or mentally unstable patients or those with uncontrolled movements due to disease.
- The pregnant uterus.
- Conditions in which haemorrhage is occurring or likely to occur. Any form of heat, by increasing the vasodilation and decreasing blood viscosity, might prolong haemorrhage but usually with other forms of heat this is confined to the surface. In the case of shortwave diathermy, heating can be induced in the deeper tissues so that enlarging haematomas or haemarthroses would be affected and therefore should not be treated. Similar concerns apply to treating the pelvis during menstruation.
- Ischaemic tissues whose blood flow cannot be increased to dissipate heat and meet the demands of the increased metabolic activity. This would be most commonly found in the feet of patients with atheroma of the femoral and popliteal arteries. Heating ischaemic tissue is entirely inappropriate because it leads to increased demand on an already precarious circulation causing pain and possibly precipitating gangrene. Reflex heating of the proximal part is safe and may have therapeutic value since it will provoke reflex vasodilation of the affected distal part. However, this may only be moving a limited blood flow from one tissue to another and may have no long-term beneficial effect.
- Malignant tumours should not be treated by any form of heat in case the increased metabolic rate leads to increased rates of growth or metastases, which it is believed could result from low heating at therapeutic levels. Similarly it is often recommended that possible precancerous tissues, such as those damaged by radiation therapy, should not be further stressed by heating since this might provoke malignant changes.
- Active tuberculous lesions should not be treated since heating may increase activity of the bacillus. Once again there seems to be no evidence on this matter but it certainly seems reasonable to avoid such lesions.
- Sites of recent venous thrombosis should be avoided in case heating loosens the clot leading to pulmonary embolism (Scott, 1957). When the vessel is fibrosed it is safe to treat.
- While the patient is pyrexic any form of extensive heating should be avoided.

PULSED HIGH-FREQUENCY ELECTROMAGNETIC ENERGY – PULSED SHORTWAVE

The output of shortwave diathermy machines can be pulsed in the same way as ultrasound (see Chapter 6). This modality is known by a profusion of different names. Besides the two above, 'pulsed electromagnetic field', 'pulsed electromagnetic energy', and appropriate acronyms, are used among many others.

Production of pulsed shortwave

The principles of production of the oscillating high-frequency 27.12 MHz continuous output have already been described earlier. By incorporating a timing circuit, the output can be turned on and off, allowing bursts of oscillations to be emitted for any length of time. Some machines give fixed-length pulses, e.g. 65 or 400 µs, but others allow a choice.

Output

The output depends on:

- peak (or pulse) power in watts
- pulse length in µs
- pulse frequency (repetition rate) in Hz.

Each pulse is a series of oscillations. As the shortwave diathermy frequency is 27.12 MHz, in 1 s there are 27.12×10^6 cycles, and in 1 µs there are 27.12 cycles. A 65 µs pulse therefore contains 1762.8 oscillations. At 100 pulses per second each complete period lasts 10 000 µs (i.e. 10 ms). The first pulse would therefore be separated from the next by an interval of 9935 µs. The duty cycle, i.e. the ratio of pulse length to total period, is in this case 0.65% and the mark space ratio is 1:152.9 (65:9935). The mean power can be found from calculating the duty cycle and taking this proportion of the peak power (see Fig. 10.14).

Possible therapeutic mechanisms

It must be said that all explanations advanced to explain the mechanisms by which pulsed shortwave acts on the tissues are entirely speculative, as is the case with other low-energy therapies such as pulsed ultrasound and laser therapy. An interesting and valuable review of this topic (Kitchen and Dyson, 1996) notes several cellular sites at which low-energy treatments might be active.

A simple but reasonable explanation is to consider that the electromagnetic energy 'stirs' ions, molecules, membranes and perhaps cells thus speeding up phagocytic activity, enzymatic activity, transport across membranes and so forth. This would

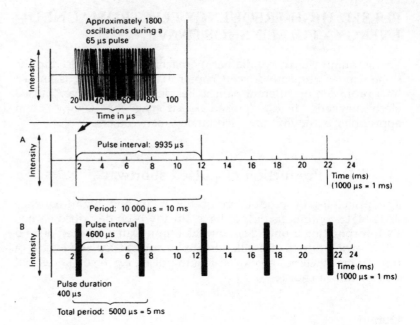

Fig. 10.14 Pulsed high-frequency oscillations. A = 65 µs pulses of 27.12 MHz oscillations repeated 100 times per second. Duty cycle = 0.65%. If peak power is 1000 W, mean power is 6.5 W. B = 400 µs pulses of 27.12 MHz oscillations repeated 200 times per second. Duty cycle = 8%. If peak power is 1000 W, mean power is 80 W. Inset: 1762.8 oscillations during a 65 µs pulse.

account for the evident acceleration of inflammatory and healing processes (Evans, 1980).

The activities of all cells are related to their ionic environment. There is a characteristic potential difference across all cell membranes (see Chapter 1). Some depolarization of the cell membrane is often associated with cell dysfunction and electrical potentials develop during wound healing (see Chapter 2). The membrane potential is also involved in the control of cell division and hence in the control of growth, development and repair. It has been proposed that the electromagnetic field could influence the flow of ions through the membrane and therefore restore the normal cell potential in some damaged cells.

Tsong (1989) postulated that cells are capable of absorbing energy from oscillating electrical fields of defined frequencies (frequency windows) and amplitudes, and making use of this energy for chemical work. Collis and Segal (1988), applying a pulsed electromagnetic field at right angles to rabbit epithelium, noted that an increase in Na^+ flux was produced in one direction, and a reduction in the other. When the epithelium was rotated through 180° the effect was reversed.

Some consider the pulsing to be an important feature; one of us has previously speculated on this (Low, 1978). As noted in Chapter 6, pulsed ultrasound has been shown to accelerate healing at different rates with different intensities and pulse lengths (Dyson and Pond, 1970). It is reasonable to suppose that both electromagnetic and mechanical pulsing have similar effects at a subcellular level, a piezoelectric link. Piezoelectric effects are known to occur in the tissues, for example mechanical stress on bone leads to a redistribution of charges (Fukada and Yasuda, 1964). It is argued that the importance of pulsing may lie in the fact that brief pulses of high intensity will not necessarily have the same effect as an identical quantity of energy applied continuously. An analogy might be drawn with hammering a nail into a piece of wood. Rapidly repeated gentle tapping has no effect but the same total energy delivered as a few stout blows can drive the nail firmly into the wood. This suggests that there is a threshold which must be exceeded to produce an effect, and which is successful in brief bursts but could be excessive if uninterrupted.

The view of many, particularly in the USA, e.g. Lehmann and de Lateur (1982), is that there are no therapeutically specific effects due to pulsed shortwave. Beneficial effects are simply due to the recognized effects of very mild heating. A trial comparing continuous shortwave with pulsed electromagnetic energy (Wilson, 1974) on 20 matched pairs of patients with ankle sprains showed clearly superior results in those treated with pulsed energy. Unfortunately more total energy was applied with continuous shortwave than with pulsed energy which leads to the contention (Lehmann and de Lateur, 1982) that the greater total heating of continuous shortwave would be contraindicated for this acute condition. Thus the same results are subject to opposite interpretations. This is in conformity with the Arndt–Schultz law, which suggests that stimulation beyond a threshold is necessary for a beneficial effect which will be dose dependent. At higher levels of stimulation the effect becomes inhibitory or progressively more damaging (see Fig. 10.15).

A pilot study comparing continuous with pulsed energy in the treatment of chronic low back pain (Wagstaff *et al.*, 1986) concluded that pulsed energy was more effective. There seems a dearth of other studies on this rather passion-provoking question.

At microscopic level, 'heat' is simply the kinetic energy of small particles and is likely to vary from place to place. Thus, the addition of small amounts of energy to the tissues could well increase local particulate motion. Whether this is called mild heating becomes something of an otiose argument.

Summary

Possible therapeutic mechanisms for pulsed shortwave:

- electromagnetic energy leads to a general increase in inter-cellular and intracellular activity
- electromagnetic energy influences cell membrane ion fluxes
- particular frequencies, pulse lengths or amplitudes of electromagnetic energy have specific cellular effects
- pulsing effect – a series of relatively high-energy pulses exceed some thresholds to produce a cellular effect which can only be tolerated because of the long interpulse intervals
- mild heating effect to conform with Arndt–Schultz law.

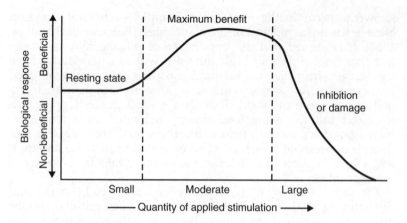

Fig. 10.15 Representation of the Arndt–Schultz law.

PHYSIOLOGICAL EFFECTS OF PULSED SHORTWAVE

There has been some research into the effects and efficacy of this therapy, both experimental laboratory work and clinical trials.

Laboratory experiments

Acceleration of tissue healing. The resolution of artificially induced haematomas in rabbits' ears was accelerated by twice daily 30-min treatments with pulsed shortwave (Fenn, 1969) and wound healing in dogs appeared more advanced after pulsed shortwave (Cameron, 1961). Muscle tissue repair in rabbits was investigated by Brown and Baker (1987) and no statistically significant difference could be demonstrated between their control and experimental groups. They did, however, note a trend toward better healing after 16 days of pulsed shortwave treatment. Krag *et al.* (1979) could find no difference between treated and control in skin flap survival area in rats. Constable *et al.* (1971) was also unable to find any benefit from pulsed shortwave for wound healing in rabbits and guinea pigs.

Enhanced nerve regeneration. This effect has been convincingly demonstrated in rats with experimental nerve lesions treated by pulsed shortwave (Wilson and Jagadeesh, 1976; Raji and Bowden, 1983; Raji, 1984).

Clinical trials

Postoperative. The rate of postoperative healing has been found to be greater with pulsed shortwave after orchidopexy (Bentall and

Eckstein, 1975), in skin graft donor sites (Goldin *et al.*, 1981) and after dental surgery (Aronofsky, 1971).

Recent tissue trauma. Acute ankle sprains have been treated by this modality with marked benefit (Wilson, 1972, 1974), some benefit (Pasila *et al.*, 1978) and no effect (McGill, 1989) – see later discussion on these studies. A large trial involving hand injuries (Barclay *et al.*, 1983) found that pulsed shortwave treatment produced very significant reductions in pain, swelling and disability in the first 7 days. This study has been criticized on methodological grounds, as have several of the others noted above.

This modality has also been applied to perineal trauma after childbirth, but a placebo-controlled trial (Grant *et al.*, 1989) found no benefit. Sports injuries are frequently treated (Wright, 1973).

Chronic lesions. Chronic back pain has been successfully treated (Wagstaff *et al.*, 1986), but in a study of pulsed shortwave applied to osteoarthritic hips no pain relief was obtained (Klaber Moffett *et al.*, 1996).

Superficial ulcers (bedsores) have been successfully treated (Seaborne *et al.*, 1996). In this study quite low energy applications (13.4 kJ per 24 h) were found to be most effective. This may be associated with the superficial site of these lesions.

THERAPEUTIC USES

It seems that pulsed shortwave is often an effective treatment for most tissue trauma, both accidental and postoperative, especially during the early stages. Thus all recent injuries, as well as acute traumatic synovites and haematomas, could be treated.

Acute infections, such as paranasal sinusitis, as well as subacute and chronic infections which it has been claimed will benefit, are also suitable for treatment. From the experimental evidence quoted above there seems to be a reasonable case for the early treatment of peripheral nerve lesions. Pain due to a variety of conditions including degenerative arthritis and neurogenic pain (phantom limb pain, causalgia, Sudeck's atrophy etc.) and pain due to osteoporosis (Wilson, 1981) seem to improve, sometimes dramatically, with this treatment.

APPLICATION OF PULSED SHORTWAVE

Pulsed shortwave can be applied to the body tissues in the same way as conventional shortwave, but several machines limit the method of application to a drum-type electrode consisting of a flat helical metal coil contained in a plastic casing (Oliver, 1984). The pattern of effects in the tissues would be the same as described for heating the tissues with continuous shortwave. Thus one would expect the drum-type electrode to cause effects principally in the skin and superficial muscle tissues, having weaker effects as it spreads out further into the tissues. The drum-type electrode is placed close to, or just touching, the skin over the area to be treated. A thermal sensation test should be carried out to ensure that there is no sensory deficit, especially when delivering pulsed shortwave at a mean power exceeding 5 W (Bricknell and Watson, 1995).

DOSAGE

There is little evidence and even less agreement concerning the treatment parameters that should be used.

Hayne (1984) suggested that one could compare the energy for different combinations of pulse widths and repetition rates by calculating the number of cycles of high-frequency energy for each. An alternative way of expressing the output is the average power in watts for each setting.

Others believe that short treatment times of 5–10 min are effective for all conditions. While an open mind must be kept on the matter, the evidence does seem to suggest that longer treatment times with high pulse repetition rates and short pulses are most effective. This is illustrated by the three studies on sprained ankles mentioned above:

- Wilson (1972) treated for 1 h/day with 600 pulses/s, 38 W mean power, which led to a good result. After 3 days the treated group had improved about twice as much as the controls.
- Pasila *et al.* (1978) gave 20-min treatments at 38 W mean power which led to the treated ankles doing marginally better than the controls.
- McGill (1989) gave 15 min of 19.6 W with no significant difference between treated and control groups.

Analysis of the energy applied per 24 h, in these and other clinical studies, showed that the threshold value for some success appeared to be 40 kJ/24 h, with the greatest success achieved with doses above 100 kJ/24 h. There were no effects at lower doses (Low, 1995). This meta-analysis conforms with the Arndt–Schultz law (see Fig. 10.15) noted above, that an appropriate quantity of energy – 'not too little, not too much' – is needed over relatively long treatment durations for efficacy. This would account for the ineffectiveness noted in a number of the studies noted above (e.g. Grant *et al.*, 1989).

CONTRAINDICATIONS

With the low average power of pulsed shortwave there is very little danger of a burn due to concentration of the field by metal or water. Thus it may be applied through wet dressings and in the presence of metal implants. However, it is important to realize that the treatment is relatively, not absolutely, athermic so that longer pulses given at higher frequencies can lead to heating and hence burning. This has been quantified in a study by Bricknell and Watson (1995) which found detectable heating at a mean power of 10.88 W delivered for some 7 min. In this case the potential dangers indicated for continuous shortwave are appropriate.

There have been no damaging effects of any kind reported to date with pulsed shortwave. However, due to the unknown mode of action discussed above it is considered prudent to avoid rapidly dividing tissues, such as the fetus or the uncontrolled growth of precancerous tissues or neoplasms. Similarly the theoretical risk of reactivating encapsulated lesions suggests that tuberculosis should be avoided. It is recommended that seriously hyperpyrexic patients should not be treated.

As cardiac pacemakers could certainly be affected in the same way as described for continuous shortwave such patients should be kept clear of pulsed shortwave sources, although there seem to have been no injuries reported. Hearing aids and other electronic equipment, such as some modern telephones, can be affected and although not dangerous to the patient can be inconvenient.

LOW-POWER PULSED HIGH-FREQUENCY ENERGY

A number of devices are available which generate pulses similar to those just described but at a tiny fraction of the power. They produce pulses of 27.12 MHz oscillations at various repeat rates but with about 0.5 W average power and 15 W peak power. There are some reports of their effectiveness in treating a variety of conditions, e.g. Debelle *et al.* (1977). These results were not substantiated in a rigorous controlled trial by Barker *et al.* (1985) involving ligament sprains.

Oedema and bruising were found to be less on the treated side during a controlled study of recovery after bilateral blepharoplasty (Nicolle and Bentall, 1982). All these sources apply energy to the tissues by means of an induction coil aerial placed on the surface of the skin. It has been claimed that the proximity to the tissues compensated for their low output. (For the blepharoplasty study the aerials were fashioned into spectacle frames worn over the dressings.) There are several reports of these low-power pulses being used successfully to encourage healing of skin wounds: it is possible to speculate that insufficient energy is reaching deeper structures to have any therapeutic effect.

Foley-Nolan *et al.* (1990) applied low-power pulsed electromagnetic energy via a cervical collar for persistent neck pain and found an increase in range of movement and a decrease in pain.

Methods of application vary but usually the small induction coil is held in contact with the skin over the lesion by a bandage or

Velcro strap. Length of treatment times suggested also vary a good deal but are often quite long, 1–2 h or even up to 6 h/day. The small battery-operated devices have been used for 16 h each day, and some continuously.

KILOHERTZ FREQUENCY DEVICES

Therapeutic sources generating frequencies of around 750 kHz and 500 kHz, with outputs up to 300 W (Indiba treatment), are available, although not widely known in the UK. These produce local heating through the application of a pair of metal electrodes to the skin (via a cream). Heating occurs throughout the intervening tissues, but is greatest close to the smaller active electrode. As noted earlier, currents of similar frequencies were at one time quite widely used, called 'longwave diathermy'. The therapeutic effects are presumably those of local deep tissue heating.

Summary of therapeutic high-frequency electromagnetic energy

- Continuous shortwave diathermy:
  - majority of sources 27.12 MHz frequency
  - output up to a few hundred watts
  - coupled to tissues inductively or capacitively
  - can give clearly detectable heating
  - usually applied for 20–30 min.
- Pulsed shortwave:
  - 27.12 MHz
  - output a few tens of watts, mean power emitting very short pulses of up to 1000 W peak power
  - coupled to tissues usually inductively; sometimes capacitively
  - heating only detected with outputs above 10 W
  - can be applied up to 60 min.
- Low-power pulsed high-frequency energy:
  - 27.12 MHz
  - output often less than 1 W mean power, peak power of a few watts, various pulsing regimens
  - coupled to tissues inductively
  - no detectable heating
  - often applied for hours a day.
- Kilohertz devices:
  - around 750 and 500 kHz frequency
  - output a few hundred watts
  - coupled to tissues capacitively via electrodes
  - detectable heating
  - applied 15–20 min.

THE USE OF MAGNETISM IN THERAPY

It has already been explained that magnetic forces are an inevitable consequence of the movement of charges so that any electric current produces a corresponding magnetic field. Having discussed high-frequency electromagnetic energy in this chapter it seems appropriate to give a brief account of the use of static and low-frequency therapies.

There is no certainty about the way in which magnetic fields react with living tissue. As has already been noted, tissues are largely transparent to a magnetic field but varying fields will induce currents in any conductors, including the tissues, that they cross. Further, the living tissues contain many moving charges due to blood or lymph flow, cell movement, nerve impulses and so forth, which could interact with any magnetic field so that the concept of a static magnetic field is too simple.

It must also be recognized that all life forms occur in a permanent magnetic field – the earth's magnetic field – which varies from place to place and has other varying (mainly man-made) magnetic fields superimposed; see later discussion on this topic.

The inexplicable forces due to ferromagnetism have provided powerful suggestions of healing properties. Thus early in the 16th century Theophrastus Bombastus Paracelsus von Honenheim had apparently used iron rodlets to 'heal fractures and ruptures, pull hepatitis out, and draw back dropsy' among other wonders (quoted by Cameron, 1983). Later Mesmer used iron magnets for treatment and ever since there have been therapies based on some form of permanent magnet.

Static magnetic fields

The most recent form of these therapies is based on the fact that modern permanent magnets are much more powerful than earlier magnets. They are alloys of cobalt, nickel and various rare earths such as yttrium, that can be up to 15 times the magnetic strength of the older steel magnets. In one therapy, called biomagnetism, small (1.5 mm) magnets are stuck on the skin in the centre of an adhesive patch about 2 cm across, often over a trigger point. Biomagnetism is also called Taiki therapy and various other sizes of magnet are used. It is claimed to be effective in a variety of vaguely specified conditions (Holzapfel *et al.*, 1981) but there appears to be no definitive evidence.

Static magnetic fields are also provided by a flexible material containing magnetic strips of alternating polarity and covered with a thin metal foil. These are bandaged or stuck to the skin over the lesion to be treated and left in place continuously, but not for more than 1 week. The local magnetic fields provided by this material are said to be relatively large (Hayne, 1984). Various other versions of this material giving a static magnetic field have been developed with different configurations of the permanent magnets, e.g. Bioflex, a circular alternating polarity magnetic foil which can be used as a pad or a tunnel.

The mode of action of static magnetic fields is said to be similar to pulsed shortwave, only much slower because the tiny induced electric currents must reach a threshold before any biological process is affected (Hayne, 1989). The main therapeutic uses are said to be for circulation, analgesia and wound healing. Post-polio pain was successfully relieved in a double-blind study (Vallbona *et al.*, 1997) using static magnetic fields of 300 or 500 gauss. This study is the most convincing evidence for the efficacy of these 'bioflex' magnets. Others have found no effect from magnetic therapy; for example, in a controlled trial, Leclaire and Bourgouin (1991) found this treatment gave no benefit in the management of periarthritis of the shoulder.

Low-frequency magnetic fields

A relatively powerful magnetic field set up in a large coil into which the part can be placed is provided by some machines. This field is oscillated, changing direction at various frequencies up to 50 Hz. Other pulsed devices use higher pulsing frequencies but much weaker magnetic fields and are placed in contact with the part to be treated. There is no objective evidence that clearly supports the therapeutic value of these therapies for many of the conditions for which they are recommended. McMeekan (1992) found that the field settings of a pulsed magnetic field machine, specified as producing vasodilation, did not do so. There is, however, good evidence of the effectiveness of low-frequency pulses applied to the tissues by electromagnetic induction in the treatment of ununited fractures (Bassett *et al.*, 1982) and Perthes' disease (Harrison and Bassett, 1984). Similar 0.38 ms pulses at around 72 Hz have been used successfully in the treatment of rotator cuff tendinitis in a double-blind trial (Binder *et al.*, 1984). All these therapies were applied for several hours each day, the patients often sleeping while the coils were active. Whether such low-frequency, single pulses applied for long periods act by a different mechanism from that of the pulsed high-frequency described earlier is not known. The terms 'pulsed electromagnetic fields' or 'pulsed electromagnetic energy' encompass both.

As to the safety of magnetic fields, there appears to be no evidence of any deleterious effects. The World Health Organization notes the absence of any adverse effects due to exposure to static magnetic fields up to 20 000 gauss (2 tesla).

EFFECTS AND SAFETY OF ELECTROMAGNETIC FIELDS

For many years there has been concern that electromagnetic radiations might constitute a health hazard in some way. This has been engendered by the realization that exposure to all kinds of electromagnetic radiations has greatly increased over the whole world during the past hundred years or so. The basic argument is that up to this time living organisms had been exposed to natural background electric and magnetic forces over millions of years and would have evolved to tolerate and perhaps benefit from these forces. Suddenly over a few decades much greater electric and magnetic forces have become a part of the environment. This is especially so close to high-voltage electric power transmission lines where the average magnetic field is somewhat higher than the average static earth magnetic field of about 0.5 gauss. The electric field close to the highest voltage lines can be 7–8 times greater than the typical natural field (Dowson, 1989). Radio waves at higher frequencies and microwaves at still higher frequencies, notably from cellular telephones, also contribute, as do domestic appliances.

McDowell and Lunt (1991) took electromagnetic field strength measurements on Megapulse units, and stated that the limits could be considered contained within a radius of 0.5 m from the applicator. They commented that, although there is a great deal of pick-up between electromagnetic fields and telephone lines in and near the treatment area, resulting in interference, the field strength is not high enough to damage equipment. They found coupling between water pipes and the electromagnetic fields, resulting in relatively high field strength at radiators. People and metal furniture near the treatment applicator can considerably distort the field.

There have been a number of studies to establish whether there is any correlation between electromagnetic exposure and disease; in the main low-frequency electromagnetic energy has been considered because this would make by far the largest contribution to electromagnetic 'pollution' – if it is pollution. These studies can be classified into four groups:

- studies in the laboratory on animals and cell cultures exposed to controlled, artificially produced electromagnetic fields
- similar studies of humans exposed to controlled electromagnetic fields
- epidemiological studies of human populations exposed to electromagnetic fields, for example those living near power transmission lines
- epidemiological studies of specific groups of people who are exposed to electromagnetic fields, e.g. in the electricity industry.

In the last two groups several detailed studies have investigated the incidence of various cancers, especially in children, to ascertain whether there was an increase among those exposed to the higher electromagnetic fields. Some found no effect while others found a slight but significant correlation between disease and exposure to strong electromagnetic radiations. (For a further account see Dowson, 1989.) Some studies found increased risk of malignant disease among electrical workers, e.g. Milham (1982).

Suggestions have been made that exposure to strong electro-magnetic fields might be associated with depression. In a study of patients committing suicide, no association was found between the relation of power lines to their place of residence (Reichmanis *et al.*, 1979). However, a later re-evaluation of the data measuring the electromagnetic fields found a significant relationship (Perry *et al.*, 1981). A study of workers at a Russian high-voltage electricity substation (Asanova and Rakov, 1966) found dysfunction of the (in particular, autonomic) nervous system associated with rather generalized complaints of headaches, insomnia, sluggishness, fatigue and other complaints in a high proportion of workers. This and other studies led to strict regulations concerning exposure of people to electromagnetic fields in the USSR. These are still the most restrictive in the world. This evidence has not been confirmed, although a recent study (Dowson and Lewith, 1988) found an association between recurrent headache and radiations from overhead high-voltage cables, especially at a particular distance of 60–80 m. These and other studies supporting the view that electromagnetic fields are hazardous, are described in an extensive account by Smith and Best (1989). Much of this evidence is disputed; some is based on correlations that do not necessarily mean there is a cause and effect relationship.

Numerous experiments have been done, mostly at low frequency, to define the effects of electric and magnetic fields on cells, tissues, organs, systems and even behaviour, in animals and humans. There is evidence for effects on the central nervous system, on fat and calcium metabolism and on circadian rhythm in humans and animals from electromagnetic fields of various strengths and frequencies amongst numerous others. For an extensive review see Sheppard and Eisenbud (1977); an earlier review and discussion by Presman (1970) or Becker and Marino (1982). Although much of these data are contradictory and confused it can be firmly stated that relatively weak electric and magnetic fields are able to evoke many neurophysiological effects. It is repeatedly suggested by these experiments that electromagnetic energy has a communicating and controlling influence on biological systems when applied at low intensities, which is lost at higher intensities. Suggested mechanisms include causing conformational changes in molecules of cell walls and the stimulation of adrenocortical responses to stress.

In summary, at the present time there is no certain evidence of significant health damage from artificial electromagnetic fields. For a full review, with comments on the physiotherapeutic implications and discussion, see Charman (1991). The beneficial effects of low-intensity fields are difficult to quantify. It is agreed by all that more research is urgently needed in this area.

REFERENCES

Aronofsky D. H. (1971). Reduction of dental post-surgical symptoms using non-thermal pulsed high-peak-power electromagnetic energy. *Oral Surg.*, **32**, 688.

Asanova T. P., Rakov A. I. (1966). *The State of Health of Persons Working in Electric Field of Outdoor 400 and 500 kV Switchyards. Hygiene of Labor and Professional Diseases 5.* Translation in special publication 10. Piscataway NJ: IEEE Power Engineering Society.

Baker R. R. (1981). *Human Navigation and the Sixth Sense*. London: Hodder & Stoughton.

Bansal P. S., Sobti V. K., Roy K. S. (1990). Histomorphochemical effects of short-wave diathermy on healing of experimental muscle injury in dogs. *Indian J. Exp. Biol.*, **28**, 766–70.

Barclay V., Collier R. J., Jones A. (1983). Treatment of various hand injuries by pulsed electromagnetic energy (Diapulse). *Physiotherapy*, **69**, 186–8.

Barker A. T., Barlow P. S., Porter J. *et al.* (1985). A double-blind clinical trial of low power pulsed shortwave therapy in the treatment of soft-tissue injury. *Physiotherapy*, **71**, 500–4.

Bassett C. A. L., Mitchell S. N., Gaston S. R. (1982). Pulsing electromagnetic field treatment in ununited fractures and failed arthrodeses. *J. Am. Med. Assoc.*, **247**, 623.

Becker R. O., Marino A. A. (1982). *Electromagnetism and Life*. New York: State University of New York Press.

Bentall R. H. C., Eckstein H. B. (1975). A trial involving the use of pulse electromagnetic therapy on children undergoing orchidopexy. *Kinderchirugie*, **17**, 380–2.

Binder A., Parr G., Hayleman B. *et al.* (1984). Pulsed electromagnetic field therapy of persistent rotator cuff tendinitis. *Lancet*, **i**, 695–8.

Bricknell R., Watson T. (1995). The thermal effects of pulsed shortwave therapy. *Br. J. Therapy Rehabil.*, **2**, 430–34.

Brown M., Baker R. D. (1987). Effects of pulsed shortwave diathermy on skeletal muscle injury in rabbits. *Phys. Ther.*, **67**, 208–13.

Cameron B. (1961). Experimental acceleration of wound healing. *Am. J. Orthop.*, **53**, 336–43.

Cameron H. U. (1983). Electromagnetic therapy: fact or fiction. *Mod. Med. N.Z.*, **16**, 17.

Charman R. (1991). Environmental currents and fields – man-made. *Physiotherapy*, **77**, 129–40.

Chartered Society of Physiotherapy. (1992). Guidelines for the safe use of continuous shortwave therapy equipment. *Physiotherapy*, **78**, 755–6.

Collis C. S., Segal M. B. (1988). Effects of pulsed electromagnetic fields in Na^+ fluxes across a stripped rabbit colon epithelium. *J. Appl. Physiol.*, **65**, 124–30.

Constable J. D., Scapicchio A. P., Opitz B. (1971). Studies of the effects of Diapulse treatment on various aspects of wound healing in experimental animals. *J. Surg. Res.*, **11**, 254–7.

Debelle M., Lorthier J., Berghmans M. *et al.* (1977). Therapeutic effect of very low powered hertzian wave transmissions. *Brux-Med.*, **57**, 551–63.

Delpizzo V., Joyner K. H. (1987). On the safe use of microwave and shortwave diathermy units. *Aust. J. Physiother.*, **33**, 152–62.

DHW (1983). *Safety Code 25 – Shortwave Diathermy Guidelines for Limited Radiofrequency Exposure*. Canadian Department of Health and Welfare, 83-EHD-98.

Dowson D. I. (1989). A review of epidemiological studies into the health effects of electromagnetic fields. *Compl. Hlth Res.*, **3**, 25–9.

Dowson D. I., Lewith G. I. (1988). Overhead high voltage cables and recurrent headaches and depression. *Practitioner*, **232**, 435–6.

Dyson M., Pond J. B. (1970). The effect of pulsed ultrasound on tissue regeneration. *Physiotherapy*, **56**, 136–42.

Evaluation Report: Shortwave Therapy Units (1987). *J. Med. Eng. Technol.*, **11**, 285–98.

Evans A. (1980). The healing process at cellular level: a review. *Physiotherapy*, **66**, 256–8.

Fenn J. E. (1969). Effects of pulsed electromagnetic energy (Diapulse) on experimental haematomas. *Can. Med. Assoc. J.*, **100**, 251–4.

Foley-Nolan D., Barry C., Coughlan R. J. *et al.* (1990). Pulsed high frequency (27 MHz) electromagnetic therapy for persistent neck pains. *Orthopaedics*, **13**, 445–51.

Forster A., Palastanga N. (1985). *Clayton's Electrotherapy: Theory and Practice*. London: Baillière Tindall.

Fukada E., Yasuda I. (1964). Piezoelectric effects in cartilage. *Jpn. J. Appl. Physiol.*, **3**, 117–21.

Goldin J. H., Broadbent N. R. T., Nancarrow J. D., Marshall T. (1981). The effects of Diapulse on the healing of wounds: a double-blind randomised controlled trial in man. *Br. J. Plast. Surg.*, **14**, 267–70.

Grant A., Sleep J., McIntosh J., Ashurst A. (1989). Ultrasound and pulsed electromagnetic energy treatment for perineal trauma. A randomised placebo-controlled trial. *Br. J. Obstet. Gynaecol.*, **96**, 434–9.

Guy A. W. (1982). Biophysics of high frequency currents and electromagnetic radiation. In *Therapeutic Heat and Cold* (Lehmann J. F., ed.) Baltimore: Williams & Wilkins, pp. 199–277.

Hansen T. I., Kristensen J. H. (1973). Effect of massage, shortwave diathermy and ultrasound upon ^{133}Xe disappearance rate from muscle and subcutaneous tissue in the human calf. *Scand. J. Rehabil. Med.*, **5**, 179–82.

Harrison M. J. M., Bassett C. A. L. (1984). Use of pulsed electromagnetic fields in Perthes disease: report of a pilot study. *J. Paed. Orthop.*, **4**, 579–84.

Hayne C. R. (1984). Pulsed high frequency energy – its place in physiotherapy. *Physiotherapy*, **70**, 459–66.

Hayne C. (1989). The healing fields. *Ther. Weekly*, March 16.

Holzapfel E., Crepon P., Philippe C. (1981). *Magnet Therapy*. Wellingborough: Thorsons.

Jones S. L. (1976). Electromagnetic field interference and cardiac pacemakers. *Phys. Ther.*, **56**, 1013–18.

Kallen B., Malmquist G., Moritz U. (1982). Delivery outcome among physiotherapists in Sweden. Is non-ionizing radiation a fetal hazard? *Arch. Environ. Hlth*, **37**, 81–4.

Kitchen S., Dyson M. (1996). Low energy treatments: nonthermal or microthermal? In *Clayton's Electrotherapy*, 10th edn (Kitchen S., Bazin S., eds) Philadelphia: W. B. Saunders, pp. 110–15.

Klaber Moffett J. A., Richardson P. H., Frost H., Osborn A. (1996). Placebo controlled, double-blind trial to evaluate the effectiveness of pulsed shortwave therapy for osteoarthritic hip and knee pain. *Pain*, **167**, 121–7.

Kloth L., Morrison M. A., Ferguson B. H. (1984). *Therapeutic Microwave and Shortwave Diathermy*. HHS Publication FDA, 85–8237. US Dept of Health and Human Services.

Krag C., Taudor F. U., Siim E., Bolund S. (1979). The effect of pulsed electromagnetic energy (Diapulse) on the survival of experimental skin flaps. *Scand. J. Plastic Reconst. Surg.*, **13**, 377–80.

Leclaire R., Bourgouin J. (1991). Electromagnetic treatment of shoulder periarthritis: a randomized controlled trial of the efficiency and tolerance of magnetotherapy. *Arch. Phys. Med. Rehabil.*, **72**, 284–7.

Lehmann J. F., de Lateur B. J. (1982). Therapeutic heat. In *Therapeutic Heat and Cold* (Lehmann J. F., ed.) Baltimore: Williams & Wilkins, pp. 404–562.

Low J. L. (1978). The nature and effects of pulsed electromagnetic radiations. *N. Z. J. Physiother.*, **6**(4), 18–22.

Low J. (1995). Dosage of some pulsed shortwave clinical trials. *Physiotherapy*, **81**, 611–16.

Mann J. (1989). Department of Health Procurement Directorate, London.

Martin C. J., McCallum H. M., Strelley S. *et al.* (1991). Electromagnetic fields from therapeutic diathermy equipment: a review of hazards and precautions. *Physiotherapy*, **77**, 3–7.

McDowell A. D., Lunt M. J. (1991). Electromagnetic field strength measurements on megapulse units. *Physiotherapy*, **77**, 805–9.

McGill S. N. (1989). The effect of pulsed shortwave therapy on lateral ligament sprain of the ankle. *N. Z. J. Physiother.*, **16**, 21–4.

McMeekan J. M. (1992). Magnetic fields: effects on blood flow in human subjects. *Physiotherapy Theory Pract.*, **8**, 3–9.

Milham S. (1982). Mortality from leukaemia in workers exposed to electrical and magnetic fields. *N. Z. J. Med.*, **307**, 249.

Nicolle F. V., Bentall R. A. C. (1982). Use of radio-frequency pulsed energy in the control of post-operative reactions in blepharoplasty. *Aesth. Plast. Surg.*, **6**, 169–71.

Nielson N. C., Hansen R., Larsen T. (1979). Heat induction in copper bearing IUDs during shortwave diathermy. *Acta Obstet. Gynaecol. Scand.*, **58**, 495.

Oliver D. E. (1984). Pulsed electro-magnetic energy – what is it? *Physiotherapy*, **70**, 458–9.

Oosterveld F. G. J., Rasker J. J., Jacobs J. W. G. *et al.* (1992). The effects of local heat and cold therapy on the intraarticular and skin surface temperature of the knee. *Arth. Rheum.*, **35**(2), 146–51.

Pasila M., Visuri T., Sundholm A. (1978). Pulsating shortwave diathermy: value in treatment of recent ankle and foot sprains. *Arch. Phys. Med. Rehabil.*, **59**, 283–6.

Perry F. S., Reichmanis M., Marino A. A., Becker R. O. (1981). Environmental power frequency magnetic fields and suicide. *Hlth Phys.*, **41**, 267–77.

Presman A. S. (1970). *Electromagnetic Fields and Life.* New York: Plenum Press.

Raji A. M. (1984). An experimental study of the effects of pulsed electromagnetic field (Diapulse) on nerve repair. *J. Hand Surg.*, **9B**, 105–11.

Raji A. R. M., Bowden R. E. M. (1983). Effects of high-peak pulsed electromagnetic field on the degeneration and regeneration of the common peroneal nerve in rats. *J. Bone Joint Surg.*, **65B**, 478–92.

Reichmanis M., Perry F. S., Marino A. A., Becker R. O. (1979). Relation between suicide and the electromagnetic field of overhead power lines. *Physiol. Chem. Phys.*, **11**, 395–403.

Schwan H. P. (1965). Biophysics of diathermy. In *Therapeutic Heat and Cold* (Licht S., ed.) Baltimore, Maryland: Waverly Press Incorporated.

Scott B. O. (1957). *The Principles and Practice of Diathermy.* London: Heinemann Medical Books.

Scott B. O. (1965). Shortwave diathermy. In *Therapeutic Heat and Cold* (Licht S., ed.) Baltimore, Maryland: Waverly Press Incorporated.

Seaborne D., Quirion-DeGiradi C., Rousseau M., Rivest M., Lambert J. (1996). The treatment of pressure sores using pulsed electromagnetic energy (PEME). *Physiotherapy* (Canada), **48**, 131–7.

Sheppard A. R., Eisenbud M. (1977). *Biological Effects of Electric and Magnetic Fields of Extremely Low Frequency.* New York: New York University Press.

Smith C. W., Best S. (1989). *Electromagnetic Man: Health and Hazard in the Electrical Environment.* London: Dent.

Taskinen H., Kyyrönen P., Hemminki K. (1990). The effects of ultrasound, shortwaves and physical exertion on pregnancy outcome in physiotherapists. *J. Epidemiol. Community Health*, **44**, 196–201.

Tsong T. Y. (1989). Deciphering the language of cells. *Trends Biol. Sci.*, **14**, 89–92.

Vallbona C., Hazlewood C. F., Jurida G. (1997). Response of pain to static magnetic fields in postpolio patients: a double-blind pilot study. *Arch. Phys. Med. Rehabil.*, **78**, 1200–3.

Verrier M., Ashby P., Crawford J. S. (1978). Effects of thermotherapy on the electrical and mechanical properties of human skeletal muscle. *Physiotherapy* (Canada), **30**, 117–20.

Verrier M., Falconer K., Crawford J. S. (1977). A comparison of tissue temperature following two shortwave diathermy techniques. *Physiotherapy* (Canada), **29**, 21–5.

Wadsworth H., Chanmugan A. P. P. (1980). *Electrophysical Agents in Physiotherapy.* Marrickville, NSW, Australia: Science Press.

Wagstaff P., Wagstaff S., Downey M. (1986). A pilot study to compare the efficacy of continuous and pulsed magnetic energy (shortwave diathermy) on the relief of low back pain. *Physiotherapy*, **72**, 563–6.

Ward A. R. (1986). *Electricity Fields and Waves in Therapy.* Marrickville, NSW, Australia: Science Press.

Whyte H. M., Reader S. R. (1952). Heating the knee joint. *Ann. Rheum. Dis.*, **11**, 54.

Wilson D. H. (1972). Treatment of soft tissue injuries by pulsed electrical energy. *Br. Med. J.*, **2**, 269–70.

Wilson D. H. (1974). Comparison of shortwave diathermy and pulsed electromagnetic energy in treatment of soft tissue injuries. *Physiotherapy*, **60**, 309–10.

Wilson D. H. (1981). PEME: the new beam for fractures. *World Med.*, 97–8.

Wilson D. H., Jagadeesh P. (1976). Experimental regeneration in peripheral nerves and the spinal cord in laboratory animals exposed to a pulsed electromagnetic field. In *Proceedings of the Annual Scientific Meeting of the International Medical Society of Paraplegia. Part III: Paraplegia*. pp. 12–20.

Wright G. G. (1973). Treatment of soft tissue and ligamentous injuries in professional footballers. *Physiotherapy*, **59**, 385–7.

11 Electromagnetic radiation

The last four chapters of this book are concerned with the therapeutic uses of radiations of one kind or another. Historically, there has always been a powerful association between the rays of the sun and healing, and from earliest times the sun has been central to religious belief. The Latin *deus* (god) is said to derive from the sun-worshipping Aryans' name for the sun. The healing effects of heat and light were widely known to the ancients and repopularized among the scientific advances of the end of the seventeenth century and onwards to the present day.

It is therefore necessary for this chapter to provide a general foundation for what follows by describing the nature and characteristics of these radiations.

All electromagnetic radiations have common features, which are described in the opening section. The interactions of radiations with matter are then considered, including reflection, refraction, scattering and, importantly, absorption.

NATURE

Electromagnetism can be considered to have three aspects: electrostatic, magnetic and radiation (see Chapter 10). Electromagnetic radiations are waves in the sense that they consist of regular sinusoidal variations of an electric and a magnetic field at right angles to one another (see Fig. 11.1). They are similar to sound and ultrasonic waves, considered in Chapter 6, in that they exhibit the features of energy transmission by any wave motion, but they differ from sonic waves in two important respects:

- the wave is a variation in the strength of both electric and magnetic fields and is thus independent of the atoms and molecules through which it passes, although it may give energy to them; sonic waves on the other hand are variations in the position (e.g. compression) of the atoms and molecules of the material through which the wave passes (see Chapter 6)
- electromagnetic waves are transverse waves, that is the variation occurs at right angles to the direction of travel; this is unlike the compressions and rarefactions of sonic waves which are longitudinal, i.e. in the direction of travel of the wave.

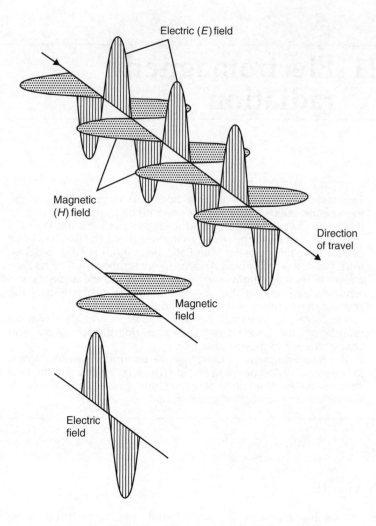

Fig. 11.1 Electric and magnetic fields.

All electromagnetic waves have a constant velocity in space. When no matter is present they travel at a speed of 300 000 000 m/s (3×10^8 m/s) in a straight line – to be strictly accurate 2.9979 × 10^8 m/s. When radiations pass through matter the velocity is decreased somewhat but for most of the radiations the effect of air is trivial.

As these waves are simply regular variations in amplitude of the electric and magnetic fields they can be described in terms of the number of times in each second they repeat that change, that is the frequency in hertz (Hz). Similarly, the distance between any point of the wave and the place where that point is repeated, say crest to crest, can be described as the wavelength, in units of length such as metres, millimetres or nanometres. The waves vary sinusoidally with both time and distance. These points are illustrated in Figure 11.1.

In spite of their constant velocity, electromagnetic radiations, differing only in wavelength and frequency, have very different interactions with matter and are therefore recognized in totally different ways. The list or spectrum of radiations, shown in the Frontispiece, includes radio waves, microwaves, infrared radiations, visible and ultraviolet radiations, X-rays, gamma and cosmic rays. The small range of radiations which are able to stimulate the retinal cells of the eye are recognized as visible light and so are by far the most familiar and best studied. In fact, much of the behaviour of electromagnetic radiations is understood and illustrated by reference to experiments done with light.

The names given to the various radiations reflect their historical discovery and uses. Thus radio waves (also called hertzian waves) are divided into long-, medium- and shortwave bands in connection with radio and television broadcasting (see Chapter 10). Microwaves are also known as radar radiations. The naming of infrared, below the red, and ultraviolet, beyond the violet, is self-explanatory of their relationship to the colours of the visible spectrum. X-rays are also known as Roentgen radiations.

There is only an arbitrary division between one kind of radiation and the next, except for the limits of the visible spectrum which can be defined fairly precisely by what the human eye can and cannot see. The naming covers wide bands of radiations so that different effects may be due to different frequencies of the same radiation, thus long ultraviolet (UVA) has rather different effects in the skin from ultraviolet B (UVB).

It will be evident that the magnitude (by analogy with water, the height of the wave) can vary. This is called the amplitude and is the strength of the electric and magnetic fields. This is not the only way in which the energy varies. It can be seen from the Frontispiece that those radiations which have the most vigorous effects on matter are those with the shortest wavelengths and highest frequencies, like X-rays and gamma rays; the energy increases with frequency. This occurs because radiations are made up of discrete units of energy called quanta which cannot be subdivided. The energy of one quantum is called a photon; it depends on the frequency of radiation. Thus higher frequency radiations carry more energy and are able to have more vigorous interactions with matter.

Ionization means that an electron has been separated from its atom. Radiation that has this effect is called ionizing radiation. Atoms can be thought of as a positively charged nucleus with a number of rapidly orbiting electrons. Electrons occupying different orbits have different energy levels and by giving energy to the atom an electron can be made to occupy higher energy levels; the atom thus absorbs a precise amount of energy. Similarly, when electrons are made to jump from a high energy level to a lower one a precise amount of energy, due to the difference in levels, is released. This is emitted in the form of electromagnetic radiation. The wavelength or frequency of this radiation depends on the energy difference. The transition between two energy levels by one electron can be made to occur due to the absorption of 1 quantum of radiation at a particular frequency and can cause the emission of 1 quantum of radiation of a particular frequency.

Electromagnetic radiations are produced whenever electrons are accelerated or decelerated. Radio waves, for example, are produced by high-frequency oscillating currents, as described in Chapter 10. It was seen in Chapter 7 that heat is molecular motion and if the rotational and vibrational movements of molecules are increased by heating, the changing electron motion leads to the emission of infrared radiations. Thus any moderately hot body emits infrared radiation (also considered in Chapter 7). With greater heating more nuclear and atomic vibration will occur leading to the emission of radiations with shorter wavelengths and higher frequencies and thus carrying more energy. The emitted photons will have a range of different wavelengths with the shortest wavelength produced depending on temperature. Thus at higher temperatures some shorter wavelengths are produced. For example, at around 400°C the shortest wavelength emitted from a heated solid is in the infrared region but at about 700°C some radiations in the red visible region are emitted. Thus the solid glows red-hot. Still further temperature rises lead to even more vigorous vibration of atoms with the emission of photons with still shorter wavelengths, including the whole of the visible spectrum so that the object appears white-hot; this can occur at temperatures around 1500°C.

A second way in which visible radiations can be produced occurs when, for example, atoms and ions are made to collide in a low-pressure gas giving energy to an outer electron which subsequently returns to a lower energy level, causing the emission of a photon of energy characteristic of that particular transition energy. Therefore particular atoms produce radiations of particular wavelengths. This forms a line spectrum which is characteristic of the particular atoms. Sodium, for example, produces typical yellow lines giving the familiar yellow light of sodium-vapour street lighting. Ultraviolet radiations are produced in a similar way but involve higher energies and therefore shorter wavelengths. X-rays are produced when high-energy transitions are made to occur either when orbiting electrons jump between inner orbits or when rapidly moving electrons are abruptly decelerated. Gamma radiations are emitted from the nuclei of certain radioactive atoms.

Summary

Electromagnetic radiations are:

- emitted whenever the constant motion of an electron is changed
- energy in the form of oscillating electric and magnetic fields perpendicular to one another and to the direction of travel (see Fig. 11.1)
- named to encompass eight bands but more precisely identified by frequency or wavelength
- able to travel at a constant velocity of 3×10^8 m/s in space (as with all wave systems, the velocity is the product of frequency and wavelength)
- emitted as quanta whose energy is proportional to the frequency of the radiation
- able to induce ionization of some atoms at higher frequencies.

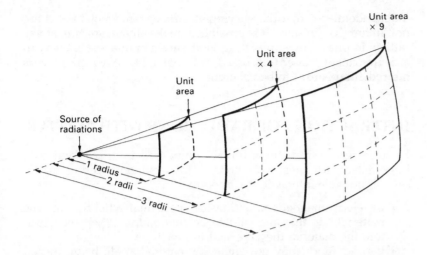

Fig. 11.2 The inverse square law. The intensity of radiation from a point source is inversely proportional to the square of the distance from the source.

FEATURES OF ELECTROMAGNETIC RADIATION

Rectilinear propagation

Electromagnetic radiations travel in straight lines in space. This is clearly evident with visible radiations since shadows are formed where the light path is interrupted by an object. Radiations are emitted from their source in all directions so that if the source is relatively small the radiations will spread out equally in all directions with the result that the energy passing through a unit area per unit time – the intensity – will decrease with distance. This is illustrated in Figure 11.2. The relationship between the distance from the source and intensity of radiation is expressed in *the inverse square law* which states that the intensity of the radiation from a point source is inversely proportional to the square of the distance from the source:

$$I \propto \frac{1}{d^2}$$

where I = intensity and d = distance.

This is, of course, only strictly true if there is no scattering or absorption of the radiations but for many radiations it is effectively true in air and of great practical importance (see later discussion on the application of infrared and ultraviolet). The consequence is that small changes of distance will cause large changes of intensity, as shown in Figure 11.2. Doubling the distance between the source and the irradiated surface will reduce the intensity to one-quarter; tripling the distance would reduce the intensity to one-ninth and so on. Similarly, halving the distance will quadruple the intensity.

Phase difference and coherence

Radiations emitted from a source consist of random bursts of radiation because each atom or molecule of the source acts independently so that the varying electric and magnetic fields are not 'in time' or 'in step'. It is possible to make all the emitting atoms radiate in phases by stimulating light emission in a special way in a device called a laser (discussed in Chapter 14). When this occurs the radiation is said to be coherent.

INTERACTIONS OF RADIATIONS WITH MATTER

Electromagnetic radiations travel unhindered in space (and to a large extent, for most radiations, in air) but on meeting matter several possible interactions can occur:

- the electromagnetic radiations can pass unaffected through the material, i.e. they are said to be *transmitted*. When they pass into the material they are said to penetrate
- the radiations may not enter the material at all, being turned back or *reflected*.

In both these cases as there is no energy lost to the material there is no effect on the material:

- radiation energy may be *absorbed*; if it is to have any effect it must be absorbed; this is an idea first proposed by Grotthus in 1820, so it is sometimes noted as Grotthus' law.

In real situations all three happen together so that some radiations are transmitted right through, some are reflected and some absorbed. The amount of each depends on the wavelength or frequency of the radiation and the nature of the material. Often one aspect predominates, for example light will be mainly transmitted through panes of window glass but it is evident that some of the light is reflected (if this were not so the glass would be invisible), also some is absorbed. In the case of a shiny metal surface reflection of visible radiations predominates.

Radiations entering a new material, a new medium, may be bent at the surface – a process called refraction – and transmitted at some angle to the original line.

In non-homogeneous materials, both reflection and refraction may occur in the bulk of the material; a process called *scattering*. This has a strong influence on where the radiation is absorbed in the material.

Reflection of radiations

When electromagnetic radiations pass through matter they interact with the electric fields of the atoms and molecules and this determines their velocity in that particular material. At the junction of two kinds of matter, say glass and air, the electromagnetic waves have to change velocity as the velocity is less in glass. The wave will not change in frequency so that only part of the wave energy can be transmitted; the rest is turned back or reflected.

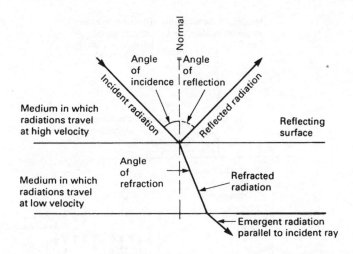

Fig. 11.3 Reflection and refraction.

- The amount of reflection depends on the:
  - nature of the radiation
  - angle of incidence
  - nature of the surface.
- The direction of the reflected radiation depends on:
  - the angle of the incident radiation.
- For a beam of radiation impinging on a plane surface:
  - the angle of incidence is equal to the angle of reflection
  - the incident and reflected beam are in the same plane as the 'normal', a line perpendicular to the surface at the point of incidence.

The last point states the two laws of reflection illustrated in Figure 11.3. They are well understood in connection with visible radiations but are equally valid for other electromagnetic radiations, e.g. microwaves bouncing off a flat metal sheet in a microwave oven or, for that matter, any other wave system such as sonic waves, as described in Chapter 6.

The reflection of visible radiations from matter is, of course, central to human perception of the visible world. The recognition of colour and form is due to the reflection of radiations from objects (except when the object is emitting visible radiations of its own). The retinal cells of the eyes are sensitive to extremely low energy levels and are able to detect a few photons and discriminate between colours with wavelength differences of only a few tens of nanometres.

When a beam of radiations strikes a surface the part of the beam that is not reflected must penetrate into the new medium; so there is a constant relationship – the more that is reflected, the less that penetrates, and vice versa. The relationship between the amount of any given radiation reflected and the amount that penetrates any particular surface depends on the angle at which it strikes the surface – the angle of incidence. This can be understood in terms of photons having a greater chance of penetrating if they meet the surface at right angles – as a dart is more likely to penetrate if it

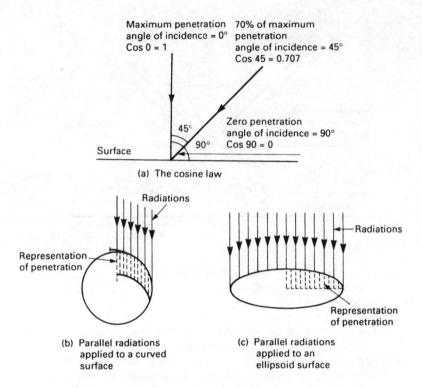

Fig. 11.4 Ratio of reflected and penetrating radiations. (a) The cosine law; (b) parallel radiations applied to a curved surface; (c) parallel radiations applied to an ellipsoid section.

strikes the board at right angles and more likely to bounce off if it strikes a glancing blow. Further, if a beam strikes a surface at right angles the area covered is the cross-section of the beam, but if angled to the surface the area covered increases so that the intensity on unit area decreases. This can be easily demonstrated by shining a torch vertically down on to the floor and comparing the circle of light with the larger oval produced when the torch is shone at an angle.

The *cosine law*, as it is called, relates the intensity of radiation falling on a surface to the cosine of the angle of incidence of the radiation (Fig. 11.4(a)). If the radiations are applied perpendicular to the surface the angle of incidence is 0°; the cosine of 0 is 1, which gives the maximum intensity of radiations per unit area, and hence the greatest penetration. At an angle of incidence of 45°, cos 45 = 0.7, it can be seen that the intensity will be 70% of maximum, thus the amount of radiation penetrating will be less. While the cosine law is inaccurate to predict the precise proportions of reflected and penetrating radiations, it nevertheless indicates the approximate pattern of this relationship. Thus, if the radiations are parallel to the surface, i.e. there is an angle of incidence of 90°, there will be no penetration of the surface because the cosine of 90 is 0. From the above it can be seen that small angular deviations from the perpendicular make very little difference; thus errors of 15 or 20° in the placing of lamps or angling of laser applications are insignificant but at large angles the absorption falls off markedly.

Thus the relationship between the amount of radiation reflected to that penetrating depends on:

- the angle of incidence
- the interaction of the radiation with the new medium (depending on the electrical properties of its microstructure).

A further important consequence of this is the effect of parallel radiation on a curved surface. It will be evident that penetration will diminish around the sides of a circular surface as the angle of incidence increases and the cosine of the angle decreases (Fig. 11.4(b)). To achieve uniform irradiation it is necessary to apply radiations from two directions at right angles. If the surface is elliptical in section (Fig. 11.4(c)) the angular changes between radiation and surface are small except at the very edge of the ellipse. Thus parallel radiations applied to such surfaces give almost uniform penetration over much of the area. Since the trunk and some limb segments of the body are approximately ovoid in cross-section most of the body is more or less evenly irradiated in just two positions, i.e. sunbathing lying down prone and supine.

Refraction

When radiation meets a boundary with a medium in which it travels at a different velocity its velocity will be altered and it will be refracted or bent unless the radiation is perpendicular to the boundary (Fig. 11.3). The part of the wave front of any radiation entering a medium in which it travels more slowly will be delayed compared to the part of the wave front still in the high-velocity medium. This will cause the wave front to be turned through an angle which depends on its relative velocities in the two media. (The velocity of waves in a medium depends on the nature of the medium and the wavelength.) Consequently radiations of different wavelengths can be made to travel different paths by being refracted to different degrees. This is how a glass prism can be used to separate the different wavelengths of the visible spectrum.

The glass–air interface is, of course, used to bend visible radiations through lenses in all kinds of optical instruments, microscopes, magnifying lenses, cameras and so forth. The specialized transparent tissues forming the lens of the eye work in the same way. If a ray enters a medium in which it will travel more slowly, it is bent towards the normal as it enters (see Fig. 11.3): similarly the reverse is true. Thus visible radiations emerging from glass into air will be refracted away from the normal. In the case of, say, a parallel-sided block of glass the emergent ray is parallel to the incident ray but displaced sideways (see Fig. 11.3). Increasing the angle of incidence at the dense–less dense interface increases the angle of refraction. At a certain angle of incidence, called the critical angle, the radiation will travel parallel to the surface. At any greater angle the radiation would be reflected back into the glass, an effect called total internal reflection.

Reflection and refraction have been described largely in terms of visible radiation but it must be understood that these are general principles which apply to all electromagnetic radiations, albeit to different degrees with different radiations and media. Microwaves are reflected from metal surfaces, thus enabling the position of aircraft and ships to be monitored by radar. Long radio waves can be reflected by an ionized layer in the outer atmosphere. Ultraviolet radiations are retained in curved quartz rods (applicators) by total internal reflection.

Absorption and penetration

The relationship between the amount of an electromagnetic radiation that is absorbed and the distance it penetrates any given material is of the greatest importance. Absorption is the reciprocal of penetration (i.e. the greater the penetration the less the absorption). For a homogeneous material the amount of any given radiation absorbed will be a fixed proportion of the total radiation present at that point. Thus the amount of radiation absorbed will fall exponentially with depth in the same way as sonic waves, described in Chapter 6. In order to describe this pattern of absorption in a convenient way a single figure is used, either:

- penetration depth – the depth at which 63% of the original radiation has been absorbed, or
- half-value depth – the depth at which 50% has been absorbed. This concept is illustrated in Figure 11.5.

Different frequencies/wavelengths of radiation have different penetration depths in any particular material, thus materials of a particular nature and thickness can be used as filters. This filtering effect is applied in many situations, e.g. filtering out the short ultraviolet (UVC) radiations but leaving the longer ultraviolet rays for some treatment or filtering out all the UVR but leaving visible radiations, as in protective ultraviolet goggles (see Chapter 15).

The concept of absorption described above and in Figure 11.5 is also important in considering the effect of radiations on the tissues. The penetration and absorption of the different modalities will be considered in the appropriate chapters. Some infrared and visible radiations may have half-value penetration depths of less than 1 mm while some microwaves have a half-value depth of several centimetres. It must, however, be emphasized that the tissues are not homogeneous so that absorption in the tissues is much more irregular than Figure 11.5 suggests.

Scattering

Radiations passing in non-homogeneous matter may be partly scattered, that is the direction of some radiations is altered,

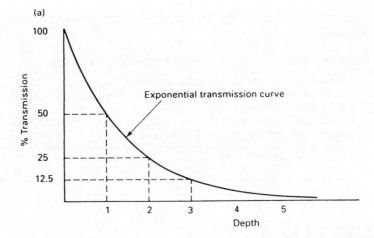

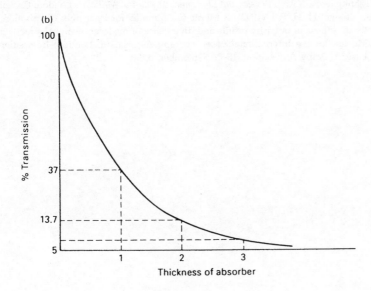

Fig. 11.5 (a) Half-value thickness; (b) penetration depth.

effectively reducing the depth of penetration. The scattered radiation may travel in a different direction and be absorbed at some point away from the main beam of radiation. Scattering is due to reflection and refraction from small particles and shorter wavelengths are more affected than longer ones. Scattering of radiations in the tissues is a highly complex matter (Van Breugel, 1992). In general, the shorter wavelengths, e.g. ultraviolet, are strongly scattered in the skin decreasing their penetration (Nightingale, 1959).

Summary

Electromagnetic radiations interact with matter by being:

- reflected – turned back from a surface
- transmitted (penetrate) – line of travel of radiation altered at junction of different materials
- scattered – direction of radiation in material altered by numerous reflections and refractions
- absorbed – energy of the radiation is converted to some other energy form.

REFERENCES

Nightingale A. (1959). *Physics and Electronics in Physical Medicine*. London: G. Bell.

Van Breugel H. H. F. I. (1992). A Monte-Carlo model for laser light distribution in tissue: effects of intensity profile and divergence of the laser beam [Abstract]. 2nd Meeting of the International Laser Therapy Association. London: International Laser Therapy Association, 18–20 September, p. 30.

12 Microwave diathermy

With shorter wavelengths than the familiar radio waves but longer than infrared radiations, microwaves are, perhaps, one of the least well-recognized group of electromagnetic radiations. The Frontispiece shows that they are sited between 1 m wavelength (300 MHz) and 1 cm wavelength (30 GHz) – or as short as 1 mm (300 GHz). This unfamiliarity, coupled with their much increased commercial usage, has possibly engendered rather more frequent suspicions about their safety than seems justified by the evidence.

The nature and production of microwave radiation for therapeutic purposes are addressed briefly at the beginning of this chapter.

The interactions and effects of microwave radiation in the tissues are then considered, with the patterns of heating which may be expected. Comment is made on the therapeutic uses followed by the principles of application and dosage. Finally, some potential dangers are noted.

INTRODUCTION

The microwave frequencies allotted for medical use are given in Table 12.1. The 2450 MHz frequency is much the most widely available but is, perhaps, not the most satisfactory to achieve therapeutic muscle heating, for reasons considered below. The heating effect of microwaves is well known with microwave ovens. They are also used in telecommunications and in tracking ships, aircraft, rockets and satellites as radar.

Microwave radiation behaves like other electromagnetic radiation, described in Chapter 11, in that it is reflected and refracted at interfaces and will be absorbed or penetrate material to varying degrees depending on the nature of the materials. It also exhibits rectilinear propagation, a necessary feature for its use as radar.

Table 12.1 Frequencies and wavelengths of microwaves used in medicine

Frequency (MHz)	Wavelength (cm)
2450	12.245
915	32.79
433.9	69.14

Europe uses all three; the USA the top two frequencies.

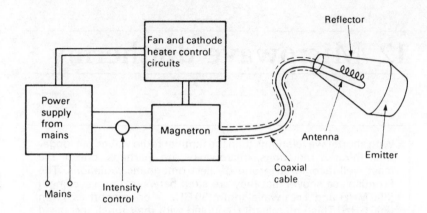

Fig. 12.1 Production of microwaves: block diagram of microwave diathermy generator.

Thus, microwaves can be directed to, and will penetrate, the tissues while being strongly absorbed by water. This makes it an effective method of tissue heating, especially muscle.

PRODUCTION OF MICROWAVES

High-frequency oscillating currents will produce electromagnetic radiations of radio frequencies (see Chapter 10) which can be radiated from suitable antennae as radio and television transmissions. At higher frequencies it becomes impossible for the electrons in the electric circuit to oscillate sufficiently rapidly because of the time needed for them to pass through a valve or transistor. For the higher frequencies of microwave at relatively high power a device called a magnetron is used which generates oscillating currents directly from high-velocity electron motion. These currents are collected and fed along a coaxial cable to the antenna or emitter which radiates microwaves. The dimensions of the coaxial cable are arranged to provide a suitable capacitance, so that microwaves of a given frequency are conveyed to the emitter with maximum efficiency. The antenna, which is simply a suitable-sized and shaped piece of wire, is mounted in front of a metal reflector so that a beam of microwaves is emitted in one direction (Fig. 12.1).

The output of microwave energy can be controlled by varying the power supplied to the magnetron. Machines have an intensity control and the output is indicated on a meter which, of course, gives no reliable indication of the heating of the tissues. The frequency of the microwaves produced depends on the structure of the magnetron and is therefore fixed. There will also be a means of switching the mains power on and off and suitable indicator lights. On some machines a delay switch may be fitted to allow time for the magnetron to reach its proper working temperature.

A standby switch may be provided. Thus successive treatments may be given or adjustment of the emitter made without having to switch off the magnetron and wait for it to warm up again.

The emitter, also called a director or applicator, gives out a beam of microwaves which diverges somewhat because it is technically difficult to produce a completely uniform beam (Ward, 1986). The effect of this divergence is to reduce the intensity of radiations considerably with distance (see the inverse square law, Chapter 11; Guy, 1982).

Microwave therapy can be in either continuous or pulsed mode.

THE PHYSIOLOGICAL EFFECTS OF MICROWAVES ON THE TISSUES

When the electromagnetic energy of microwave radiation is absorbed in the tissues it provokes ionic movement, rotation of dipoles and electron orbit distortion (as already described for shortwave diathermy in Chapter 10) which leads to heating. The amount of heating will be proportional to the amount of absorbed radiation. The effects of heating on the tissues have been fully considered in Chapter 7.

Since microwaves are being applied from outside the tissues and 'beamed in' and are strongly absorbed by water it would be expected that heating would be greatest at the surface and diminish exponentially with depth (see Fig. 11.5). While this is a useful simple generalization it needs further elucidation.

The pattern of microwave absorption in the tissues

In Chapter 11 it was noted that when any radiation meets the surface of a different medium it may either be reflected or penetrate. Those radiations that do penetrate will only have an effect if they are absorbed (Grotthus' law); thus they will be ineffective if they pass right through. In the case of microwaves there is considerable reflection at the air–skin boundary and at skin–fat and fat–muscle boundaries in the tissues. The percentage of microwave radiation (at 2450 MHz) reflected varies with thickness of fat and skin from 50 to 75% (Scowcroft *et al.*, 1977). (Tissue thickness makes a great difference at this frequency. Some radiations that are reflected from the fat–skin interface and other interfaces in the tissues can be radiated out of the body.) At the other frequencies in therapeutic use some 60–70% of the energy is reflected but it is much less affected by variations in skin tissue thickness (Ward, 1980).

The relationship between the amount of radiation absorbed and that which penetrates is shown in Figure 11.4 as an exponential relationship in which the half-value depth for microwave is often given as 3 cm (penetration depth 4.3 cm). This smooth change would only be true if the tissues were homogeneous, which they are definitely not.

Calculations can be made for an approximate model of the tissues, consisting of a 2 cm layer of fat over muscle and bone, by using the dielectric constants and conductivities of these tissues to give a pattern of energy absorption, shown in Figure 12.2. This pattern

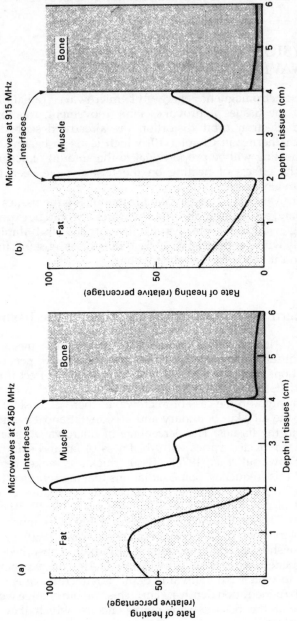

Fig. 12.2 Proportional heating of 2450 MHz and 915 MHz microwaves through tissues. Continuous line represents the heating pattern predicted for a 3-layer model of fat–muscle–bone as a percentage of the maximum at the fat/muscle interface.

occurs because absorption of microwaves is much lower in fat (half-value about 3.5 cm) and higher in the vascular muscle tissue (half-value about 0.7 cm). There is also reflection from the fat–muscle and fat–bone interfaces causing standing waves which lead to 'peaks' in the middle of each tissue layer (Fig. 12.2). These theoretical patterns, calculated by Ward (1980), are likely to be much less clearly defined in real tissue because of the irregularities of the interfaces, the heat-distributing effects of the blood flow, especially in muscle tissue, and also the effects of conduction. These calculations do not give actual temperature changes, just the relative energy absorption.

When the same calculations are made for microwaves at 915 MHz (Fig. 12.2(b)), the relatively better heating of muscle compared to fat is illustrated; microwaves of lower frequencies penetrate further. For this reason, and due to unpredictable reflection from the surface, noted earlier, it is considered by some that 915 MHz (and 434 MHz which gives a similar pattern) are more suitable frequencies for therapeutic heating than the widely used 2450 MHz. Although it is not shown in Figure 12.2, the skin would be heated to a greater degree than the deeper tissues in most circumstances. This ensures the safety of microwave treatments under normal circumstances, since excess heating will be felt by heat receptors in the skin.

Morphological effects

The shape of the tissues to which the microwave beam is being applied will have significant effects due to both reflection and refraction:

- There is considerable reflection of therapeutic microwave radiation from skin which is greater when it is not being applied perpendicularly to the surface (see cosine law, Chapter 11 and Fig. 11.4).
- Microwave radiation passing in the tissues will be subject to refraction as the wave velocity decreases from air to skin and fat and then to muscle. The radiations are bent towards the normal (see Fig. 11.3), hence converging and giving relatively greater heating than would otherwise occur (Guy, 1982; Ward, 1986).

These effects are illustrated in Figure 12.3 and both will be greater where the tissues have a small radius of curvature, e.g. forearm or leg. Treating tissue concavities, such as the palm with semi-flexed fingers or the popliteal space, would have opposite effects.

While the generalizations described above are valid, it must be emphasized that the tissues are very irregular and microwave absorption is influenced by other factors such as the thickness of the fat layer. Consequently, absorption patterns cannot be predicted with certainty. Furthermore, the heating in the tissues depends not only on microwave absorption but also on the rate of heat transfer within and between the tissues.

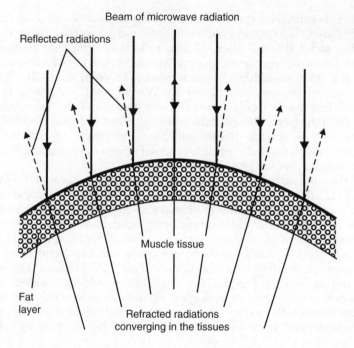

Fig. 12.3 How refraction of microwave radiation at tissue junctions can cause convergence.

Effect of emitter shape

The distribution of energy over the body surface will depend on the size and shape of the emitter. Circular emitters usually give a somewhat ring-shaped pattern (but if close it may be more or less circular). Other emitters are available which are rather longer in one direction and give an oval pattern; still other emitters of apparently similar shape may give the greatest output at the central axis, diminishing outwards. This is often the situation in practice since many body areas are convex so that the centre of the area is nearest to the emitter. Some emitters are designed to focus the radiation into the tissues and thus achieve better depth of heating. All the emitters described so far are distance emitters, that is they are applied to the tissues with an air gap. It is also possible to have contact emitters.

Contact emitters

Microwaves are markedly reflected from skin and in Chapters 6 and 11 it was explained that reflection depends on the different impedances encountered when waves – whether sonic or electromagnetic – pass from one medium to another. To achieve better transmission to skin and to enable the emitter to be made much smaller a suitable ceramic dielectric material is used. This will enable a better match to be made between the applicator and the tissues. These contact emitters can be made quite small, 1.5 or 3.5 cm diameter, and will radiate microwaves directly into the tissues away from the surface of the emitter. Other small emitters can be placed in body cavities – rectum, vagina and external auditory meatus – emitting radially to heat the walls of the cavity.

As microwave transmission is better with these contact emitters the power that can be applied may be limited to a low level (25 W); see later comment on cooled emitters. Small contact emitters are not widely used; they have been described as ineffective (Forster and Palastanga, 1985) and if hand-held are considered potentially hazardous (Scowcroft *et al.*, 1977), but no evidence is given. Special sandbags can also be used with some distance emitters to prevent the microwave radiations diverging so far and so giving greater intensity. They act like the ceramic dielectric emitters.

Heating effect

McMeeken and Bell (1990), applying microwave at doses used clinically, substantially increased the skin temperature (10°C) and the deep and superficial blood flow in the forearm and hand of normal subjects. The response was localized to the area of irradiation and lasted up to 20 min after treatment. They postulated that this was likely to be caused by a local increase in metabolic rate in the heated tissues and that microwave appeared to be particularly effective in heating deep muscle. Heating of the superficial musculature is supported, at least under some conditions, by experiments in which human tissue temperatures were measured (Lehmann and de Lateur, 1982).

Conradi and Pages (1989) showed decreasing temperature with depth using microwave on the gluteal region of the minipig. The maximum temperature was achieved subcutaneously at approximately 10 min and in muscle and periosteum at 20 min, this being 30–40% of that subcutaneously. There was no difference in the temperature reached between continuous and pulsed microwave, as long as the energy delivered was identical. Fadilah *et al.* (1987) found that synovial membrane was heated preferentially in rabbit joints using microwave, and attributed this to its high water content.

The more rapid resolution of artificially induced haematomas in pigs using 915 MHz microwaves has been demonstrated (Lehmann *et al.*, 1983).

Summary

Of microwave interaction with the tissues:

- the approximate half-value depth of penetration is 3 cm
- much radiation is reflected from the skin
- the theoretical absorption pattern indicates absorption in skin, fat, muscle (especially at interfaces) and very little in bone
- refraction in the tissues could influence the degree and depth of absorption
- the widely used 2450 MHz has a less satisfactory absorption pattern for therapeutic purposes than lower frequencies
- the shape and size of the emitter influences the energy distribution onto the tissues
- good transmission to the skin can be achieved with contact emitters
- generally, microwave heating has been found to occur in the first few centimetres of tissue traversed, especially in muscle.

THERAPEUTIC USES

The indications are those of heating. Like shortwave, some debate surrounds the issue of whether there are any specific therapeutic effects due to microwave. There seems to be no clear supporting evidence of any effect except heat. Microwaves can be pulsed and the effects are claimed to be those of pulsed shortwave (see Chapter 10).

Microwave heating is suitable for superficial tissue heating, both muscle and articular structures close to the surface such as the wrist joint or anterior aspect of the knee, but it is not likely to affect deeply placed structures covered with muscle tissue like the hip joint. Perhaps it should be emphasized that heating patterns are highly irregular and probably vary considerably from patient to patient. A comparison might be made with ultrasound (see Chapter 6) which has similar penetration but is usually applied with a continuously moving treatment head which evens out the distribution of energy in the tissues.

One of the major uses of microwave therapy is for heating muscle tissue to achieve, amongst other things, an increase in intramuscular blood flow. This, it is believed, only occurs if the temperature is significantly raised. It has been shown in dogs that 15 min of microwave can cause a considerable rise in intramuscular temperature followed by an 85% increase in blood flow (Richardson, 1954). This increased flow only occurred after a critical threshold temperature had been reached. It has already been pointed out that 915 MHz microwave is much more efficient at heating the deeper tissues than the more usual 2450 MHz microwave (Fig. 12.2). Weinberger *et al.* (1989), using 915 MHz microwave, found the pain from articular effusions reduced and walking time increased.

Heating is limited by the skin surface heating so that greater total heating and thus deep heating can be achieved if the heated surface is deliberately cooled. This can be done by passing cold air over the skin surface. Therapeutic applicators have been made which work at 915 MHz; these have contact emitters which contain a dielectric material with apertures through which cooling air is blown. As the emitter is used in contact with the skin the amount of scattered radiation is also diminished. These are considered by some to be an efficient way of generating even heating in the deep tissues. However, with the thermal receptors in the skin deliberately cooled there is an increased risk of a burn, and extreme caution is required with this technique.

The therapeutic effects of heat are considered in Chapter 7, with further discussion on low-energy heating due to pulsed application in Chapter 10.

PRINCIPLES OF APPLICATION

Preparation of patient. The nature of the treatment should be described to the patient, explaining how the microwave energy is dissipated in the body so that only a small temperature rise will occur, unlike the situation of a microwave oven in which the temperature can be made to rise to cooking levels because the heat and reflected microwaves cannot escape. The thermal sensitivity of the skin to which the microwaves are to be applied should be tested, as described in Chapter 7. The patient is given a pair of microwave goggles (see below) if radiation could enter the eye.

Preparation of apparatus.   The choice of emitter is dictated by the size of tissue area to be treated. The power should be switched on, the machine given time to warm up after which it can be left on a standby switch.

Preparation of part to be treated.   The patient should be positioned so that the part to be treated is comfortably supported and sufficiently exposed. Microwave should not be applied through clothing or where there is metal in the field. Wooden furniture should be used and care should be taken that the treatment head does not irradiate any large metal surfaces that could reflect the beam.

Setting up.   The emitter should be positioned so that the radiations strike the surface at right angles, bearing in mind that as distance emitters have diverging beams, only the axial radiations will be strictly at right angles while the peripheral radiation will strike at small incident angles. While this may not make much difference (see cosine law, Chapter 11) when the emitter is 'square on', slight angling of the emitter increases the already considerable reflection from the skin surface, making the treatment ineffective.

Instructions and warnings.   The degree of heating required must be described to the patient, as for shortwave (see Chapter 10). Like other heat treatments the only information about the intensity and site of heating in the tissues is derived from the patient's sensations. The meter only indicates the output of the machine so it is essential to have the patient's full co-operation. He or she must also be warned to call if the heating becomes more than a comfortable warmth or if discomfort or pain is felt, and to remain still.

Application.   The microwave output is switched on for the predetermined length of time.

Termination.   After switching off and removing the apparatus, the treated area is examined, and the skin surface temperature and presence of any erythema are noted and recorded.

Practical point
The distance between the emitter and the skin determines both the area treated and the intensity because of the diverging beam. Thus if a small area is to be treated the emitter should be placed close to the skin, say 2–5 cm, and the appropriate heating regulated with the intensity control on the machine. If larger areas are to be heated the spacing can be increased, to 10 or 15 cm, and the intensity control advanced to give sufficient heating. Distances of about 10 cm are commonly utilized for most treatments.

DOSAGE

Treatment is usually given for 20 min as this is considered to be the optimum time because the vascular adjustments have become 'steady' by this time. However, it is evident that the deeper tissues take rather longer to reach a maximum steady temperature (de Lateur *et al.*, 1970). At depths greater than 2 cm the temperature is still rising after 10 min (Conradi and Pages, 1989). If significant muscle heating is required it would be reasonable to apply the microwave treatment for rather longer, say 30 min.

The intensity is regulated by the patient reporting the sensation of heat. It seems to take an absorbed dose of some 200 mW/cm^2 to give detectable heating (Knauf, 1968). What matters is the rate of energy that is absorbed per unit of tissue mass in both microwave and shortwave heating. This can be quantified as the specific absorption rate (SAR) in W/kg. SARs of 50–170 W/kg are used therapeutically, the upper limit being close to the tolerable maximum (Kloth, 1986).

POTENTIAL DANGERS

Microwave absorption leads to heating and if the heating is excessive a burn can result in the same way – but not due to the same mechanism – as from any other form of heat. Investigation of microwave burns in living tissue, in piglets, showed a characteristic pattern called 'layered tissue sparing' in which the skin and muscle tissues were burned but the intervening subcutaneous fat was relatively spared (Surrell *et al.*, 1987). This is in conformity with the pattern of microwave heating described earlier and with what would be expected.

Some points need to be considered specifically in connection with microwaves.

Effects of metal

As microwaves are strongly reflected from metal surfaces any metal placed on the tissue surface will act as a shield preventing radiations reaching the underlying tissues; this may lead to ineffective treatment. Metal may also distort and concentrate the microwave field causing local overheating which could be dangerous. If metal is so placed that it could reflect microwave energy into the tissues it is again possible that overheating could occur. If, for example, the hand is rested on a metal surface and microwave radiation applied some would pass through the hand and be reflected back into it again. With normal sensory awareness there is no reason why this should lead to burning but it would be an undesirable and uncontrolled pattern of heating. Metal embedded in the tissues, due to accident or surgery, could also cause reflections in the tissues which might lead to overheating. Since there are no heat receptors in the deep tissues the patient would only be aware of deep pain when the damage had occurred. Such an effect does not seem to have been reported and would probably only be likely with superficially placed metal. However, it is generally advisable to avoid treating the region of metal implants with microwaves. It should be noted that the reason for avoiding them is rather different from that in shortwave applications (see Chapter 10).

Effects of surface moisture

Perspiration must be allowed to evaporate freely. If moisture appears on the surface from any source, e.g. open wounds or wet dressings, it will absorb radiations, so treatment should be stopped and the moisture removed.

Cardiac pacemakers

These could be affected if microwaves were directly applied to the region (see Chapter 10) but there is little, if any, risk from scattered radiation.

The eyes

Due to its structure (a water-filled sphere) the eye selectively absorbs microwaves and is not easily able to dissipate heat and thus can become overheated. Although cataracts in laboratory animals have been produced with high doses of microwaves there is no evidence that they have been caused in humans (Lehmann and de Lateur, 1982). It is considered wise to avoid exposing the eyes directly to high doses of microwave energy. If the treatment is such that radiation may enter the eye, when treating the anterior aspect of the shoulder with a distance emitter for example, the patient should be given goggles which are impervious to microwaves. Such goggles are of two kinds – either a metal mesh which reflects practically all microwave radiation but allows sufficient light between the mesh to see clearly, or a thin layer of metal supported on glass which again reflects microwave radiations but interferes little with visible light. However, it is difficult to make goggles totally effective because of diffraction (Delpizzo and Joyner, 1987). It is important that microwave goggles do not become confused with ultraviolet or laser goggles in busy physiotherapy departments as they can look similar but have different functions. Closing the eyes would not prevent the transmission of microwaves but would diminish them. However, McMeeken and Stillman (1996) have suggested that metal goggles should not be used as they have the potential to burn adjacent skin.

The testes

While quite small temperature rises can interfere with spermato-genesis in mammals, which is why the testes are located outside

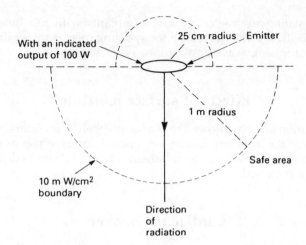

With an indicated output of 100 W

25 cm radius — Emitter

1 m radius

Safe area

10 m W/cm² boundary

Direction of radiation

Fig. 12.4 Safe distances from a micro-wave source.

the abdominal cavity, there is no evidence that mild heating has any damaging effect although marked heating can cause damage, albeit reversible. It is felt that heating of 100 mW/cm² could possibly produce testicular damage in humans (Watson, 1971); therefore direct irradiation of the testes should be avoided and care taken to prevent large amounts of reflected or scattered radiation reaching the region.

The testes are more susceptible because of their exposed position and possibly their structure. The same does not apply to the deeply placed ovaries which are unlikely to be heated by microwave treatment.

Pregnancy

It is recommended that microwave should not be given to the pregnant uterus or patients attempting pregnancy (Elder *et al.*, 1989).

General safety with microwaves

Patients undergoing microwave treatment are in a controlled situation, their thermal perception is checked and dosage regulated. For uncontrolled exposure fairly low levels of microwaves are recommended (Medical Research Council, 1971). Thus standards have been set for exposure of the public to microwave. These vary a good deal from one part of the world to another. In the UK the Medical Research Council has set 10 mW/cm² as a safe level for continuous exposure and for higher doses it considers that the total should not exceed 1 mW/cm². The Standards Association of Australia recommends a lower limit of 1 mW/cm² at 2450 MHz (Delpizzo and Joyner, 1987).

Measurements made by the National Radiological Protection Board on typical physiotherapy treatments with microwave indicate that the safe level of radiation is not exceeded under almost any conditions at more than 1 m in front or at the side of the emitter and 25 cm behind the emitter (Health Equipment Information, 1980; Fig. 12.4). If powers of more than 100 W are used the dimensions of the zones are increased, e.g. for 200 W it is increased to 1.4 m. However, it must be noted that many emitters give out a very irregular beam of microwave radiation (Brown and Johnson, 1975). In order to obtain effective heating for treatment purposes these levels must be exceeded at the treatment site. However, for the short times involved in treatment there is no evidence of hazard to the patient.

CONTRAINDICATIONS

- Diminished thermal sensation.
- Defective arterial circulation.
- Acute inflammation.
- Recent haemorrhage.
- Metal in the area under treatment.
- Malignancy.
- Implanted cardiac pacemakers.
- Intrauterine devices when using a vaginal electrode – a practice not recommended by the preliminary report of the Chartered Society of Physiotherapy working party (Scowcroft *et al.*, 1977).
- Eyes and testes, due to poor heat dissipation.
- Pregnant uterus.

REFERENCES

Brown B. H., Johnson S. G. (1975). Microwave diathermy (treatment note). *Physiotherapy*, **61**, 117.

Conradi E., Pages I. H. (1989). Effects of continuous and pulsed microwave radiations on distribution of heat in the gluteal region of the minipig. *Scand. J. Rehabil. Med.*, **21**, 59–62.

de Lateur B. K., Lehmann J. F., Stonebridge J. B. *et al.* (1970). Muscle heating in human subjects with 915 MHz microwave contact applicator. *Arch. Phys. Med. Rehabil.*, **51**, 147–51.

Delpizzo V., Joyner K. H. (1987). On the safe use of microwave and shortwave diathermy units. *Aust. J. Physiother.*, **33**, 152–61.

Elder J. A., Czerski P. A., Stuchly M. A. *et al.* (1989). Radio frequency radiation. In *Non-ionising Radiation Protection*, 2nd edn. (Suess M. J., Benwell-Morison D. A., eds) Geneva: WHO Regional Publication, European Series 25.

Fadilah R., Pinkas J., Weinberger A. *et al.* (1987). Heating rabbit joints by microwave applicator. *Arch. Phys. Med. Rehabil.*, **68**, 710–12.

Forster A., Palastanga N. (1985). *Clayton's Electrotherapy: Theory and Practice*. London: Baillière Tindall.

Guy A. W. (1982). Biophysics of high frequency currents and electromagnetic radiation. In *Therapeutic Heat and Cold* (Lehmann J. F., ed.) Baltimore: Williams & Wilkins, pp. 199–277.

Health Equipment Information (1980). No. 188, September. London: DHSS.

Kloth L. (1986). Shortwave and microwave diathermy. In *Thermal Agents in Rehabilitation* (Michlovitz S. L., ed.) Philadelphia: Davis.

Knauf G. M. (1968). Biological effects of microwave radiations. *Arch. Ind. Hlth*, **17**, 48.

Lehmann J. F., de Lateur B. J. (1982). Therapeutic heat. In *Therapeutic Heat and Cold* (Lehmann J. F., ed.) Baltimore: Williams & Wilkins, pp. 404–562.

Lehmann J. F., Dundore D. E., Esselman P. C. *et al.* (1983). Microwave diathermy: effects on experimental muscle haematoma resolution. *Arch. Phys. Med. Rehabil.*, **64**, 127–9.

McMeeken J. M., Bell C. (1990). Microwave irradiation of the human forearm and hand. *Physiother. Pract.*, **6**, 171–7.

McMeeken J., Stillman B. (1996). Microwave diathermy. In *Clayton's Electrotherapy*, 10th edn (Kitchen S., Bazin S., eds) Philadelphia: W. B. Saunders, pp. 179–96.

Medical Research Council (1971). *Recommendation MRC 70/1314*, January 8.

Michaelson S. M. (1982). Bioeffects of high frequency currents and electromagnetic radiations. In *Therapeutic Heat and Cold* (Lehmann J. F., ed.) Baltimore: Williams and Wilkins, pp. 278–352.

Oleson J. R., Gerner E. W. (1982). Hyperthermia in the treatment of malignancies. In *Therapeutic Heat and Cold* (Lehmann J. F., ed.) Baltimore: Williams & Wilkins, pp. 603–35.

Richardson A. W. (1954). Effects of microwave-induced heating on the blood flow through peripheral skeletal muscles. *Am. J. Phys. Med.*, **33**, 103–7.

Scowcroft A. T., Mason A. H. L., Hayne C. R. (1977). Safety with microwave diathermy: preliminary report of the CSP working party. *Physiotherapy*, **63**, 359–61.

Surrell J. A., Alexander R. C., Cohle S. D. *et al.* (1987). Effects of microwave radiation on living tissues. *J. Trauma*, **27**, 935–9.

Ward A. R. (1986). *Electricity Fields and Waves in Therapy*. Marrickville, NSW, Australia: Science Press.

Watson P. (1971). Microwaves – their effects and safe use. *N.Z. J. Physiother.*, **4**, 20–24.

Weinberger A., Fadilah R., Lev A. *et al.* (1989). Treatment of articular effusions with local deep microwave hyperthermia. *Clin. Rheumatol.*, **8**, 461–6.

13 Infrared and visible radiations

Of all radiations, perhaps the most 'natural' from a human perspective are those infrared radiations constantly emitted and absorbed by all humankind. Therapeutically, only the shorter infrared wavelengths are utilized.

The nature and definition of infrared radiations are described, also the way those radiations are produced for therapy. Discussion of the absorption and penetration of IR and visible radiations in the tissues follows.

The physiological effects and therapeutic uses of these radiations are then described and considered. The therapeutic application and dangers of IRR conclude this chapter.

INTRODUCTION

Infrared radiations are those whose wavelengths are longer than that of visible red light extending to the microwave region, i.e. from 760 nm to 1 mm (Harlen, 1982). Other authorities suggest the longer radiations only extend to wavelengths of 0.1 or 0.4 mm.

These infrared radiations can be subdivided into three regions or bands, A, B and C (Harlen, 1982), approximately distinguished by their absorption characteristics. A and B are utilized therapeutically and correspond roughly to an older classification of 'near' and 'far' infrared (Table 13.1).

Infrared radiations are produced in all matter by various kinds of molecular vibration. When atoms move further apart or closer together without breaking free from one another, the molecules formed by them alter shape and infrared radiations are emitted. Any given molecule is already in a state of vibration and rotation and this can be altered by absorbing heat which leads to the emission

Table 13.1 Classification of infrared radiation

Type	Wavelength
IRA	760–1400 nm
IRB	1400–3000 nm
IRC	3000 nm–1 mm (not used in therapy)
Former classification	
Near or short IR	760–1500 nm
Far or long IR	1500–15 000 nm

of many different wavelengths of infrared. The result is that *any* heated body emits infrared radiations; indeed any material that is at a temperature above absolute zero emits infrared. Although the radiations will be of a whole range of different frequencies, the frequencies at which the maximum intensity of radiation is emitted are proportional to temperature. Thus the higher the temperature the higher the frequency and hence the shorter the wavelength. At the higher temperatures generated by a tungsten filament light bulb the peak emission is about 960 nm, i.e. in the near infrared, with plenty of emission in the visible region (see Fig. 14.3). The human body also emits a whole range of infrared radiations, mainly type C, with a peak around 10 000 nm. Absorption of all these radiations causes similar kinds of molecular vibrations.

The shorter, visible radiations not only cause molecular and atomic motion but can also break chemical bonds when they are absorbed. It is this that provokes chemical changes in the retinal pigments which are detected via the optic nerve as sight. These and other chemical changes do not directly result in heat, unlike the atomic and molecular motion induced by infrared.

Summary

Infrared radiations:

- are emitted from any heated body
- are divided into long and short wavelength for therapeutic purposes
- produce heat when absorbed.

Visible radiations may produce some chemical changes as well as heat when absorbed.

PRODUCTION OF INFRARED

Any heated material will produce infrared radiations, the wavelength being determined by the temperature. If short infrared is to be produced efficiently the material must not be oxidized (burnt) by the higher temperatures used. The most convenient method is to heat a resistance wire by passing an electric current through it. An ordinary household electric fire can be made of a coil of suitable resistance wire, such as nickel-chrome alloy, wound on a ceramic insulator.

Therapeutic infrared lamps

Various kinds of infrared lamps are used for therapy.

Non-luminous generators

One type is made in a similar way to an electric fire. In these heaters the wire glows red thus giving some radiations in the visible region but peak emission in the short infrared. The ceramic material, being heated to a lower temperature than the wire, gives only infrared and no visible radiations.

Some infrared lamps for therapy have the wire embedded in the insulating ceramic (or porcelain or fireclay) so that no visible radiations are given out.

The heater wire can also be mounted behind a metal plate or inside a metal tube which does not become red-hot but emits infrared in the same way. As such a lamp becomes hotter all the parts – the emitter, the metal plate on the end of the emitter, the protective wire mesh and the reflector – become heated, giving off a range of wavelengths from near to far infrared.

The infrared emitter is placed at the focus of a hemispherical or parabolic reflector to reflect the radiations into an approximately uniform beam (see Fig. 13.1). However, the beam does diverge somewhat due to the relatively large size of the emitter compared to the reflector, and this serves to reduce the risk of 'hot spots'. The reflector and emitter are mounted on a strong, firmly supported metal stand which can be adjusted to alter the height and angle of the reflector/emitter. When such lamps are switched on they require some time to warm up because of the thermal inertia of the considerable mass of metal and insulating material that has to be heated; thus small lamps may take about 5 min but larger ones may take up to 15 min to reach maximum emission (Forster and Palastanga, 1985).

In spite of the fact that lamps with an exposed coil will give off a red glow they are collectively designated as 'non-luminous' sources to distinguish them from those that emit visible as well as infrared radiations; these are called 'luminous' lamps.

> **Practical point**
> Because of thermal inertia, this type of lamp must be switched on for a sufficient time before it is needed for treatment.

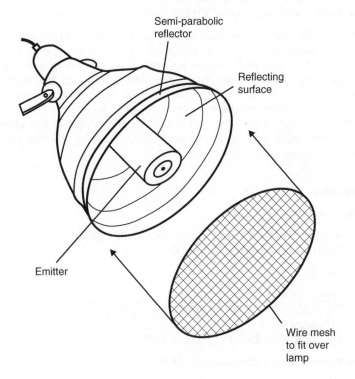

Semi-parabolic reflector

Reflecting surface

Emitter

Wire mesh to fit over lamp

Fig. 13.1 Parabolic reflector of a typical non-luminous infrared lamp.

Luminous generators

Luminous generators (incandescent lamps) consist of a tungsten filament in a large glass envelope which contains inert gas at low pressure. Part of the inside of the glass bulb is often silvered to provide a reflector. These lamps work on the same principle as a simple electric light bulb; the filament is heated to a high temperature (around 3000°C) by the current passed through it and so gives off a continuous spectrum in the infrared and visible regions. Oxidation of the filament does not occur because there is no oxygen present, only a trace of some inert gas. The peak emission occurs at near 1000 nm but radiation extends from the long infrared throughout the visible to the ultraviolet (see Fig. 14.4). These latter radiations are absorbed by the glass and are not therefore transmitted by the lamp (Ward, 1986). Sometimes the glass is reddened, absorbing some of the green and blue rays to give a red visible emission; this is believed to make little difference therapeutically (Lehmann and de Lateur, 1982). Luminous generators are sometimes called 'radiant heat' generators, indicating that heating is by both infrared and visible radiations.

Power

The power of infrared sources can broadly be described as:

- smaller lamps (luminous and non-luminous), usually 250–500 W
- large, non-luminous, 750–1000 W
- large, luminous, 600–1500 W.

Generally, the larger lamps are used to treat extensive areas but the same effect can be achieved by mounting three smaller luminous bulbs, which can be separately controlled in one holder. In this way a large area can be covered with all the bulbs in use and a small area using only one or two. In the interest of safety, large lamps are fitted with wire-mesh screens over the front of the reflector to prevent accidental contact with the hot emitter. The screen will also diminish any remote risk of the hot emitter element falling out.

Emission

Non-luminous:

- mainly 3000–4000 nm (long IR), with about 10% between 1500 nm and visible (short IR)

Luminous

- approximately 70% short IR
  5% visible
  24% long IR
  1% UVR absorbed by glass of bulb.

(Wadsworth and Chanmugan, 1980).

Summary

Infrared sources for therapy are:

1 Non-luminous lamps
  • produced by electrically heated wire embedded in ceramic and backed by an external reflector
  • giving off long IR radiations around 3000 or 4000 nm (some give off a little red visible radiation)
  • small lamps have power of 250–500 W
  • larger lamps have power of 750–1000 W.

2 Luminous lamps
  • produced by electrically heated filament in an evacuated glass bulb, often with silvered inner surface to provide a reflector
  • giving off both IR and visible radiations mostly in the short IR band (peak around 1000 nm)
  • small lamps have power of 250–500 W
  • large lamps have power of 600–1500 W.

ABSORPTION AND PENETRATION OF INFRARED AND VISIBLE RADIATIONS

Some radiations striking the surface of the skin will be reflected and some will penetrate, to be scattered, refracted and ultimately absorbed in the tissues. The amount of reflection of visible radiation varies with skin colour but, for therapeutic infrared, is negligible. Close to 95% of the radiation applied perpendicular to the skin is absorbed (Ward, 1986). Small amounts of radiations in some circumstances may actually be transmitted, not only through the skin, but through the underlying tissues and even through a part of the body. Skin (epidermis and dermis) is not, of course, a single homogeneous tissue but a complicated multilayered structure full of irregular forms, such as hair follicles and sweat glands. In general, water and proteins are strong absorbers of infrared. What happens, therefore, to any radiation entering the skin is highly complex, depending on the

  • structure
  • vascularity
  • pigmentation of the skin
  • wavelength of the radiation, most crucially.

This accounts for the difficulty of determining the pattern of penetration and absorption of radiation in the skin; see, for example, Van Breugel (1992) and also for discrepancies in the quoted figures (see Table 13.2).

Penetration

The usual method used to describe the overall penetration of radiations is to give the penetration depth. Confusion sometimes

Table 13.2 Penetration depths of infrared from different authors

Source	Penetration depth (mm)	Wavelength (nm)
King (1989)	2–4	800–900
Harlen (1982)	3	'short IR'
Ward (1986)	'few'	1200
Nightingale (1959)	0.36	1100
Gourgouliatos (1990)	5–10	1200
Laurens (1933)	1–2.5	'near IR'

arises from a failure to appreciate that this term has a specific, clearly defined meaning (see Chapter 11, and Fig. 11.5).

The penetration depth is the depth at which approximately 63% of the radiation energy has been absorbed and 37% remains.

It is neither the depth to which *all* radiations penetrate nor the depth beyond which *none* penetrate.

The effects are summarized in a simplified way in Figure 13.2, which shows how scattering and refraction decreases the penetration depth and can modify the pattern of absorption.

Looking at the whole spectrum of infrared and visible radiations from the microwave to the ultraviolet (see Frontispiece), some very different patterns of penetration/absorption emerge. Very long wavelength infrared (around 40 000 nm) behaves like microwave and penetrates several centimetres. However, the long infrared used therapeutically is absorbed at the surface, much of it by the water on the skin surface. At around 3000 nm, penetration depth is about 0.1 mm (Ward, 1986). From here there is increasing penetration with decreasing wavelength in the short infrared region, to a maximum penetration depth of about 3 mm around the 1000 nm wavelength

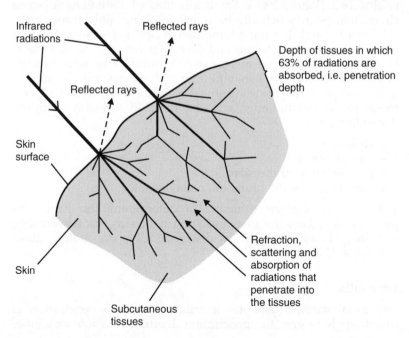

Fig. 13.2 Representation of the influence of refraction and scattering on the penetration/absorption of radiations entering the skin.

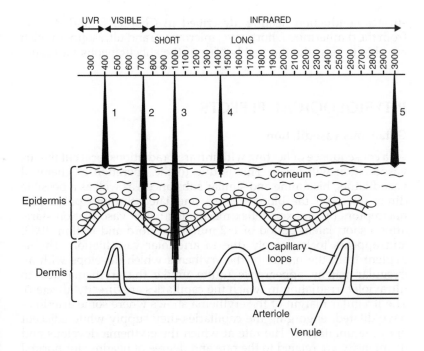

Fig. 13.3 Representation of penetration and absorption of some infrared and visible radiations into the skin.

	Bands of radiations of wavelengths around (nm)	Appropriate penetration depth (mm)
1	400	0.07
2	730	1.5
3	1030	3.0
4	1430	0.3
5	3000	0.1

region (see Table 13.2). The very short infrared and red visible radiations have penetration depths of about 1 or 2 mm, while those of the rest of the visible spectrum penetrate much less (see Fig. 13.3). In fact, at the blue end of the visible spectrum, the penetration depth is about 0.07 mm and decreases uniformly with wavelength through the ultraviolet region. The much greater penetration of red light is easily demonstrated by putting a small torch in the mouth and seeing that only red light emerges through the cheek. Only a tiny proportion of the original radiation is being transmitted, but it is evident because the eyes are such highly efficient photon detectors.

Summary

- Infrared radiation is strongly absorbed near the skin surface.
- Little infrared is reflected from the surface if it is applied perpendicular to the skin.
- The only infrared radiation to penetrate the tissues to any significant extent is a band approximately between 650 nm in the red visible and 1500 nm in the short infrared.

The effect will therefore be marked heating of the skin. Some of this heat will be conducted more deeply into the subcutaneous tissues, both due to simple conduction and to increased local circulation of heated blood. This is the same as the situation of surface conduction heating, described in Chapter 8, and distinct from the diathermies (shortwave, microwave and ultrasound) which are able to pass the thermal barrier of the subcutaneous fat tissue.

PHYSIOLOGICAL EFFECTS

Cutaneous vasodilation

As a consequence of heating with infrared radiations local cutaneous vasodilation will occur. This is due to the liberation of chemical vasodilators, histamine and similar substances, as well as a possible direct effect on the blood vessels (mediated through polymodal nociceptors by an axon reflex mechanism). The vasodilation starts after a short latent period of 1–2 min (Crockford and Hellon, 1959) and appears to be largely due to arteriolar vasodilation. This is evident from the nature of the erythema which develops with an irregular patchy appearance (quite unlike the erythema due to ultraviolet irradiation in which the capillaries are directly affected). The irregular margin of the erythema shows where some arterioles have dilated, engorging the capillaries they supply while adjacent ones are unaffected. The rate at which the erythema develops and its intensity are related to the rate and degree of heating; for normal individuals heating the skin to about core temperature (37°C) over some 20 min will lead to very mild erythema; heating to around 42°C will lead to marked erythema. Reflex dilation of other cutaneous vessels will also occur in order to maintain a normal body heat balance, as discussed in Chapter 7. For mild heating the vasodilation of other parts, which could only be detected by a skin thermometer, is likely to begin after some 10 min or so. The local erythema lasts for about 30 min after irradiation has stopped (Crockford and Hellon, 1959).

Sweating

With prolonged or intense heating, sweating will start to occur. This will absorb some of the applied infrared irradiation and leads to surface cooling as it evaporates; see Chapter 7 for discussion on thermal control. This does not necessarily lead to inefficiency since cooling the surface may allow better penetration (Fig. 13.4).

Sensation

Thermal heat receptors will be stimulated in the skin so that the patient is aware of the heating.

Increase in metabolism

Where the temperature is raised there will be an increase in metabolism.

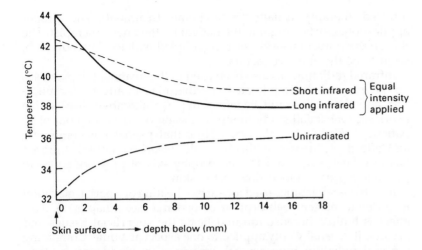

Fig. 13.4 Temperature gradient in the tissues due to heating with long and short infrared radiation. Modified from Nightingale (1959).

Summary

Physiological changes due to heating (discussed in Chapter 7):

- increased metabolic rate
- decreased viscosity
- increased collagen extensibility
- stimulation of sensory nerves
- consequent vascular changes.

Chronic changes

Excessive and prolonged infrared application can cause the destruction of erythrocytes, releasing pigments and causing brown discoloration of the skin. This rarely occurs as a sequel to normal treatment; it usually results from prolonged exposure of the legs to domestic fires.

THERAPEUTIC USES OF INFRARED

Therapeutically, infrared has been used as a form of heat for the purposes discussed in Chapter 7. These include:

- pain relief
- reduction of muscle spasm
- acceleration of healing and repair.

An increase in sensory nerve conduction might influence sensory responses via an increase in endorphins, which could affect the pain gate mechanism (Kitchen and Partridge, 1991).

Fungal infections which are difficult to control and thrive in moist conditions, e.g. paronychia, are sometimes treated with regular infrared therapy, usually as a home treatment. The proper application may be taught to the patient by the physiotherapist. The thorough drying of the skin surface, coupled with local vasodilation, seem to be the effective factors.

Infrared radiation has also been used in the treatment of psoriasis, on the grounds that moderate hyperthermia can affect cell replication and therefore could benefit a hyperproliferative disease like psoriasis. One small study found remission occurred in 8 out of 10 patients (Westerhof *et al.*, 1987). Note that psoriasis is commonly and effectively treated with ultraviolet (see Chapter 15). Infrared has also been suggested for the prophylaxis of pressure sores, to promote a greater blood flow in the skin.

Infrared is sometimes used for surface heating of a part in elevation in order to hasten reabsorption of oedema (see Chapter 7). This effect is limited because infrared heats the superficial tissues and because it is usually only applied to one aspect at a time. Combining infrared radiation from several aspects with conduction heating, placing the elevated hand in a hot-air cabinet for example, is likely to be a more effective treatment. Heating the whole hand exploits the large surface area to volume ratio of the hand.

Infrared is sometimes chosen as a form of heat prior to stretching, mobilization, traction, massage and exercise therapy, as discussed in Chapter 7. There is, however, no evidence that muscle temperature or blood flow is increased to any significant extent by infrared radiation, unlike the diathermies. It may also be used prior to electrical stimulation, testing or biofeedback to warm the skin, making it more vascular and hence a better conductor. This is done before wetting the skin to lower its electrical resistance further. A warm soak would seem preferable for circumstances in which it is practical and possible.

EFFECTS AND USES OF VISIBLE RADIATIONS

Visible radiations are, by definition, able to stimulate the retinal cells of the eye. It is hardly surprising that simple exposure to light is considered to have some therapeutic effect. Some forms of depression have been found to be more evident during the darker winter months (seasonal affective disorder) and successful treatment consists of exposure to bright fluorescent lighting for a period every day (Wehr *et al.*, 1985).

Red light has been used to stimulate healing since ancient times and there is now some experimental evidence for this effect (Karu, 1989).

The bile pigment, bilirubin, formed by the breakdown of haemoglobin, can reach high levels in the blood of newborn babies leading to brain damage. This is called neonatal jaundice and is successfully treated by exposing the baby to blue light – ordinary fluorescent tubes may be used – in the region of 400–450 nm. Any ultraviolet radiation is screened out. The beneficial effect seems to be due to the conversion of bilirubin to compounds which can be easily excreted.

Colour therapy, in which particular colours are applied or viewed for particular conditions, has a long history as alternative medicine in various forms. While there is no direct evidence of significant therapeutic effect an interesting association has been shown using electromyographic activity between viewing red light and greater maximum voluntary (hand-grip) contraction (Hasson *et al.*, 1989). It is speculated that seeing red light leads to arousal in the central nervous system and/or sympathetic stimulation (red for danger) and that the use of red in the treatment environment may increase muscle tone. Although blue light has been considered to have a calming effect, the study quoted above found no significant difference between the blue light and the controls.

Summary

Thus, infrared and visible radiations may be used therapeutically to:

- relieve pain and muscle spasm
- promote superficial healing and repair
- promote tissue flexibility and reduce stiffness
- treat some skin conditions
- increase the vascularity of the skin.

CHOICE OF LUMINOUS (RADIANT HEAT) OR NON-LUMINOUS SOURCES

- The luminous heat source is a more efficient tissue-heating source since it penetrates further (because peak emission is in the short infrared) and therefore the energy is distributed in a larger volume of tissue.

- Non-luminous radiation, with peak emission around 4000 nm, is absorbed almost entirely in the skin.

As the total heating is limited by the sensation felt by the patient, and thermal sense organs are close to the skin surface, it is evident that the non-luminous radiation will reach the limit of tolerable heating with a lower intensity than the luminous. These ideas are illustrated in Figure 13.4.

If the desired effects are due to:

- heating – the luminous shorter infrared source is preferred
- sensory stimulation – the non-luminous is most satisfactory.

It is possible to achieve more even, deeper penetration by cooling the surface with a draught of cool air but the risks of burning may also be greater. Compare the similar mechanism for microwave (Chapter 12).

APPLICATION OF INFRARED RADIATION

Preparation of apparatus. If a non-luminous lamp is chosen it should be switched on up to 15 min before application to allow time for it to reach its maximum emission.

Preparation of patient. The patient is placed in a suitable, well-supported position with the area to be treated exposed.
Explanation: The nature and effects of the treatment are explained to the patient.

Examination and testing. The skin to be treated is examined and the thermal sensation tested.

Setting up. Any object or garment that might obstruct the infrared or impede the blood flow, such as a tightly rolled-up sleeve, is removed. If the eyes could be irradiated they are shielded.

The lamp is positioned so that the radiations strike the surface at or near right angles to achieve maximum penetration, as described in Chapter 11. It is recommended (Wadsworth and Chanmugan, 1980) that the lamp is never positioned directly over the patient in case it tips over on to the patient or the element falls out. Both are unlikely with properly maintained lamps and reasonable care in positioning. Modern lamps are fitted with a protective mesh across the front to prevent contact with the bulb or element. The lamp is sited at an appropriate distance: about 60–75 cm for large 750 or 1000 W lamps and about 45–50 cm for the smaller ones. The luminous lamp is now switched on.

Instructions and warnings. The heat sensation is described to the patient who is asked to indicate the amount of heat and the area in which it is felt. The patient is warned to report immediately if heating becomes more than a comfortable warmth as otherwise a burn could occur, and also not to touch any part of the lamp or to move during treatment.

Application. The intensity of heating is controlled by altering the position of the lamp, or on some by altering a resistance and hence the current to the element. In spite of the reflector, radiations diverge considerably so that small changes of distance lead to quite large changes of intensity on the skin surface, described in Chapter 11 as the inverse square law. Adjustments are made to achieve the appropriate mild or moderate heating as reported by the patient. Once the correct skin temperature is achieved the treatment is usually continued for about 20 min. It should be checked periodically as many lamps increase in output gradually over this time and may need to be adjusted. The 20-min treatment length is determined by the fact that it takes about this time for the vascular adjustments, noted in Chapter 7, to become complete.

Termination of treatment. At the end of treatment the skin should feel mildly or moderately warm and a moderate erythema should be evident. Skin temperatures of 36–38°C would be considered a mild treatment; the more usual moderate warmth gives skin temperatures of 38–41°C. The intensity of erythema does not necessarily parallel the skin temperature: some vasolabile individuals show a vivid erythema at quite moderate skin temperatures.

DANGERS WITH INFRARED TREATMENT

Burns

The most obvious danger is of a heat burn which occurs if the patient is unaware of the heat by reason of defective sensation or reduced consciousness. Rarely, a mentally abnormal or perhaps masochistic patient may stoically tolerate painful and damaging levels of heat. Occasionally patients accidentally touch the hot element if there is no protective guard. These dangers can be avoided by:

- careful application
- adequate warnings to the patient
- checking the effects on the skin (which is easily visible with this treatment) several times during the application.

The suggestion which is sometimes made that the patient could be burnt if he or she fell asleep during treatment is dubious. People have slept in front of powerful sources of infrared – coal, gas and electric fires – over the centuries without being burnt except when consciousness was impaired, by alcohol or an epileptic episode, for example.

Burns can, of course arise if the infrared lamp sets fire to some combustible material. Highly inflammable materials should not be in the region. Poor positioning of the lamp can lead to blankets or pillows being charred, but these should be of low flammability and thus relatively safe.

It has been suggested (Wadsworth and Chanmugan, 1980) that metal on the surface could cause a burn in the underlying skin. This will only be a danger if the metal itself becomes heated to the point at which contact with it is injurious. This is unlikely with the intensity and duration of most infrared treatments. Metal will reflect radiations and for that reason could lead to irregular application of infrared, so is often removed from the irradiated area.

Skin irritation

Most acute inflammatory skin conditions are made worse by heating. Some chemical irritants on the skin have their effects increased by heating, sometimes to the point of irritation or inflammation. For this reason liniments which cause mild erythema (rubifacients) should be removed prior to treatment.

Lowered blood pressure

As infrared treatment causes marked cutaneous vasodilation it may lead to temporary lowering of blood pressure, particularly in elderly people who have less effective vasomotor control. This may lead to faintness especially on standing up immediately after treatment. It may also cause headache.

Areas of defective arterial blood flow

Areas in which the arteries and arterioles cannot respond by adequate vasodilation to the demands of additional heating should not be treated. Such areas would be those affected by arterial disease such as atherosclerosis, arterial injury or after skin-grafting. The possible result of heating such tissue would be tissue necrosis (gangrene).

Eye damage

Prolonged and extensive exposure to infrared, such as occurs in furnacemen, has been associated with eye damage. Long-term irradiation can cause corneal burns from far infrared, and retinal and lenticular damage from near infrared (Moss *et al.*, 1989). This is not a significant danger for the usual lengths of treatment time. However, infrared applied to the eyes causes surface drying, hence irritation, and should be avoided.

Dehydration

Prolonged and intensive treatment to large body areas could cause sweating, sufficient to provoke dehydration if the water is not replaced. Local dehydration of open wounds is also thought to be deleterious.

CONTRAINDICATIONS

- Impaired cutaneous thermal sensation.
- Defective arterial cutaneous circulation.
- Patients whose level of consciousness is markedly lowered by drugs or disease.
- Acute skin disease, e.g. dermatitis or eczema.
- Skin damage due to deep X-ray therapy or other ionizing radiation.
- Defective blood pressure regulation.
- Acute febrile illness – additional heating is not helpful and possibly dangerous to patients whose heat regulation system is under stress.
- Tumours of the skin may be stimulated to increased growth.

REFERENCES

Crockford G. W., Hellon R. F. (1959). Vascular responses of human skin to infra-red radiation. *J. Physiol.*, **149**, 424–32.

Forster A., Palastanga N. (1985). *Clayton's Electrotherapy: Theory and Practice*, 9th edn. London: Baillière Tindall.

Gourgouliatos Z. (1990). Application of the Monte Carlo model in the investigation of the direct penetration of light produced by single and multiple wavelength diode cluster probes. The 4th International Biotherapy Laser Association. Seminar on Laser Biomodulation, Guy's Hospital, London.

Harlen F. (1982). Physics of infrared and microwave therapy. In *Physics in Physiotherapy* (Docker M. F., ed.) London: Hospital Physicists Association Conference report series 35, p. 18.

Hasson S. M., Williams J. H., Gadberry W., Henrich T. (1989). Viewing low and high wavelength light. Effect on EMG activity and force production during maximal voluntary handgrip contraction. *Physiother. Canada*, **41**, 32–5.

Karu T. I. (1989). Photobiology of low-power laser effects. *Health Phys.* **56**, 691–704.

King P. R. (1989). Low level laser therapy – a review. *Laser in Medical Science*, **4**, 141–50.

Kitchen S. S., Partridge C. J. (1991). Infra-red therapy. *Physiotherapy*, **77**, 249–54.

Laurens H. (1933). *The Physiological Effects of Radiant Energy*. New York: Chemical Catalog.

Lehmann J. F., de Lateur B. J. (1982). Therapeutic heat. In *Therapeutic Heat and Cold* (Lehmann J. F., ed.) pp. 404–562. Baltimore: Williams & Wilkins.

Moss C., Ellis R., Murray W., Parr W. (1989). *Infrared Radiation: Nonionising Radiation Protection*, 2nd edn. WHO Regional Publications, European Series, No. 25. Geneva: World Health Organization.

Nightingale A. (1959). *Physics and Electronics in Physical Medicine*. London: G. Bell.

Van Breugel H. H. F. I. (1992). A Monte Carlo model for laser light distribution in tissue: effects of intensity profile and divergence of the laser beam [abstract]. *2nd Meeting of the International Laser Therapy Association*, London: International Laser Therapy Association, 18–20 September, 33.

Wadsworth H., Chanmugan A. P. P. (1980). *Electrophysical Agents in Physiotherapy: Therapeutic and Diagnostic Use*. Marrickville, NSW: Science Press.

Ward A. (1986). *Electricity Fields and Waves in Therapy*. Marrickville, NSW, Australia: Science Press.

Wehr J. A., Rosenthall N. E., Sack D. A. (1985). Role of light in the cause and treatment of seasonal depression. *Photochem. Photobiol.*, **41** (suppl), 45.

Westerhof W., Siddiqui A. H., Cormane R. H. (1987). Infrared hyperthermia and psoriasis. *Arch. Dermatolog. Res.*, **279**, 209–10.

14 Laser therapy

The roots of the laser mechanism are very modern. In 1900 the great German physicist Max Planck presented an explanation of why the colours of a glowing hot body change with temperature. He proposed that radiation comes in discrete quantities ('quanta'). So radiation was not only a series of waves but, at one and the same time, a stream of particles ('photons'). By 1917, Einstein had outlined the principles underlying the production of laser radiation as part of quantum theory.

The earliest medical lasers, developed in the 1960s and 1970s, were used for tissue destruction and coagulation. Some beneficial effects were noted in sites at which low energy had been applied. This led to the therapeutic use of low-energy lasers.

In this chapter the nature and principles of the production of lasers are explained. Several types of lasers are briefly noted, each with some account of how the laser energy is produced and classified.

The effect of laser irradiation on living tissues is considered, followed by discussion of the therapeutic uses and value of lasers. The principles of application and dosage follow. Finally there is consideration of the dangers and contraindications.

INTRODUCTION

The word *laser* is an acronym for light amplification by the stimulated emission of radiation. It refers to the production of a beam of radiation which differs from ordinary light in the following ways:

- *Monochromaticity*: lasers are of a single specific wavelength and hence of a defined frequency. In the case of visible lasers a single pure colour is produced, e.g. ruby lasers give a red light at 694.3 nm (Table 14.1). Single-wavelength laser radiation is also referred to as monochromatic in the infrared and ultraviolet regions, despite being invisible.
- *Coherence*: laser radiation is not only of the same wavelength but also in phase, that is to say the peaks and troughs of the electric and magnetic fields all occur at the same time. This is called 'temporal coherence'. Furthermore they are all travelling in the same direction; this is called 'spatial coherence' (see Fig. 14.1). The distance over which the wavelengths stay in phase is called the coherence length. It varies from less than a millimetre to hundreds of metres.

Table 14.1 Examples of lasers

Laser type		Wavelength (nm)	Radiation
Ruby		694.3	Red light
Helium–neon		632.8	Red light
Gallium aluminium arsenide diodes	Continuous wave	650	Red light
		750	Red light
		780	Infrared
		810	Infrared
		820	Infrared
		850	Infrared
		1300	Infrared
	Pulsed injection	860	Infrared
		904	
Carbon dioxide		10 000	Infrared

- *Collimation*: as a consequence of spatial coherence lasers remain in a parallel beam. Because the radiations do not diverge the energy is propagated over very long distances. This property makes it invaluable for measurement and aiming purposes.

The analogy may be made that ordinary visible (non-coherent) radiations are like a crowd of people all in different clothing, walking in different directions out of step. Laser radiation is like a column of soldiers all marching in step (in phase) in the same direction (spatial coherence) and wearing the same uniform (monochromatic).

When laser radiations interact with matter the effects are the same as any other equivalent electromagnetic radiation – reflection, refraction, absorption and hence scattering. In this way collimation and coherence are diminished or lost. The extent to which this happens will depend on the nature and density of matter present so that laser radiations will pass unaffected through space and be only slightly altered in air (for visible radiations) but be markedly altered on entering a more dense material such as the tissues.

Lasers can be both pulsed and focused. They can therefore be used to deliver large amounts of energy to a small region over a very short time.

When laser radiation is absorbed by the tissues it will cause heating if it is of sufficient intensity, but it is also considered to have specific biological effects due to the special nature of laser radiation.

Principles of lasers

It will be recalled that electrons of an individual atom exist as a 'cloud' of negative charges circling the positively charged nucleus. According to quantum theory; electrons can only occupy certain energy levels or 'shells' around the nucleus. The electrons in the outermost orbit or shell are most easily affected by outside forces. If the atom is given additional energy, say by heating, these outer electrons can be made

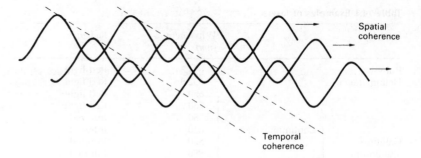

Spatial coherence

Temporal coherence

All 3 waves are travelling in the same direction – spatial coherence
in step at the same time – temporal coherence

Fig. 14.1 Coherence.

to occupy higher energy levels and, if enough energy is added to the atom, an outer electron may gain sufficient energy to free itself from the pull of the nucleus. The atom then becomes a positively charged ion and the electron a free negative charge.

When the outer electrons are in one of the higher energy states, they will tend to return to a lower energy state, sometimes to the most stable or ground state. An electron may do this either by cascading down from one energy level to the next or it may jump directly to the ground state. In both cases the additional energy must be given up and this is done by giving off a photon (quantum) of radiation (Fig. 14.2(a) and (b)). Each step from one energy level to the next is known as a transition and the wavelength (and thus the frequency) of the emitted photon depends on the energy difference between the two energy levels; the more the energy difference, the shorter the wavelength and higher the frequency.

While an electron is in a higher energy state the atom is said to be excited and this state will last a very short time, characteristically about 10^{-8} s, before the electron falls to a lower energy level emitting a photon. There are some excitation levels in all atoms from which electrons cannot easily leave spontaneously but need to give up their energy on collision with other atoms. Such electrons remain in their higher energy state for much longer average times, e.g. 0.001 s (10^{-3} s) and are referred to as being metastable states (Silfvast, 1973).

Energy can be introduced into matter in various ways. Heat, for example, leads to molecular collisions which alter the complex energy

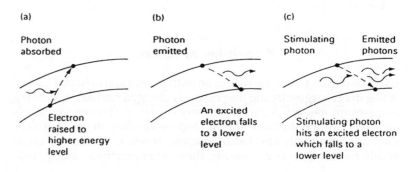

(a)

Photon absorbed

Electron raised to higher energy level

(b)

Photon emitted

An excited electron falls to a lower level

(c)

Stimulating photon   Emitted photons

Stimulating photon hits an excited electron which falls to a lower level

Fig. 14.2 Absorption and emission of photons. (a) absorption; (b) spontaneous emission; (c) stimulated emission.

levels sustained by molecular interaction causing excitation. Electrons falling back to their stable states emit photons at numerous different wavelengths giving a continuous spectrum in the infrared and visible spectrum (i.e. the way infrared lamps work (see Fig. 14.4).

An electric charge applied to a gas of a single element may cause certain permitted transitions only. Thus only photons of a few characteristic wavelengths are emitted, hence a line spectrum.

Photons themselves, if absorbed, can give energy to an atom; this causes excitation. For absorption of the photon to occur its wavelength must correspond exactly to the difference in energy between the existing state of the electron and a possible higher energy level. Similarly if the electron is already in a higher energy state and can move to a lower level with a difference that corresponds to the energy of the stimulating photon it may do so by giving out a photon of its own identical to that of the colliding photon. This process is called stimulated emission (Fig. 14.2(c)).

A large number of atoms with electrons in the excited state can lead to amplification since one photon releases a second and these two can release two more and so on – a kind of cascade or avalanche effect. Such a system can only emit photons if there are more electrons at a higher energy level than in the ground state. If this does not occur all the photons released from electrons falling from high-energy states are absorbed in the molecules, raising the energy of electrons in the low-energy (ground) state. Having more atoms in the upper energy state than the lower is called 'population inversion', simply because it is the reverse of the usual situation in which there are more electrons in the ground state and at lower energy levels.

Such a population inversion can be achieved by forcing the electrons of many atoms into their metastable state. As electrons remain in this state for a relatively long time it is possible, with an intense energy input, to have more electrons entering the metastable state than leaving it. Hence a temporary population inversion is achieved.

Summary

Laser radiation:

- is monochromatic, i.e. of a single wavelength
- is coherent in both
  - phase – temporal coherence
  - direction – spatial coherence
- is collimated, i.e. a parallel beam
- behaves like all radiations
  - reflected
  - refracted, hence can be focused or scattered
  - absorbed
- is produced by the emission of large numbers of identical photons from suitably energized material.

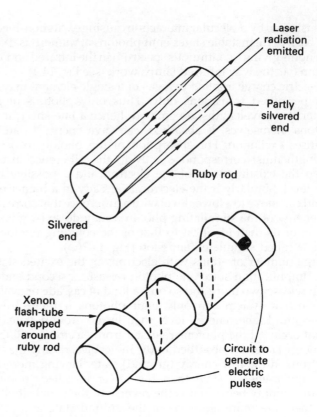

Fig. 14.3 A ruby laser.

TYPES OF LASERS

The application of the foregoing principles will be illustrated by an initial description of the ruby laser.

The ruby laser

This consists of a small synthetic ruby rod made of aluminium oxide. A helical xenon flash tube, wound around it, gives an intense flash of white light. Both ends of the rod are made flat and silvered, one end being totally reflecting and the other partially transparent so that some radiation can be emitted (see Fig. 14.3).

This brief light pulse (0.5 ms) excites the ruby molecules and raises many electrons to higher levels which they occupy for very short average times before falling to the metastable level where they remain for much longer average times. Thus, for a time, there are more electrons in the metastable level than the ground level and so population inversion has occurred. When the transition from metastable to ground state does occur a photon with a wavelength of 694.3 nm is emitted. This photon would have exactly the right energy to raise a ground state electron to the metastable level and be reabsorbed but as there are relatively few ground-state electrons the photon is much more likely to interact with other metastable

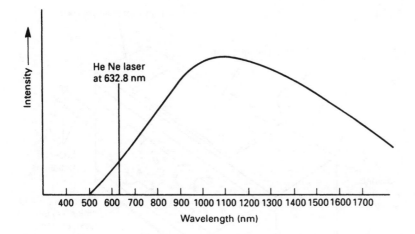

Fig. 14.4 Comparison of laser output with infrared lamp. (Infrared and visible radiations were emitted from typical luminous infrared lamp giving radiations at a range of wavelengths; peak emission around 1000 nm.)

electrons, causing them to return to the ground state and so emitting an identical photon. The process rapidly accelerates as more and more photons are released; i.e. stimulated emission of radiation occurs. The photons, having a wavelength of 694.3 nm, which is of course red light, are reflected up and down the short ruby rod (see Fig. 14.3), rapidly increasing the effect. Thus all the energy stored in the ruby molecules is released in a very brief time, as a pulse of red light of identical photons and so of a single wavelength of coherent radiation: this emerges from the rod at the partially transparent end (see Holwill and Silvester, 1973).

Helium–neon lasers

Helium–neon lasers consist of a long tube containing these natural gases at low pressure surrounded by a flashgun tube, as described for the ruby laser. Excitation of these atoms leads to different energy levels between them and the transfer of energy, giving off a photon of wavelength equivalent to the energy gap. The photons are reflected to and fro along the tube giving rise to further photon emission and emerging as a narrow beam (of about 1 mm diameter) from the partially transparent end. Helium–neon lasers give radiation in the red visible region at 632.8 nm. See Figure 14.4 for comparison of helium–neon laser output with the infrared lamp. The output is usually applied to the tissues via an optical guide – a fibreoptic cable – the end of which is held in contact with the tissues. There are, of course, some energy losses in the glass fibre of the cable and the laser beam may diverge somewhat as it emerges at the end of the optical fibre.

Diode lasers

These are specialized light-emitting diodes, based on semiconductor p–n junctions. They are of various kinds, involving gallium

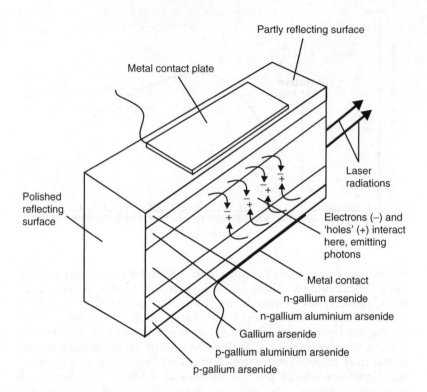

Fig. 14.5 The structure and principle of a semiconductor laser diode.

aluminium arsenide (GaAlAs). In these, electrons can flow more readily in one direction than in the other. The electrons are excited by the application of a suitable electrical potential and their occupation of 'holes' in the crystal lattice arrangement may lead to the emission of a photon which may then stimulate identical photons in the manner already described. The photons are reflected to and fro and emitted as a laser beam from one partially transparent end (see Fig. 14.5). These are conveniently small, relatively cheap and robust devices. By varying the ratio of gallium to aluminium such devices can be built to emit specific wavelengths (see Table 14.1).

Semiconductor laser diodes can give either a continuous or a pulsed output. Continuous wave diode lasers are usually of relatively low power. Alternatively they can be pulsed electronically. On some machines the pulse frequency can be varied.

Superluminous diodes. Making diode lasers fully coherent is difficult. It is cheaper to produce superluminous diodes (SLDs) which are fully monochromatic and collimated but non-coherent. It is argued that coherence is therapeutically superfluous (Karu, 1987) and in any case is rapidly lost as radiations enter the tissues. While SLDs are not strictly lasers, they are widely used in therapy.

Due to their small size semiconductor lasers can be applied directly to the tissues in a hand-held applicator. Sometimes several laser diodes of assorted wavelengths are mounted together to form an

Table 14.2 Classification of lasers

Class	Power	Effect	Usage
1	Low	None on eye or skin	Blackboard pointer Supermarket barcode reader
2	Low CW→1 mW	Safe on skin Eye protected by aversion responses	
3A	Low–medium (mid) CW→5 mW	Direct intrabeam viewing with optical aids may be hazardous	Therapeutic – physiotherapy models
3B	Medium (mid) CW→500 mW	Direct intrabeam viewing may be hazardous	
4	High CW−500 mW+	Hazardous to skin and eye	Destructive – surgical models

CW = continuous wave.

emitter which can be used to treat a larger area. These are known as 'cluster probes'. They may also contain SLDs.

For all these forms of low-power laser a suitable electronic circuit is provided to generate appropriate currents to power the diodes. Pulsing and timing are also controlled electronically.

Summary of laser devices

- Ruby laser
- He–Ne laser
- Diode lasers (GaAlAs lasers)
  - of various wavelengths
  - continuous or pulsed emission
- Superluminous diodes (non-coherent)
- Cluster probes
  - groups of laser diodes and SLDs of different wavelengths.

MEASUREMENT OF LASER ENERGY

- The amount of energy falling on a surface is expressed in joules per square metre (J/m^2) or joules per square centimetre (J/cm^2). It is often called **energy density**.
- The rate at which energy is produced or absorbed is measured in joules per second, i.e. in watts ($1\,W = 1\,J/s$) and called power.
- Most lasers used in physiotherapy have output powers of milliwatts (see Table 14.2). The average power per unit area can be expressed as irradiance or **power density** in W/cm^2.

If the laser is pulsed the temporal average power must be distinguished from the temporal peak power. The temporal peak power is that of each pulse but the average or mean power depends on the pulse length and the pulse frequency. The very short individual pulses may be a few watts, but the mean power will be a few milliwatts.

- The laser beam is not perfectly collimated and the divergence may be expressed in terms of an angle.

EFFECTS OF LASER RADIATION ON THE TISSUES

Like all radiations laser may:

- be reflected from the surface
- penetrate the tissues in proportions that depend on the:
  - wavelength
  - nature of the tissue surface
  - angle of incidence.

Having entered the tissues laser radiation is scattered by:

- divergence
- reflection
- refraction

and further attenuated by absorption (see Chapter 11).

The penetration depth of red visible and short infrared radiation is considered to be a few millimetres, 1–2 mm for red light and 2–4 mm for IR of 800–900 nm in soft tissue (King, 1989).

It has been suggested (Basford, 1995) that a dose of as little as $0.01 \, J/cm^2$ can alter cellular processes and that such a dose may be achieved at 6 penetration depths from a $4 \, J/cm^2$ surface application, e.g. at 1.2 cm depth for radiation of 2 mm penetration depth. However, the effects of scattering in the tissues are much more complex than indicated in Figure 13.2. This can lead to local intensities actually higher than the applied beam at a point just below the skin surface (Van Breugel, 1992).

Due to this marked scattering in the tissues, it is considered that areas between the diodes of a cluster probe are also treated (Gourgouliatos, 1990). Scanning lasers can be used to treat larger areas.

Any energy absorbed by the tissues will inevitably lead to greater kinetic energy at molecular and cellular level.

Absorption in the tissues

Visible radiations are markedly absorbed in haemoglobin and melanin (chromophores), while infrared is strongly absorbed by water (Diamantopoulos, 1994).

It is thought that red light is absorbed by cytochromes in the mitochondria of the cell. All cells have these cytochromes, so all may be stimulated by red light. This, in turn, possibly affects cell membrane permeability. In this way, laser is affecting the membrane from within (cf. ultrasound). Various types of cells have different photo-acceptors in their membranes. Because of this, different wavelengths could have an all-or-none effect on specific cells, which may provide a way, in future, of targeting these cells.

As with ultrasound, the key factor seems to be the transport of calcium ions across the cell membrane. This sets in train a whole sequence of events necessary to restore the cell to its normal function. As long as an energy threshold at cellular level is reached, an effect can occur. Mester *et al.* (1985) suggested that $4 J/cm^2$ was an appropriate dose, but a range of $1–32 J/cm^2$ has been used.

It is possible that there is a 'window' for effective photo-biostimulation, above threshold but below a level that causes inhibition. This concept, described as the Arndt–Schultz law (see Chapter 10 and Fig. 10.15), has been invoked to perhaps account for the conflicting results of laser studies (Baxter, 1994).

Macrophages, which have an important role in controlling the inflammatory response (see Chapter 1), can be influenced by laser radiations (Young *et al.*, 1989). This would only occur if the radiations were able to reach the macrophage cell at the site of the lesion.

THERAPEUTIC USES OF LASERS

The terms 'low-reactive level laser therapy' (LLLT) and 'low-intensity laser therapy' (LILT) are sometimes used to distinguish the low-energy applications used in physiotherapy, from the high-energy applications used therapeutically for tissue destruction. The terms 'photobiomodulation' and 'photobiostimulation', describing the effect, are also used.

There are two major areas for which laser therapy is used: tissue healing and pain control. Within these two broad categories, laser therapy is widely used in the treatment of all kinds of soft tissue injuries, such as muscle tears, haematomas and tendinitis. Laser acupuncture is also applied and the laser treatment of some arthropathies has been reported.

Tissue healing

The use of radiations of all kinds to accelerate wound healing has a long history but radiations in the red part of the visible spectrum have been particularly employed and found to be effective. In fact it is suggested (Karu, 1987) that the advent of the helium–neon laser led to the rediscovery of the therapeutic benefit of 'red light therapy', at least in respect of accelerating tissue healing. The observed benefit of laser therapy has been attributed to its coherence but this idea is not supported by the evidence (Karu, 1987). However, Colver and Priestley (1989) found a failure of the helium–neon laser to affect components of wound healing *in vitro*.

Wavelength.   The evidence relating wavelength of radiation to specific biological effects is extensive, covering tissue and cellular experiments in the laboratory, but it is inconsistent. However, Young *et al.* (1989) showed that 660, 820 and 870 nm wavelengths encouraged macrophages to release factors that stimulated fibroblast proliferation above the control levels whereas the 880 nm wavelength was inhibitory. Only the 820 nm wavelength was coherent and polarized, showing that at certain wavelengths coherence and polarization are not essential. In general, it seems that responses to visible radiations occur at both cellular and organismal levels; that laser stimulation is of a photobiological nature and that effects are due to both coherent and non-coherent radiation (Karu, 1987).

Pulse frequency.   Dyson and Young (1986) found that when using a Space Mix 5 laser (combined infrared at 904 nm 200 ns pulses and helium–neon at 632.8 nm) on surgical skin lesions of mice, there was greater wound contraction at 700 Hz infrared pulse frequency compared to 1200 Hz. By 11 days after injury there was greater cellularity and more and better organized fibroblasts in the 700 Hz group. King (1989) draws attention to the fact that no significant differences in contraction were found on many days in the time series. There is a suggestion that 16 Hz is an effective pulse frequency for tissue healing.

Additional factors involved in the acceleration of wound healing by laser may include a marked increase in collagen formation, vasodilation and DNA synthesis (Mester *et al.*, 1985) and an increase in RNA production (Gamaleya, 1977).

Laser treatment is recommended for the treatment of indolent wounds and trophic ulcers to promote more rapid healing and it is considered that low-intensity visible radiation has an effect in accelerating or stimulating cell proliferation. In such wounds cell proliferation may be inhibited by low oxygen concentration, abnormal pH or other abnormality such as deficiency of nutrients. In these circumstances light may act as a signal to increase proliferation. Any physiotherapeutic effect may be much less evident, or non-existent if the wound is healing at the optimum rate (Karu, 1987). For an extensive discussion of the wound healing related to laser stimulation see Shields and O'Kane (1994).

Pain control

Musculoskeletal.   Laser therapy is used for the relief of pain in many conditions, both acute and long-term (England, 1988). Rheumatoid arthritis, osteoarthritis, bursitis and various aspects of back pain (nerve inflammation, muscle spasm) are found to have benefited from laser treatment (Seitz and Kleinkort, 1986). The laser treatment of rheumatoid arthritis has also been studied by Colov *et al.* (1987) and was found to have a significant pain-relieving effect and reduction of joint swelling as well as objective improvement in hand function (Goldman *et al.*, 1980). Vasseljen (1992) found that 47% of patients treated (with a cluster head, 3 times a week, for 8 treatments) for tennis elbow were pain free or, at least, less painful 1 month after treatment. Grip strength also increased significantly. A double-blind trial on patients with supraspinatus tendinitis (Saunders, 1995) found improvement in pain and weakness in the treated group. Fracture consolidation has been found to be accelerated (Trelles and Mayayo, 1981) and post-traumatic nerve degeneration prevented (Nissan *et al.*, 1986; Schwartz *et al.*, 1987).

Neurogenic. Neurogenic pain (trigeminal, postherpetic neuralgia and others) has been found to be relieved in some patients by laser applications (Walker, 1983). This was thought to be due to the laser affecting serotonin metabolism.

Trigger/acupuncture points. Pain is also often treated by application of the laser source to trigger or acupuncture points (Ong, 1986), both on their own and in conjunction with local treatment. Such points show a lower than normal skin resistance when tested with a small current (see Chapter 3). It is further considered that resolution of the condition is associated with a return to normal skin resistance. A randomized, double-blind study (Snyder-Mackler *et al.*, 1986) of the skin resistance over trigger points before and after three successive treatments of helium–neon laser showed a statistically significant increase in skin resistance after treatment. This suggests that the laser treatment has some therapeutic effect on the underlying musculoskeletal trigger point and may aid resolution of the pathological condition. In two groups of healthy subjects given therapy to auricular acupuncture points, an increase in pain threshold at the wrist was found only in those treated with laser (King *et al.*, 1990).

Nerve conduction rate. There have been a number of studies on nerve conduction rates that have produced conflicting evidence, but particularly careful and valuable work (Baxter *et al.*, 1991a) has repeatedly shown that laser irradiation over the median nerve of normal subjects increases nerve conduction latencies. Similar results have been obtained by others (Snyder-Mackler and Bork, 1988). It is not known how the laser application (of $1.2\,J/cm^2$ in one study by Baxter *et al.*, 1991b) would affect the underlying nerve or how this might lead to pain modification. Kramer and Sandrin (1993) found that conduction rates were about 1% slower with a helium–neon laser and 1% faster with white light, but there was no significant difference with placebo or infrared. They speculated that these results were unlikely to be clinically meaningful.

An investigation of nerve conduction latency, amplitude and temperature around the nerve (Greathouse *et al.*, 1985) could find no change as a consequence of either 20- or 120-s infrared laser application. However, studies by Baxter *et al.* (1990) found a small but reproducible increase in nerve conduction latency due to laser irradiation at therapeutic doses in humans. Such an effect can hardly be due to heating – which would decrease nerve latency – and could perhaps account for the analgesic effects claimed for laser therapy.

EFFECTIVENESS OF LOW-INTENSITY LASER THERAPY

In spite of considerable interest and research into the application of laser energy for non-surgical therapies, including the publication of several books (e.g. Oshiro, 1991; Baxter, 1994), there is still uncertainty about whether it is effective, and little agreement over the mechanisms that might underly any effects.

Several reviews of collected clinical trials have been unable to resolve this uncertainty. For example, Kitchen and Partridge (1991) say therapeutic effects are far from clear, and Seichert (1991) concludes that it cannot be recommended, from either a scientific or a clinical point of view. However, a meta-analysis of 36 randomized clinical trials (Beckerman *et al.*, 1992) found that no conclusions could be drawn about the efficacy of laser therapy for skin disorders; but for musculoskeletal disorders the efficacy seems to be better than for a placebo treatment. For rheumatoid arthritis, post-traumatic joint disorders and myofascial pain, laser therapy seemed to have a substantial therapeutic effect.

Baxter *et al.* (1991a), in a study of the use of laser therapy in clinical practice, found that over 50% of respondents felt that soft tissue injuries and wound healing including burns responded particularly well to treatment.

PRINCIPLES OF APPLICATION

Most low- or medium-power laser sources are applied to the skin by a hand-held applicator about the size of a large marker pen. The laser diode is close to the tip, which is a small lens. Direct application to the skin ensures maximum transfer of laser energy and light pressure; squeezing blood from superficial vessels can increase the penetration further (Baxter, 1994).

In other types of laser the applicator may be held in a rigid but mobile stand and applied about 30 cm away from the patient. This latter type may provide several sources of laser output to cover a relatively large area.

Some versions use laser diodes, called cluster diodes, which all emit at different wavelengths to take advantage of any different effects that may ensue from the use of different wavelengths.

Preparation of the patient.   The nature of the treatment and the need to wear goggles or spectacles are explained to the patient.

Preparation of the apparatus.   The laser apparatus is conveniently positioned. Protective goggles, designed for the particular wavelength being used, are worn to obviate any risk of accidental application of the laser beam into the eye (see below).

Preparation of the part.   The surface of the skin to be treated is cleaned with an alcohol wipe in order to remove any material on the surface that might absorb or scatter the radiation. The part is supported in such a way that any pressure of the laser applicator does not cause movement or discomfort.

Application.   A key usually activates the machine and ensures that unauthorized people do not switch the laser on. The laser applicator is applied to the surface before switching on. There is sometimes a switch on the applicator itself and usually an indicator light to show that the infrared laser – which is, of course, invisible – is on. It is important to maintain the laser applicator in contact with the tissues so that the beam is applied at right angles in order to achieve maximal penetration.

If contact is not desired, for example because of an infected wound, the applicator may be held just off the surface or covered with transparent non-reflective film. In all other circumstances firm contact should be maintained throughout treatment but should not provoke pain where tenderness is present. The position is maintained for the necessary time. If a larger area is to be treated the applicator is removed and repositioned on a new site, turning off the output during the transfer.

Termination.   The device is switched off before removing the applicator from skin contact. The details of dosage and any patient response, such as immediate increase or decrease of pain, are noted and recorded, plus the parameters of dosage.

DOSAGE

An inevitable consequence of uncertainty about the therapeutic effects of laser radiation is an equivalent uncertainty regarding the dosage. In general:

- the wavelength
- the area of application

are fixed by the type of laser apparatus used. The energy density can be varied by the time of a single application of the probe or applicator and/or by varying the pulsing parameters. The size of the area treated can be adjusted by the number of discrete applications made and also by the use of cluster probes.

Wavelength

Visible red laser is recommended for superficial conditions, such as wounds, ulcers and skin conditions, and infrared for deeper, musculoskeletal structures.

Energy density

The treatment dose is usually given in J/cm^2 (or mJ/cm^2) and called energy density or sometimes radiant exposure.

1   The mean power output in milliwatts is usually fixed (it can be varied on some machines by altering the pulsing regimen).
2   When divided by the (fixed) area of the beam it gives the power density or irradiance in mW/cm^2.
3   When multiplied by the number of seconds for which the treatment is applied, it gives the number of joules/cm^2 or energy density.

Example

1   Mean power $= 10\,mW$
     Beam area $= 0.125\,cm^2$
2   Therefore power density
$$= \frac{10}{0.125} = 80\,mW/cm^2$$
3   If the treatment is applied for 50 s,
     the energy density $= 80\,mW/cm^2 \times 50\,s$
$$= 4000\,mJ/cm^2$$
$$= 4\,J/cm^2.$$

There is wide variation in the recommendations for the optimal energy for different conditions. The usual ranges are from 1 to $10\,J/cm^2$ but doses as low as $0.5\,J/cm^2$ and up to $32\,J/cm^2$ have been suggested. Mester *et al.* (1985) suggested that there was a 'saturation energy density of $4\,J/cm^2$' in open wound experiments. Higher doses are usually recommended for subcutaneous tissues. The existence of a therapeutic 'window' for laser dosage has been suggested as between $0.5\,J/cm^2$ and $4\,J/cm^2$ (Laakso *et al.*, 1993).

It should be recognized that the dosages indicated above, and elsewhere, are those applied to the tissue surface. The dose at depth in the tissues is unknown. With the uncertainties pertaining to penetration depth, noted earlier, any estimate is extremely unreliable.

Pulsed output

On some machines the mean power output is always the same regardless of pulse frequency. This is achieved by adjusting the pulse duration so that the low pulse rates have long pulse lengths and the high rates have shorter pulse lengths. It is generally recommended that the low pulse frequencies and long pulse durations are used for acute conditions and higher pulse repetition rates and short pulse durations for chronic conditions but note that

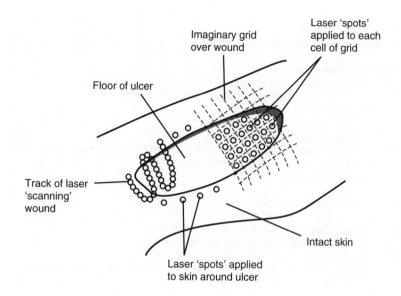

Floor of ulcer

Imaginary grid
over wound

Laser 'spots'
applied to each
cell of grid

Track of laser
'scanning'
wound

Intact skin

Laser 'spots' applied
to skin around ulcer

Fig. 14.6 The treatment of an open wound by laser 'spots' on a grid and an intact skin, as well as the continuous movement of a scanning technique.

on machines where the mean power output is said to be constant the energy introduced into the tissues will not be altered by this pulsing difference.

Where the duty cycle (percentage of time the laser is on) varies, the mean power will also vary as the same proportion (i.e. as the duty cycle) of peak power.

The arguments for pulsed versus continuous beam lasers are similar to those for ultrasound. There is some evidence that particular pulsing frequencies have specific effects at a cellular level (Rajaratnam *et al.*, 1994).

Area of treatment

Discrete lesions should be treated directly over the affected part. For wounds and large areas, the part is divided into centimetre squares (like a grid) and each area is separately stimulated, or a scanning technique may be used in which the laser is moved continuously over the wound surface. Adequate dosage is achieved, it is suggested, because granulation tissue has higher absorption than intact skin (Ohshiro and Calderhead, 1988). Alternatively the healthy skin at the edge of the wound can be stimulated with a series of applications at 1–2 cm lengths (see Fig. 14.6). While the applicator is pressed firmly onto normal skin, for the treatment of open wounds it should be held just off contact.

Painful areas are usually treated at the point of maximal pain, for example a trigger or acupuncture point (Ong, 1986).

Progression of treatment

If there is no response to treatment the dose should be increased. Five to six treatments are said to be sufficient to establish some response to treatment.

There is no consensus about the optimum frequency of treatment.

Summary of dosage parameters

- wavelength
  - fixed for a given laser
  - choice can influence depth of penetration
- area treated
  - cross-section of single beam
  - repeated applications of single beam
  - continuous movement of single beam (scanning)
  - collection of lasers (cluster diodes)
- mean power (in mW)
  - fixed
  - variable – by laser control
    - by pulsing
- duration of application (in seconds)
  - determines the energy density in J/cm^2
- pulsing (in Hz) – may have special effects
- frequency of treatment – usually limited and regulated by results.

DANGERS AND CONTRAINDICATIONS

The main danger involving low-level laser therapy is a risk of eye damage if the beam is applied directly into the eye. As therapeutic lasers have very little power there is normally no thermal effect when it is applied to the skin. However, if it passes through the lens of the eye, the beam can become focused on a very small area, causing intense heating. Various reported studies on rabbits and monkeys (Seitz and Kleinkort, 1986) have indicated that this mechanism does cause burns of the retina but that at least 7 mW power at the cornea was needed to produce irreversible damage in monkeys. Although the risk to humans would seem to be small, shining a laser into the eye or looking directly into the laser beam should be strictly avoided.

Reasonable precautions.   Although any risk to the eye is small, the following are often advised:

- using laser devices only in specially designated areas
- avoiding reflecting the laser beam from shiny surfaces
- only switching the laser on when the applicator is in contact with the skin
- using appropriate protective goggles.

It must also be recognized that the laser beam can be almost totally reflected from any shiny surfaces. It is recommended that reflecting surfaces should be removed from the area or covered. The laser beam should only be switched on when the applicator is in contact with the skin; some units have a switch on the applicator itself to facilitate this. Further precautions include wearing protective goggles. Some authorities require a notice to be on display outside the immediate treatment area warning that a laser is in use.

Direct treatment of neoplastic tissue should be avoided on the grounds that cell stimulation may occur, leading to increased rates of growth or metastases.

In the interests of prudence the use of lasers over the unclosed fontanelle of infants and over the pregnant uterus should be avoided (Seitz and Kleinkort, 1986) but there is no evidence that damage could occur in either brain or fetal tissue.

If the applicator is used in contact with infected skin areas it will need to be cleaned and sterilized with a suitable solution after use.

Contraindications

These include the direct treatment of:

- neoplastic tissue
- pregnant uterus (Seitz and Kleinkort, 1986)
- haemorrhage and infected tissue. These are among the contraindications given by some (e.g. Baxter, 1994).

REFERENCES

Basford J. R. (1995). Low intensity laser therapy: still not an established clinical tool. *Lasers Surg. Med.*, **16**, 331–42.

Baxter G. D. (ed.) (1994). *Therapeutic Lasers: Theory and Practice*. Edinburgh: Churchill Livingstone.

Baxter G. D., Bell A. J., Allen J. M. *et al.* (1990). Laser mediated increase in median nerve conduction velocities. The 4th International Biotherapy Laser Association. Seminar on Laser Biomodulation, Guy's Hospital, London.

Baxter G. D., Bell A. J., Allen J. M., Ravey J. (1991a). Low level laser therapy: current clinical practice in Northern Ireland. *Physiotherapy*, **77**, 171–8.

Baxter G. D., Bell A. J., Allen J. M., Ravey R. (1991b). Laser medicated increases in nerve conduction latencies: long term effects. *WCPT 11th International Congress Proceedings, Book II*, London: World Confederation for Physical Therapy, 747–9.

Beckerman H., de Bie R. A., Bouter L. M. *et al.* (1992). The efficacy of laser therapy for musculoskeletal and skin disorders: a criteria-based meta-analysis of randomized clinical trials. *Phys. Ther.*, **72**, 483–91.

Colov H. C., Palmgren N., Jenson G. F. *et al.* (1987). Convincing clinical improvement of rheumatoid arthritis by soft laser therapy. *Lasers Surg. Med.*, **7**, 77.

Colver G. B., Priestley G. C. (1989). Failure of a helium–neon laser to affect components of wound healing in vitro. *Br. J. Dermatol.*, **121**, 179–86.

Diamantopoulos C. (1994). Bioenergetics and tissue optics. In *Therapeutic Lasers: Theory and Practice* (Baxter G. D., ed.) Edinburgh: Churchill Livingstone, pp. 67–88.

Dyson M., Young S. (1986). Effects of laser therapy on wound contraction and cellularity in mice. *Lasers Med. Sci.*, **1**, 125.

England S. (1988). Introduction to mid laser therapy. *Physiotherapy*, **74**, 100–2.

Gamaleya N. F. (1977). Laser biomedical research. In *Tae-MSSR Laser Applications in Medicine and Biology*. New York: Plenum Press.

Goldman J. A., Chiapella J., Casey H. (1980). Laser therapy on rheumatoid arthritis. *Lasers Surg. Med.*, **1**, 93–101.

Gourgouliatos Z. (1990). Application of the Monte Carlo model in the investigation of the direct penetration of light produced by single and multiple wavelength diode cluster probes. The 4th International Biotherapy Laser Association. Seminar on Laser Biomodulation, Guy's Hospital, London.

Greathouse D. G., Currier D. P., Gilmore R. L. (1985). Effects of clinical infrared laser on superficial radial nerve conduction. *Phys. Ther.*, **65**, 1184–7.

Holwill M. E. J., Silvester N. R. (1973). *Introduction to Biological Physics*. London: John Wiley.

Karu T. I. (1987). Photobiological fundamentals of low-power laser therapy. *I.E.E.E. J. Quant. Electronics, QE23*, **10**, 1703–17.

King P. R. (1989). Low level laser therapy: a review. *Lasers Med. Sci.*, **4**, 141–50.

King C. E., Clelland J. A., Knowles C. J., Jackson J. R. (1990). Effects of helium–neon laser auriculotherapy on experimental pain threshold. *Phys. Ther.*, **70**, 24–30.

Kitchen S. S., Partridge C. J. (1991). A review of low level laser therapy. *Physiotherapy*, **77**, 161–8.

Kramer J. F., Sandrin M. (1993). Effect of low-power laser and white light on sensory conduction rate of the superficial radial nerve. *Physiotherapy* (Canada), **3**, 165–70.

Laakso L., Richardson C., Cramond T. (1993). Factors affecting low level laser therapy. *Aust. J. Physiother.*, **39**, 95–9.

Mester E., Mester A. E., Mester A. (1985). The biomedical effect of laser application. *Lasers Surg. Med.*, **5**, 31–9.

Nissan M., Rockind S., Ralon N., Bartal A. (1986). He-Ne laser irradiation delivered transcutaneously: its effect on the sciatic nerve of rats. *Lasers Surg. Med.*, **6**, 435–8.

Ohshiro T. (1991). *Low Reactive-Level Laser Therapy: Practical Application*. Chichester: Wiley.

Ohshiro T., Calderhead R. G. (1988). *Low Level Laser Therapy: A Practical Introduction*. Chichester, Wiley.

Ong K. L. T. (1986). Handling the patient in pain. *Physiotherapy*, **72**, 284–8.

Rajaratnam S., Bolton P., Dyson M. (1994). Macrophage responsiveness to laser therapy with varying pulsing frequencies. *Laser Therapy*, **6**, 107–12.

Sanders L. (1995). The efficacy of low-level laser therapy in supraspinatus tendinitis. *Clin. Rehabil.*, **9**, 126–34.

Schwartz M., Doron A., Erlich M. *et al.* (1987). Effects of low energy He-Ne laser irradiation as post-traumatic degeneration of adult rabbit optic nerve. *Lasers Surg. Med.*, **7**, 497–505.

Seichert N. (1991). Controlled trials of laser treatment. In *Physiotherapy: Controlled Trials and Facts* Rheumatology, Vol. 14 (Schlapbach P., Gerber N. J. eds) Basel: Karger, pp. 205–17.

Seitz L. M., Kleinkort J. A. (1986). Low-power laser: its application in physical therapy. In *Thermal Agents in Rehabilitation* (Michlovitz S. L., ed). Philadelphia: F. A. Davies, pp. 217–37.

Shields D., O'Kane S. (1994). Laser photobiomodulation of wound healing. In *Therapeutic Lasers: Theory and Practice* (Baxter G. D., ed.) Edinburgh: Churchill Livingstone, pp. 89–138.

Silfvast W. T. (1973). Metal-vapor lasers. *Sci. Am.*, **228**, 89–97.

Snyder-Mackler L., Bork C., Bourbon B., Trumbore D. (1986). Effects of helium–neon laser on musculoskeletal trigger points. *Phys. Ther.*, **66**, 1087–90.

Snyder-Mackler L., Bork C. E. (1988). Effect of helium–neon laser irradiation on peripheral sensory nerve latency. *Phys. Ther.*, **68**, 223–5.

Trelles M., Mayayo E. (1981). Bone fracture consolidates faster with low power laser. *Lasers Surg. Med.*, **7**, 36–45.

Van Breugel H. H. F. I. (1992). A Monte Carlo model for laser light distribution in tissue: effects of intensity profile and divergence of the laser beam [abstract]. *2nd Meeting of the International Laser Therapy Association*, London: International Laser Therapy Association, 18–20 September, 33.

Vasseljen O. (1992). Low-level laser versus traditional physiotherapy in the treatment of tennis elbow. *Physiotherapy*, **78**, 329–34.

Young S. R., Bolton P., Dyson M. *et al.* (1989). Macrophage responsiveness to light therapy. *Lasers in Surgery and Medicine*, **9**, 497–505.

Walker J. (1983). Relief from chronic pain by low power laser irradiation. *Neurosci. Lett.*, **43**, 339–44.

15 Ultraviolet radiation

Invisible radiations beyond the violet end of the visible spectrum were termed 'ultravioletten' by Johann Ritter in 1801. They are well recognized as the wavelengths that cause sunburn and tanning of the skin on exposure to the sun.

The benefit of natural sunlight for healing has been documented over many years. It can, perhaps, be traced to the worship of sun gods in almost all ancient cultures (Licht, 1983). However, there is a distinct paucity of accounts of the therapeutic usage of sunlight emanating from the period of the Middle Ages. Licht (1983) ascribes this to the rise of Christianity which suppressed 'all pagan practices including sun worship and sun bathing' in many European cultures.

About the middle of the 19th century a very great interest developed in the use of heliotherapy. Later, artificial sources of ultraviolet radiation (UVR) became available, so that therapeutic usage increased further.

In the early 20th century the relative success of UVR treatment for tuberculosis, rickets and infections led to therapeutic applications for a plethora of pathologies. By the middle of the 20th century the advent of antibiotic and other drug treatments had superseded UVR therapies for many purposes.

In recent years, the application of UVR therapy within physiotherapy has diminished as it has become a less 'fashionable' therapy. This decrease has appeared to parallel an increase in the application of UVR in dermatology clinics.

The nature and production of therapeutic UVR is considered in brief, followed by a description of the physiological effects.

Some comment on the therapeutic uses is followed by an important discussion on the factors affecting and means of adjusting the dosage of UVR.

The principles and some account of the methods of application are considered with the contraindications. Finally, comment is added on the use of heliotherapy, sunbeds and ionozone therapy.

NATURE OF ULTRAVIOLET RADIATION

Ultraviolet radiations (UVR) behave in a similar way to visible radiations in the way they are reflected, refracted or absorbed, except that they are more strongly absorbed in air, in particular the short-wavelength ultraviolet. A further difference, of course, is the fact that UVR transmit much more energy than visible radiations (see Chapter 11) so that they are able to provoke chemical changes and not simply heat at sites where they are absorbed.

Table 15.1 Classification of ultraviolet radiation

Region	Wavelength	Other names
		Biotic
UVA	400–315 nm	Long UV, blacklight
UVB	315–280 nm	Medium UV, erythemal UV
		Abiotic
UVC	280–100 nm	Short UV, germicidal UV

(The frequency therefore ranges from 0.75×10^{15} at 400 nm to 3×10^{15} at 100 nm.)

As already noted, UVR are usually defined in terms of their wavelengths, extending from the violet end of the visible at 390–400 nm to the soft X-ray region; the division here is variably defined. The ultraviolet spectrum is divided into three regions: A, B and C. The wavelengths limiting these regions are internationally agreed and are those endorsed by the National Radiological Protection Board in the UK (Table 15.1). Some variations are given in other sources. Oxygen and ozone in the stratosphere screen out UVC and much UVB from the sun's radiation.

Radiations of wavelengths between 200 and 100 nm, and sometimes below, are often called 'vacuum UV' because, being rapidly absorbed in air, they can only be effectively passed in a vacuum.

The meaning and derivation of certain terms used in UVR are summarized in Table 15.2.

Table 15.2 The meaning and derivation of certain terms

	Derivation	Meaning
Radiation	Probably from Aton Ra, Egyptian Sun god	Emission of any waves or particles; usually applied to EM spectrum
Heliotherapy	Helios: Greek god of the Sun	Treatment by means of the sun's radiation
Actinic radiation		Radiations that can cause a photochemical reaction, visible, UVR, X-ray and near IR
Actinotherapy	*Aktis* = a ray (Greek)	Treatment with actinic radiations
Phototherapy	*Phos* = light (Greek)	Treatment with UVR and visible radiation
Photobiomodulation		Biological effects of light on tissues

PRODUCTION OF UVR

Incandescent sources, like the sun, can produce UVR if the temperature is high enough. However, it is usually produced by the passage of a current through an ionized vapour – often mercury

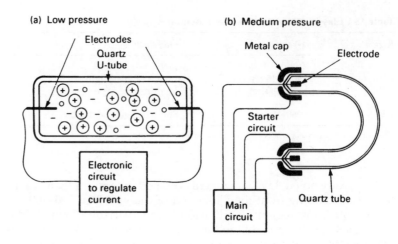

Fig. 15.1 Mercury vapour gas discharge tubes.

vapour. Gases do not conduct current well at normal temperatures and pressures but can be made to do so at low pressure or high temperatures.

Principle of working of a mercury vapour lamp

Applying a voltage across a pair of electrodes sealed into a UV transmitting quartz tube containing a little mercury vapour will cause collisions between electrons and mercury atoms. This causes the formation of free mercury ions and electrons. As these recombine, a steady current flows with electrons being added at one electrode and removed at the other. This process needs a high voltage to start it but will continue with a lower voltage and is regulated by limiting the current that is allowed to pass through the tube. As mains alternating voltage is applied the process reverses 100 times every second (see Fig. 15.1).

When free electrons are being accelerated in the tube, many collisions with neutral mercury vapour atoms will occur:

- by elastic collisions not affecting the atom
- by knocking an electron off the atom – ionization
- by moving an electron to a higher energy level – excitation.

When these excited electrons return to their normal energy level the energy they lose is emitted as a photon of a characteristic wavelength for that particular transition (see Chapter 14). Similarly electrons recombining with ions will give the same effect. The characteristic photon wavelengths given off by mercury atoms are in the green–blue–violet end of the visible spectrum and in the ultraviolet. The line spectrum produced and its intensity may be modified at different lamp pressures and by the addition of traces of metal halides, such as lead iodide. It is also filtered by the quartz or special glass envelope.

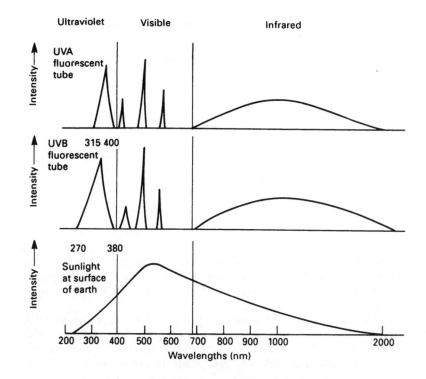

Fig. 15.2. Spectra distribution of UVA and UVB fluorescent lamps and sunlight (not in proportion).

Fluorescent lamps

These are low-pressure mercury discharge tubes with a phosphor coating on the inside. This layer absorbs short UVR, notably the spectral line at 254 nm, which causes excitation of the phosphor atoms and re-emission at a longer wavelength, i.e. fluorescence. The particular wavelengths and the amount of each emitted will depend on the composition of the phosphor used. (These phosphor coatings are actually mixtures of phosphates, borates and silicates.) The output of these lamps also varies with their temperature. Most give an optimal output with the outside of the tube at about 40°C. Such tubes are familiar as standard fluorescent lighting tubes. The tubes used for ultraviolet treatment in physiotherapy are identical in size and shape but have a special phosphor coating in the tube that makes it produce a continuous spectrum between 250–280 nm and 380 nm (with a peak at 313 nm) and lines in the blue and green visible (Fig. 15.2; Diffey, 1982b). This gives a considerable UVA and UVB output but no UVC.

For whole body treatments long fluorescent tubes can be mounted in semi-cylindrical tunnels, bed and canopy arrangements or cylindrical cubicles. Shorter tubes are mounted in other configurations for local treatments. The Theraktin tunnel, consisting of four 120 cm length tubes mounted in a semicircular assembly, which can be raised or lowered over a couch or wheeled into position, has been much used by physiotherapists. However, it gives low irradiance and is inclined to give uneven skin exposure, especially

Table 15.3 Some of the major spectral lines emitted by medium-pressure mercury vapour arc lamps

Wavelength (nm)	Radiation
578	Visible
546	Visible
436	Visible
405	Visible
365	UVA
334	UVA
313	UVB
302	UVB
297	UVB
265	UVC
254	UVC

From Diffey (1982).

at the sides of the trunk. More recently 'narrow band' output fluorescent tubes have been developed whose wavelength is limited to a range of a few nanometres; one is available with a wavelength around 311 nm.

The same type of tube is used to produce large amounts of UVA radiation for use in the treatment of psoriasis in conjunction with a psoralen sensitizer (see below) as PUVA treatment. In these the phosphor coating is different and leads to emission from 315 to 400 nm and several lines in the blue and green visible region (Fig. 15.2). A reflecting layer is applied between the glass envelope and the phosphor layer over more than half the circumference of the tube along its length. This ensures that the radiations are largely directed forwards and when several of these tubes are packed together side by side they provide an approximately uniform emission. A number of tubes (48 in one type) are fixed in the walls of a treatment cabinet in which the patient stands to receive all-round body irradiation.

All these fluorescent lamps emit visible radiation giving a bluish-white light when the tube is operating but it must be realized that the visible emission has no relation to the ultraviolet being emitted. All fluorescent tubes have a slight fall in output during their working lives. This is trivial for fluorescent lighting tubes but the ultraviolet lamps use less stable phosphors so that their useful life is usually limited to about 1000 h. Forced air cooling or air conditioning achieves a more stable output from the lamp and increased patient comfort.

Medium-pressure mercury arc lamp – Alpine sunlamp

This lamp once widely used in physiotherapy departments is in the form of a U-shaped tube (Fig. 15.1(b)). The spectral lines emitted in the UV and visible regions are shown in Table 15.3. By analogy with sunlight they are called 'high-altitude' lamps (*Höhensonne* in German), hence Alpine sunlamp. They operate in the manner described above. As well as the spectral lines noted in Table 15.3, they emit a continuous spectrum of visible and infrared radiations. This precludes placing them close to the skin unless they are cooled.

The U-tube of the Alpine sunlamp is set at the centre of a parabolic reflector made of a special aluminium alloy supported on a strong stand. As a U-tube it acts more like a point source of radiation. The reflector and tube can be easily raised and lowered on the vertical stand because there is a counterweight system and can be adjusted at two pivotal points as well as rotated about the vertical stand to allow it to be suitably positioned. It is usually applied at a distance of 45 or 50 cm.

All mercury vapour lamps contain a small quantity of the inert gas argon to facilitate starting up the lamp and help control electron mobility. It also helps to prolong the life of the metal electrodes.

In order to start up the medium-pressure burner a high voltage is applied to metal caps (Fig. 15.1(b)) fitted outside the quartz envelope by means of a separate step-up autotransformer. Pressing a button on the control panel applies a charge of 400 V or so to the metal caps, causing ionization of the argon atoms. The high charge displaces an outer orbital electron from several argon atoms, leaving them as positive ions. The presence of sufficient free positive ions and electrons allows the flow of a convection current in which positive ions gain electrons from the negative electrode and electrons move to the positive at the (lower) mains voltage. The small quantity of mercury – which is a drop of liquid at normal temperature – is rapidly vaporized due to the heat generated by the passage of current. Mercury atoms of the vapour become ionized, giving the spectral emission described above. This process takes about 5 min.

Short UVR react with oxygen in the air to produce a small quantity of ozone (O_3), which is evident from its smell, even at low concentrations. Ozone is toxic at high concentrations so ventilation should be adequate around these lamps. The time-weighted average threshold limit for exposure to ozone is 0.1 ppm by volume in air (Diffey, 1982b). In some modern lamps the burner envelope is modified so that it does not emit ozone-producing ultraviolet below 270 nm.

The Kromayer lamp

The Kromayer lamp is a medium-pressure mercury vapour ultraviolet lamp designed to be used in contact with the tissues, both on the skin surface and in body cavities. This is achieved by enclosing the emitting tube in a water jacket which cools it and filters out the infrared which would otherwise cause a heat burn, but allowing the visible and ultraviolet to pass. The use of this lamp has become less common.

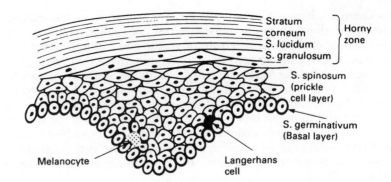

Fig. 15.3 Cross-section of the epidermis.

Summary

UVR for therapy is produced by excitation of mercury atoms in:
- fluorescent tubes – output determined by nature of phosphor coating; various configurations, usually for whole body irradiation in vertical cabinets or horizontal 'beds'
- medium-pressure mercury arc lamps:
  - Alpine sunlamp
  - Kromayer lamp.

Measurement of UVR

The energy transmitted by UVR can be measured to investigate the output of UVR lamps and quantify treatment. Photodiodes are most widely used as they are rugged and relatively cheap. Coupled to a suitable electronic circuit they register the photon emission and with added filters can determine the output of different wavelengths. The measurement is of the power of the radiation or intensity of radiation at a specific point (more properly called the irradiance) measured in watts per square metre or watts per square centimetre. The amount of energy applied is the irradiance (in W/cm^2, say) multiplied by the time of exposure in seconds giving a dose or 'radiant exposure' in joules per square centimetre (J/cm^2) (see Appendix):

Radiant exposure (J/cm^2) =
$$\text{Irradiance } (W/cm^3) \times \text{Time of exposure(s)}$$

NORMAL SKIN – REVIEW OF STRUCTURE AND ACTIVITY

Keratinization

The epidermis is supported on, and receives nutrition from, the vascular dermis which provides a strong flexible base (see Fig. 7.4). It consists of various layers (see Fig. 15.3). The stratum germinativum, or basal layer, is where cell division, or mitosis, continuously takes place, and where keratin is formed.

After mitosis in the basal layer each daughter cell or keratinocyte may:

- grow through the prickle cell layer, lose its nucleus, die and become converted to a piece of flattened keratin; these pieces of keratin are steadily lost from the skin surface, especially when the surface is rubbed or washed
- enter a resting phase, becoming inactive for a time
- proceed to another cycle of mitosis to form two daughter cells.

The time taken from mitosis to mitosis is known as the cell turnover time and is, on average, about 6 days. The average time taken for a cell to pass from the basal layer to be shed as a keratin flake at the surface is called the epidermal transit time and may be about 28 days (Burton, 1979) or longer – 45–70 days. If the transit time remains constant but the rate of mitosis speeds up, i.e. the cell turnover time is decreased, the skin will be thickened. The rate of basal cell division seems to be controlled by a variety of factors, some of which must be local since friction on the surface or the loss of some epithelial surface provokes keratinocyte synthesis, as does UVR.

Keratin itself is formed of folded, cross-linked polypeptide chains; it also forms hair and nails. Keratinized epithelium is pliable while it is wet but becomes harder and more brittle on drying. Trapping moisture in the surface by putting oils or grease on the skin, as described in connection with wax treatment in Chapter 8, will therefore make the epithelium soft and pliable by keeping it moist.

Pigmentation

The pigment melanin is produced by melanocytes in the basal layer of the epidermis. It is formed from the amino acid tyrosine by special organelles, called melanosomes, in the cell. These melanosomes are able to pass along dendritic processes of the melanocytes to enter the neighbouring keratinocytes. In the keratinocytes they cluster over the nucleus forming a protective cap – a sort of umbrella – which absorbs UVR before it can reach the DNA of the nucleus (Fig. 15.4). As the keratinocytes migrate to the surface the melanosomes and their contained melanin disintegrate and are lost with the keratin flakes from the skin surface. In darker skin there are the same number of melanocytes but they produce larger, longer-lasting and more widely dispersed melanosomes.

Melanocyte activity is stimulated by ultraviolet. The mechanism is not fully understood but involves enzymic activity and hormones, melanocyte-stimulating hormone from the pituitary, adreno-corticotrophic hormone and oestrogen. Immediate tanning occurs in some (usually type IV, V or VI, see p. 398) individuals, as a result of effects on pre-existing melanin after exposure to UVA or UVB. This may occur within minutes of exposure. Later tanning

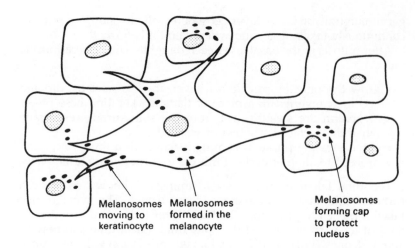

Melanosomes
moving to
keratinocyte

Melanosomes
formed in the
melanocyte

Melanosomes
forming cap
to protect
nucleus

Fig. 15.4 A melanocyte.

occurs following resolution of the erythema, due to increased melanocyte activity, and is commensurate with both the dose of ultraviolet applied and the pigmentation proclivity of the individual.

Sebaceous glands

Sebum is produced in sebaceous glands by the complete breakdown of cells in the gland turning into fatty material which passes via the sebaceous duct to the hair follicles and thence to the skin surface. This 'greasing' of the skin helps waterproofing and is mildly fungicidal. The rate of sebum production is controlled by hormones, being increased by androgens. Sebaceous glands are found with hair follicles all over the body but are particularly large and active on the face, neck, upper chest and back.

Langerhans cells

These cells are scattered in the base of the prickle cell layer. They are similar to connective tissue macrophages and are derived from bone marrow cells. They appear to be involved in cell-mediated immunity and cellular defence mechanism. They are damaged by UVR and it is suggested that this might be a reason for the carcinogenic effects of prolonged overdosage with UVR (Williams *et al.*, 1989).

PHYSIOLOGICAL EFFECTS OF ULTRAVIOLET

The well-known acute effects of the sun, i.e. sunburn, are really the effects of UVB radiations. Under normal physiological conditions it takes huge doses of UVA to provoke any kind of reddening and UVC is not normally found in significant quantities in the sun's radiation reaching the earth's surface. UVR is largely absorbed in the outer layer of the skin so that the direct effects are limited to those on the skin and the eyes. The penetration depth of UVC is approximately 40–50 μm, while 10% of UVB and 40–50% of UVA penetrates to the basal layer. These effects can be considered in two groups: the immediate or acute effects occurring within hours, days or weeks and the long-term chronic effects noted only after years.

The immediate, acute effects of ultraviolet on the skin

An erythema, or reddening, appears some time after the application of the ultraviolet. This is often a matter of hours and is called the latent period. Over some hours the erythema increases and then fades during the subsequent hours or days. Oedema and irritation of the skin are evident if the application of ultraviolet is sufficiently intense, as well as desquamation (peeling) of the superficial epidermis. If the same dose of UVB is repeated after these changes have recovered it provokes a less strong reaction due to the pigmentation (tanning) and skin thickening that occurs. This protective pigmentation and thickening can last 30–40 days and occurs not only as a result of a single erythematous exposure but also after a series of exposures each insufficient to provoke visible reddening (Nonaka *et al.*, 1984), hence called suberythemal doses.

The degree to which these effects occur depends on the amount of UVB energy applied, the radiant exposure, and the reactivity or sensitivity of the skin of the subject. Thus the fair-skinned person will exhibit a more marked reaction than the dark-skinned given the same radiant exposure. These changes are summarized in Table 15.4. During the recovery period after strong applications some itching of the skin may occur.

The erythema due to ultraviolet radiation

The redness of sunburn is familiar and unmistakedly different from that due to heat in that the redness is uniform, not mottled, and there is a sharp distinct edge at the junction with an unexposed area. This indicates that it is capillaries in the dermis that primarily dilate and not the arterioles. Since UVB and C are largely absorbed in the epidermis it is considered that the reaction is due to the release of chemical substances. Histamine substances are invoked especially during the early development as are certain prostaglandins which may be released from epidermal keratinocytes (De Leo *et al.*, 1984) as well as prostacyclin from epidermal cells in the blood vessels of the dermis. Another important cutaneous vasodilator, nitric oxide, has recently been shown to contribute to the maintenance of erythema due to UVB (Leslie, 1994, personal communication). The histamines, kinins and other agents associated with the inflammatory response are released from mast cells and probably other sites in the dermis.

Table 15.4 Description of degrees of erythema

Degree of erythema	Approximate latent period	Appearance	Approximate duration of erythema	Skin oedema	Skin discomfort	Desquamation of skin	Relation to dose causing E_1
E_1	6–12 h	Mildly pink	<24 h	None	None	None	1
E_2	6 h	Definite pink-red Blanches on pressure	2 days	None	Slight soreness, irritation	Powdery	2.5
E_3	3 h	Very red Does not blanch on pressure	3–5 days	Some	Hot and painful	In thin sheets	5
E_4	<2 h	'Angry' red	A week	Blister	Very painful	Thick sheets	10

It has been explained in the past that these chemicals were formed by a long chain of reactions and diffused slowly from the epidermis, which would account for the latent period. However, it has been clearly shown that the latent period is an artefact because the early, very slight erythema cannot be seen by the eye (Diffey and Oakley, 1987). Vasodilation appears to begin very soon after the irradiation is applied.

The erythema appears to differ somewhat depending on the ultraviolet wavelength. This has led to descriptions of an 'action spectrum', that is a graph of wavelength against erythemal effectiveness, e.g. Sayre *et al.* (1966). For discussion of this see Diffey (1982a). It seems probable that, in general, the effectiveness of the radiation in provoking erythema increases with decreasing wavelength, as might be expected, conforming with the energy carried. However, there is evidence that the mechanism producing erythema due to short UVC may be different from that due to longer UVB (Farr and Diffey, 1985).

The erythema due to UVA seems to be rather different in several respects. There is some immediate erythema merging into a much later developing erythema which may last several days. It is considered that UVA may directly affect blood vessels in the dermis. It takes about 1000 times the dose of UVA to give an erythema equivalent to that of UVB.

About 20 mJ/cm^2 of 300 nm UVB are required to produce minimal erythema in a fair-skinned individual.

Pigmentation

Pigmentation of the skin occurs as a result of both the formation of melanin in the deep region of the epidermis and the migration of melanin already formed into more superficial layers. This process takes a little time and is usually noticeable about 2 days after exposure. In already pigmented individuals some immediate tanning may occur within as little as 10 min of exposure, due to darkening of existing melanin by photo-oxidation, it is believed. Pigmentation is strongly stimulated by erythema-producing UVB at about 300 nm and also, to a lesser extent, by longer wavelengths in UVA and even into the visible (Diffey, 1982b). Thus sunbeds which emit UVA and visible radiations are able to induce a tan without the erythema, although an erythema will occur at sufficiently high doses or if the patient has taken a sensitizer (see PUVA later). The increased melanin content of the skin affords protection by preventing UVR reaching the lower layers of the epidermis where the dividing keratinocytes are situated. This protective effect is aided by the skin thickening that also occurs.

Increased skin growth

Stimulation by UVR provokes increased keratinocyte cell turnover so that the skin grows more rapidly for a time, leading to shedding of the most superficial cells at an earlier stage in their development than usual so that they remain in pieces, or even sheets, and can be peeled off. This peeling or desquamation varies with the intensity of applied UVR (see Table 15.4). As the skin recovers the growth continues so that the final result is skin thickening which adds to the protection due to pigmentation. Both these protective effects fade over 4–6 weeks if there is no further ultraviolet application.

Vitamin D production

UVB is able to convert sterols in the skin, such as 7-dehydro-cholesterol to vitamin D (calciferol, cholecalciferol) which, after changes in the liver and kidneys, is able to facilitate the absorption of calcium from the intestine. (Insufficient vitamin D coupled with undernourishment leads to rickets in babies and osteomalacia in adults.) The UVB radiations most effective in producing vitamin D are in the 280 and 300 nm regions. Suberythemal doses of UVB are adequate to promote vitamin D synthesis but otherwise healthy individuals living in higher latitudes may have insufficient vitamin D in winter, as may the bed-bound both in hospital and at home.

Immunosuppressive effects

UVR appears to trigger immunosuppressive effects, both locally and systemically. This probably occurs because UVB destroys Langerhans' cells and stimulates the proliferation of suppressor T cells. When organisms invade the skin, the macrophage-like Langerhans cells gather some of the pathogen and transport it to the lymph nodes, which send out specific killer T cells. Suppressor T cells (lymphocytes) are regulatory in that they inhibit antibody production and suppress the action of other T cells. This immunosuppressive effect is believed to be a protective response to prevent an autoimmune attack on the skin cells that have been altered by UVR. This response is necessary until cell repair has occurred. Both the nature and cause of this response to UVR by the immune system are ill-understood. It is uncertain whether an enzyme released as a consequence of DNA damage in the cell, or some photoreceptor chemical – such as urocanic acid found in the epidermis – is the responsible agent. Immunosuppressive effects may contribute to the development of skin cancer.

The immediate acute effects on the eye

Strong doses of UVB and C radiation to the eyes can lead to conjunctivitis (inflammation of the tissue over the cornea and lining of the eyelids) and to photokeratitis (inflammation of the cornea). This results in irritation of the eye, a feeling of grit in the eye, watering of the eye and aversion to light (photophobia). In severe cases intense pain and spasm of the eyelid may be present. This is also known as 'snow blindness' when it arises due to solar UVB and C reflection from the snow. It can also occur due to reflection from sand and from using welding arcs without eye protection.

The condition usually recovers in about 2 days without permanent damage but the eye, unlike the skin, does not develop tolerance to ultraviolet radiation. In fact the reverse seems to occur in that subsequent applications seem to provoke conjunctivitis more readily, but this may simply be that initial recovery is apparent but not complete for several days longer. Although all UVB and C radiations will produce these effects the most damaging seem to be those of 270 nm.

While UVB and C are absorbed in the cornea, UVA can pass through to be absorbed mainly in the lens of the eye. It has been suggested that strong doses of UVA may be implicated in the formation of cataracts.

Long-term chronic effects of ultraviolet on the skin

Prolonged exposure over many years to strong solar radiation can lead to premature ageing of the skin; this is especially so in the fair-skinned. The skin becomes wrinkled, dry and leathery and there is decreased function of sebaceous and sweat glands with loss of elastic tissue. Such changes are most often seen in those who have spent much of their working lives in strong sunlight, such as farmers, fishermen or other outdoor workers. It is a particular problem in locations where fair-skinned populations have emigrated to sunnier climates, such as Australia, South Africa or Israel. Yaar and Gilchrest (1990) noted that all the cellular manifestations of ageing were more pronounced in photodamaged skin.

Exposure to high levels of UVR over many years also increases the risk of certain skin cancers, basal cell and squamous cell carcinomas. This is evidenced by the fact that these develop on body areas exposed to sunlight, and that the incidence is higher in outdoor workers and fair-skinned people working in places that have much sunshine, as well as from laboratory studies on mice. For a given genetic susceptibility to non-melanoma skin cancer it has been shown that age and annual ultraviolet exposure are the two most important risk factors; in fact the risk is proportional to age^5 times annual dose of UV^2 (Fears *et al.*, 1977). Diffey (1989) states that the occupational risks associated with working with UVR are small provided that good working practices are adopted so that acute erythema develops no more than once or twice a year. Yoshikawa *et al.* (1990) concluded that certain individuals are 'UVB-susceptible', whereas others are 'UVB-resistant', and that this susceptibility may be a risk factor for the development of skin cancer.

> **Summary of physiological effects of UVR**
>
> - Acute effects
>   - on skin
>   - erythema
>   - pigmentation
>   - increased growth
>   - vitamin D production
>   - immunosuppression
>   - on eyes
>   - conjunctivitis
>   - photokeratitis.
> - Chronic effects on skin
>   - ageing
>   - increased risk of certain skin cancers.

THERAPEUTIC USES AND INDICATIONS

The principal therapeutic uses of UVR are for skin diseases.

Psoriasis

Psoriasis is a chronic skin disease of unknown cause affecting 2% of the population. Because it is broadly symmetrical, there is a suggestion that it is a neurogenic disorder of cutaneous nerves. A predisposition to it may be inherited. Chronic discoid psoriasis is the commonest form with thick pink or red plaques, sharply demarcated and covered with silvery scales. There are several other types: guttate, in which small lesions are scattered over the trunk; pustular psoriasis (the pustules are sterile); generalized pustular and erythrodermic psoriasis which are serious medical emergencies, and flexural psoriasis.

The epidermal transit time is reduced to about 5 days so that the keratinocytes do not change in the usual way. They keep their nuclei and tend to stick together forming the plaques. There is also increased mitosis and dilation of the dermal capillaries, which accounts for the redness.

The mechanism by which UVR affects psoriasis is obscure, but must be, at least in part, systemically mediated, since the psoriasis improves following treatment of unaffected skin. Further, areas not directly affected by UVR (e.g. the scalp), also improve. Suggestions to explain the mechanism naturally include the immunosuppressive effect of UVR. The aim is to induce a remission by the inhibition by UVR of DNA synthesis.

The effectiveness of UVR in clearing psoriasis approximates to the erythema action spectrum (the effectiveness of the different

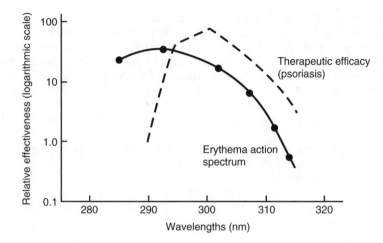

Fig. 15.5 Action spectrum for erythema compared with graph of therapeutic efficacy for psoriasis (After Parrish and Jaenicke, 1981).

wavelengths at causing erythema) (see Fig. 15.5). However, in the UVC wavelengths, while a marked erythema is provoked there is no beneficial effect on psoriasis.

Therapeutic regimens

The Goeckerman regimen. This consists of coal tar applications 2 or 3 times a day with general (total body) UVB radiation given once a day as a suberythemal or E_1 (MED) dose.

The Ingram or Leeds regimen (Ingram, 1954). The patient has a coal tar bath before being irradiated with a minimal erythema dose of UVB; the psoriatic lesions are covered with dithranol (a cytotoxic substance that inhibits DNA synthesis). Next day the dithranol is cleaned off and the process is repeated (Klaber, 1980). Although sensitizers such as coal tars have been considered an essential component of the treatment, controlled studies have shown that UVB is the effective element (e.g. Le Vine *et al.*, 1979).

Acland *et al.* (1995) suggest a wavelength of 311 nm is the most beneficial. The aim is to produce a minimal erythema by using an initial dose of 80% of MED and increasing by 15–20% each time until an erythema occurs.

Thus courses of whole-body UVB treatment are successfully employed for psoriasis, although several regimens involving adjuncts are in use, e.g. fish oil therapy (Gupta *et al.*, 1989).

Photochemotherapy for psoriasis. Psoriasis can be treated with radiations of UVA accompanied by a sensitizer. If a psoralen-type drug is given to the patient some 2 h previously, he or she will become sensitive to UVA radiations which will produce an erythema at lower intensities than normal. The drug 8-methoxy-psoralen is used making the patient highly reactive to UVA once it has been absorbed, for some 6–8 h. Topical applications of psoralen are also used. Irradiation during this time leads to an erythema similar to, but not identical with, that of UVB in that the major erythema arises later and lasts longer and may not reach a peak for 2–4 days.

As the peak of PUVA erythema occurs at 48–72 h, treatment should be given twice a week until clearance. This should be approximately 12–18 exposures (British Photodermatology Group, 1994). The UVA dose, measured in J/cm^2, is initially determined according to skin type and phototesting. While UVA consists of a range of radiations, the peak output of conventional lamps is around 350 nm.

Using a combination of psoralen and UVA gives this treatment its popular name of PUVA. It has been shown to be very successful in controlling the disease.

Long-term use leads to skin damage and there is an increased risk of squamous cell carcinoma and cataract formation. Hence, maintenance therapy is rarely used.

Acne vulgaris

This is a chronic inflammatory condition of the pilosebaceous unit especially affecting the face, chest and back. Mild acne arising at adolescence is so common as to be considered a normal feature. However, the more severe and long-lasting forms are disfiguring and cause serious distress. The sebaceous glands become more active at puberty being stimulated by androgens which, coupled with infection by the acne bacillus (*Propionibacterium acnes*), provokes the formation of blackheads or comedones. These are clumps of keratin, sebum and bacteria which block the follicle. Subsequently an inflammatory response occurs which leads to the familiar papules and pustules.

UVR given in doses such as to cause significant peeling or desquamation – usually E$_2$ – are used. The effects of the ultraviolet are to:

- accelerate skin growth because peeling of the surface will remove the lesions and open the blocked ducts
- produce a non-specific inflammatory reaction to help control infection
- sterilize the skin surface temporarily
- cause some pigmentation which may serve to make the papules less obvious.

Improvement, which can sometimes be dramatic, is temporary but repetitions at intervals of a few months may enable the patient to remain reasonably clear during the worst year or so.

Eczema

Eczema is an inflammatory response in the skin, with associated oedema. The patient suffers marked itching with redness, scaling, vesicles and exudation of serum on the skin. While it may be caused by external agents (contact dermatitis), a large group of patients have atopic eczema. It is often these who can benefit from mild UV treatment.

Chronic infection

Infected open wounds such as pressure sores are sometimes treated with high doses of UVR. The doses given must be such as to kill surface bacteria and therefore an E_4 is used. While the lethal effects of UVC on bacteria, especially the 254 nm peak, have been well known for many years the effect of the usual clinically used doses given with a standard Kromayer lamp have, surprisingly, only been quantified in the last 20 years. Thus High and High (1983) found that the radiation from the Kromayer was universally successful in killing bacteria in vitro and the reduction in colony numbers correlated with the intensity used to the point where E_4 doses totally inhibited colony growth. Similarly Burger *et al.* (1985) cultured swabs from some pressure sores before and after an E_4 ultraviolet dose given with the Kromayer. The result was a dramatic and extensive reduction in bacterial numbers.

These studies support the clinical impression that UVR is an effective, safe and convenient way of controlling surface infection. This may be particularly valuable in circumstances where antibiotics cannot reach the area in adequate proportions, if the infection is resistant to them or if they are contraindicated.

Dodd *et al.* (1989) have shown that skin oxygenation is increased for some 48 h after treatment. However, subsequent return of vasoconstriction lowers the skin oxygen tension for some 2 weeks so that treatment of the normal skin surrounding the wound is not beneficial.

Vitiligo

Vitiligo is a condition in which destruction of melanocytes in local areas causes white patches to appear on the skin. It is not uncommon and is considered to be an autoimmune disease (anti-melanocyte antibodies have been found). For the fair-skinned this disease may be of little consequence except for the need to protect the depigmented patches from excessive sunburn. In the darker-skinned it becomes a serious cosmetic problem which can be treated with topical psoralens and UVR to try to induce repigmentation. In climates with reliable natural sunshine, advice on gradual exposure may be sufficient but in higher latitudes artificial UVR is used to effect pigmentation. Both UVA and B stimulate melanocyte activity but there seem to be some differences. UVA seems to provoke a darker and longer-lasting tan (at least in normal skin) although the protective effects do not seem to be so marked, perhaps because UVB provokes more thickening. It would seem sensible to apply graded doses of either or both UVA and B. The surrounding normally pigmented area should be protected since darkening the contrasting area must be avoided.

Protection for hypersensitive skin

Normal tolerance to increased sunlight develops slowly as the seasons change, increasing over a 6-month period. However, modern air travel allows a complete climatic change over a few hours. The very fair-skinned and those hypersensitive to UVR who need to go to work (or even holiday) out of doors in regions of strong sunshine can have the risk of sunburn much reduced by a course of general UVB (UVA is not satisfactory because although it provokes tanning other features of skin protection do not develop).

Photodermatoses

Polymorphic light eruption is the commonest of these and increased tolerance to sunlight can be achieved by a course of UVB, starting with a very low dose and gradually progressing.

Treatment of vitamin D deficiency

As explained earlier, cholecalciferol (vitamin D_3) is formed in skin by the action of UVB and UVC on 7-dehydrocholesterol. This vitamin is also taken in the diet, notably in animal fat products. It has been understood for many years that exposure to either artificial UVR or, if available, natural sunlight is curative for vitamin D deficiency diseases. The dietary improvement, especially the consumption of fats, in developed countries over the past century has almost, but not quite, eliminated this disease. People moving to countries like the UK with less natural sunlight and retaining customary dietary habits sometimes show vitamin D deficiency. Further, some bed-bound elderly patients, it is thought, may benefit from artificial UVB to maintain vitamin D and calcium levels to counteract senile osteoporosis (Corless *et al.*, 1978).

Treatment for mild hypertension

It has now been shown that general (whole-body) suberythemal doses of UVB can significantly lower blood pressure (Krause *et al.*, 1998). Since this effect occurred with UVB and not with UVA, it was considered to be mediated by calcium regulating hormones associated with increased vitamin D production.

Treatment of pruritus due to biliary cirrhosis or uraemia

The intractable and serious itching that can occur due to raised bile acid level can be successfully treated by suberythemal whole-body

UVB either alone or in combination with the drug cholestyramine (Cerio and Low, 1987; Cerio *et al.*, 1987). Pruritus due to uraemia in patients with chronic renal failure has also been successfully treated by suberythemal UVB (Gilchrist *et al.*, 1977). In this study some patients were also treated with UVA at somewhat higher doses but with little effect; UVB appears to be the effective radiation. It has been suggested (Diffey, 1982b) that this useful effect of UVB may be worth trying in other situations where pruritus is a significant problem.

Psychological benefit

Considerable psychological benefit has been claimed as an effect of UVR (Scott, 1983) on the grounds that patients expect to feel better and the consequent tanning makes them look better. (Such an effect is certainly exploited by the makers of sunbeds.)

Summary of therapeutic uses of UVR

- Psoriasis – treatment regimens include
  - Goeckerman
  - Ingram
  - photochemotherapy using UVA – PUVA.
- Acne.
- Eczema.
- Chronically infected open areas.
- Vitiligo.
- Protection for hypersensitive skin
  - photodermatoses.
- Vitamin D deficiency
  - mild hypertension.
- Pruritus
  - biliary cirrhosis
  - uraemia.

DOSAGE

The skin response to UVR depends on:

- the quantity of ultraviolet energy applied to unit area of the skin
- the biological responsiveness (sensitivity) of the skin to which it is applied.

The first can be measured, or at least controlled to keep it constant, but the second can only be adequately assessed by trial applications of ultraviolet.

The quantity of energy

Typically about $20\,mJ/cm^2$ of UVB at a wavelength of 300 nm will produce minimal erythema on the moderately fair-skinned (Diffey, 1982b; Nonaka *et al.*, 1984). The response of skin alters very dramatically with wavelength, for example, at 300 nm the skin is 100 times more sensitive than at 320 nm (Diffey, 1994) (see Fig. 15.5). The amount of energy – the radiant response – depends on the:

- output of the lamp
- distance between the lamp and the skin
- angle at which radiations fall on the skin
- time for which radiations are applied.

This last factor is used to regulate dosage, for if the intensity falling on the skin is constant then the effects are directly proportional to the time of exposure. This is in accordance with the Bunsen–Roscoe reciprocity law which states that the same photochemical effect will occur if the product of the intensity and time are constant; thus low intensity for a long time can produce the same effect as high intensity for a short time.

The output of the lamp

The output of the source includes the:

- nature of the radiations, i.e. the principal wavelengths emitted
- intensity.

Even lamps of the same make and type are likely to have slightly different outputs due to ageing and other effects. It is, therefore, necessary to use the same source throughout a course of treatment.

The distance from the skin

The distance between the source of ultraviolet and the skin is critical. It is usual to calculate the effect by presuming that the ultraviolet is emitted from a point source so that the inverse square law can be used to calculate the relationship of intensity and distance when using lamps with small burners and large parabolic reflectors (see Chapter 11). Thus if the distance is doubled the intensity would be reduced to one-quarter, so, to achieve an equivalent effect, the time of application must be four times the original. For example if the desired effect was achieved in 1 min at a distance of 50 cm, the time needed at a distance of 100 cm would be four times that (4 min). The dose or effect depends on the intensity of the irradiation and the time for which it is given, as noted above.

$$\text{Effect} = \text{I}t$$

From the inverse square law:

$$I \propto \frac{1}{d^2}$$

So:

$$\text{Effect} = \frac{t}{d^2}$$

If the same effect is required, but either time or distance is altered:

$$\frac{t_1}{d_1^2} = \frac{t_2}{d_2^2}$$

For example, if an E_2 is produced in 60 s at 50 cm, at 10 cm it is produced in 2.4 s:

$$\frac{60}{50 \times 50} = \frac{t_2}{10 \times 10}$$

Since ultraviolet emitters are hardly a point source and are backed by a reflector it may be wondered why the inverse square law can be used. There are, of course, losses other than the spreading out of radiations due to absorption and scattering in air. These are approximately compensated by the reflector so that the inverse square law can be used as a satisfactory rule of thumb. It has been established for the Alpine sunlamp that at distances between 50 and 150 cm the intensity conforms with that predicted by the law (Goats, 1988). At distances less than 50 cm the intensity is apparently a little less than that predicted.

The angle at which the radiations fall on the skin

The effective intensity of radiation on the skin depends on the cosine of the angle of incidence of the radiation (see Chapter 11). Thus the lamp is normally applied at or near a right angle to the skin to achieve maximum and consistent effects. It follows that the intensity of radiation will 'fall off' around the curved body surfaces (see Chapter 11).

The biological response

The severity of the response to UVR depends on the nature of the skin to which it has been applied. Physiotherapists and dermatologists often classify patients by skin, eye and (natural!) hair colour as well as the patients' own account of how easily they burn in the sun. A system based on the burning and tanning history given by patients with observation of their pigmentation has been described (Wolff *et al.*, 1977) and is widely used for broad classification:

Type I: always burn, never tan.
Type II: always burn, tan slightly.
Type III: sometimes burn, always tan.
Type IV: never burn, always tan.
Type V: pigmented skin – mongoloid.
Type VI: heavily pigmented skin – negroid.

Coarse distinctions between light- and dark-skinned and their differing tolerance to UVR are fairly easily made. The amount of melanin in the skin contributes to both skin colour and protection against ultraviolet so it is hardly surprising to find that there is a strong correlation (Olson et al., 1973; Shono *et al.*, 1985). However, the response to UVR is so variable that it has proved extremely difficult to make accurate predictions of the response. Sayre *et al.* (1966), for example, were unable to find significant relationships between the energy needed to produce erythema and the colouring of the subject. There seems to be very little evidence concerning the reliability of these judgements of sensitivity of skin to ultraviolet. One of us (JL) ranked two small groups of 8 and 5 subjects for estimated response to UVR and subsequently ranked the ultraviolet dose for each subject needed to produce a minimal erythema. The rankings for each group were compared using the Spearman ranked correlation coefficient (Croucher and Oliver, 1979) resulting in correlations of 0.786 and 0.9 respectively ($p > 0.05$), indicating good but not perfect agreement. Recent previous exposure to UVR, by increasing skin thickness and pigmentation, will alter the biological response for any individual, raising the MED time. Avoidance of UVR will have the reverse effect (tanning due to UVA is not fully protective against UVB radiation).

Summary of factors that determine the skin response to UVR

- Quantity of UV energy applied to unit area of skin which depends on the:
  - output of the UV source
  - distance of the source from the skin
  - angle at which radiations fall on skin
  - time for which radiations are applied.
- Biological response of the skin which depends on:
  - genetic nature of the skin
  - recent history of exposure to UVR.

Assessing the response to UVR

The features used to assess the acute response to UVR include:

- the duration of the latent period in hours

- the intensity of erythema – how red it is
- the duration of the erythema in hours or days
- the severity of any irritation
- the presence of oedema or blistering
- the extent and type of desquamation.

Subjective judgement is used to grade the skin reaction. Typical descriptions are shown in Table 15.4 together with the recognized relationships.

The following are all equivalent terms:

- MED, minimal erythemal dose – widely used.
- E_1, first-degree erythema.
- MPD, minimal perceptible dose or minimal phototoxic dose.
- MPE, minimal perceptible erythema.

This last term (MPE) would seem to be the most accurate since it appears that the latent period is an artefact as changes occur when ultraviolet is applied but are undetected by the eye (Diffey and Oakley, 1987).

It will be noticed that the relationship between the erythema doses – E_1, E_2, E_3, E_4 – has an approximately log/linear relation with the duration of erythema (Low, 1986); see Table 15.4. There is a similar relationship between these doses and the latent periods shown by measurement of the actual erythema intensity by light reflectance spectrophotometry (Farr and Diffey, 1984).

It is most important to understand that the terms 'first-degree erythema' (E_1) and 'minimal erythemal dose (MED)' refer to the *response* used to define a dose. The terms are also used to indicate the dose. This customary practice is followed here but it must be realized that these terms refer to the individual *patient*. Thus referring to 'the E_1 of the lamp' is meaningless. What is being indicated is the likely erythemal response on, say, average caucasian skin at a given distance after a specified time of irradiation.

Test doses

The only way to assess the effect on any given individual is by a test. This is either applied to find the E_1 or MED response or to find the appropriate erythema for the dose to be given. An estimate is made of the time needed to produce the erythema at the intended distance with a given lamp by assessing the likely skin response based on skin colour, eye colour etc., as considered above. Some knowledge of the effect of the lamp on average skin is also needed (see below). For the Alpine sunlamp this is about 30–90 s at 50 cm from the burner and for a typical Theraktin about 4–5 min at 50 cm.

Three (or five) holes of at least $2 \, cm^2$ are cut in a piece of lint, paper or other suitable material. The test dose area (see below) is cleaned to remove surface grease and the template fixed to it securely. The rest of the patient is screened and thus protected from the UVR by suitable material; ultraviolet goggles are worn. Robson and Diffey (1990) suggested that tightly woven fabrics offered the

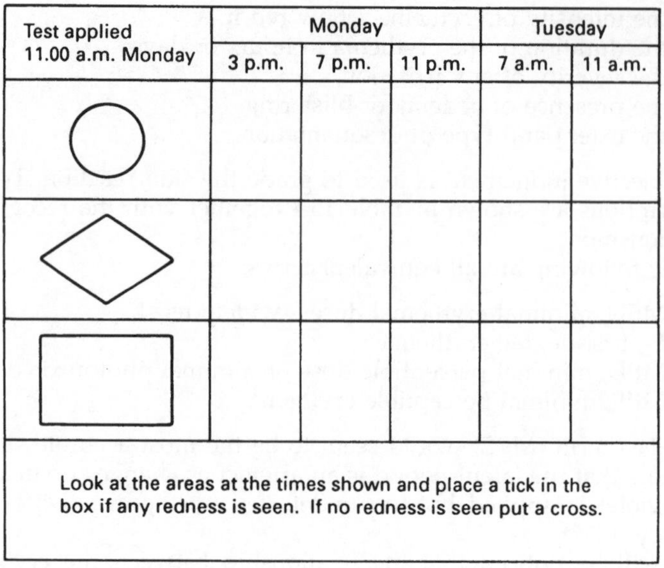

Test applied 11.00 a.m. Monday	Monday			Tuesday	
	3 p.m.	7 p.m.	11 p.m.	7 a.m.	11 a.m.
◯					
◇					
▭					

Look at the areas at the times shown and place a tick in the box if any redness is seen. If no redness is seen put a cross.

Fig. 15.6 An example of a card given to a patient to record the result of a UVR test dose.

best protection. Wood and Reed (1990) investigated the UVR that was transmitted through various thicknesses of commonly used screening material. One type of paper allowed 10% of the UVR output to be transmitted through one thickness. A single thickness of lint allowed 13% of the UVR to be transmitted, increasing to 23% when the lint was wet.

The central hole is exposed to the estimated 'best-guess' dose and the holes on each side to a greater and lesser dose. Some suggest as much as 50% larger and smaller respectively or with the use of five holes, doses 33 and 66% above and below the best estimate. Obviously greater confidence in the estimate would encourage the use of smaller differences. It is sensible to cut the holes as different sizes and shapes (Fig. 15.6) in order to make identification of the erythema easier for the patient. The smallest should not however be less than 1 cm^2 because more ultraviolet energy has been found to be needed (Olson *et al.*, 1965). It is suggested that this effect is simply due to the thickness of the shield material (Low, 1986). It is best if the test is conducted at the same distance as that to be used for treatment.

After exposure to the UVR the patient is given a card similar to Figure 15.6 (which may be the shield itself) and instructed to report the presence or absence of erythema. It is probably best to ask only for the recognition of erythema and not trouble the patient with judgement of intensity. The 24-h reading – the key one – can often be read by the physiotherapist if the patient returns for treatment at the same time on the next day. From this information the E_1 or other dose can be deduced. By definition the E_1 or minimal erythemal dose is the shape that appeared last and disappeared first, i.e. the least visible response.

The area chosen for this test is of importance. If the patient is to inspect the part at regular intervals a convenient, visible site is essential. It should be clear of skin disease and not significantly more pigmented than the area to be treated. The anterior (flexor) surface of the forearm is the most usual but the abdomen, medial aspect of the arm or thigh are also possible sites that are not usually excessively exposed to natural sunlight. The skin of the limbs is more variable in its response than that of the trunk but the difference is small (Olson *et al.*, 1966). A thorough explanation of the test and its purpose should be given to the patient, including the warning that two or three red marks will probably be visible for a day and for those who tan readily a slight pigmented mark could be left for a week or so.

Another purpose of a test dose is to determine the output of a lamp in terms of time required at a given distance for a specified erythema reaction on average skin. This is necessary for new lamps or if the output has been altered. Three staff members volunteer for the test – preferably one of average sensitivity, one slightly more sensitive (but not hypersensitive) and one slightly less so. A test dose is given to each subject in turn, as described above, and the average result determined. As already discussed, an E_1 is the minimum visible response and E_2 and E_3 responses can be judged by reference to Table 15.4.

Sensitization

Sensitization of the patient can occur with a variety of drugs, both ingested and applied topically. Testing the response would take account of this effect but care needs to be exercised if a patient's drug regimen has been altered during a course of ultraviolet treatments.

So many chemicals can act as sensitizers to ultraviolet in varying degrees that a comprehensive list would be prohibitively long. Commonly encountered groups can be:

- psoralens – used as sensitizers
- sulphonamides – antibiotics
- tetracyclines – antibiotics
- griseofulvin – antifungal agent
- phenothiazine – tranquillizer
- chlorthiazide – diuretic
- hypnotic drugs (such as Veronal)
- barbiturates
- gold therapy
- various hormones
- aspirin and derivatives.

Also substances applied to the surface:

- coal tar
- dithranol
- psoralens
- eosin.

(See Wadsworth and Chanmugan, 1980; Griffin and Karselis, 1988 for more extensive lists.)

It has also been found that neurological defect (hemiplegia) may lower the E_1 in the affected region (Cox and Williams, 1985). These writers found a mean reduction of about 16% in the MEDs of 7 of 10 patients on their hemiplegic sides. They suggested this might be due to altered vasomotor control, reduced skin thickening, or both, consequent upon the neurological defect. This has important implications for the application of UVR to such patients.

Progression of ultraviolet dosage

Even the smallest dose of ultraviolet which has no evident immediate effect causes a change in the skin due to pigmentation, allowing greater tolerance of ultraviolet. Thus, if the same erythemal effect is to be achieved repeatedly the dose must be increased to compensate each time. Table 15.5 provides guidance but it must be understood that the increased dose needed is dependent on the pigmentation and thickening, so that patients who pigment easily will need the full increase whereas those who do not will need less.

Table 15.5 Increased dose of UVR to compensate for increased tolerance

Original dose	Earliest time at which the dose can be repeated	Increase (%)
Suberythemal E_0	24 h	12.5
MED E_1	2 days	25
E_2	3–4 days	50
E_3	1 week	75

MED = minimal erythemal dose.

Advice on the increases used to repeat suberythemal doses varies; 10, 12.5 and 15% of the E_1 have all been suggested. This probably reflects different perceptions of what proportion the suberythemal dose is with respect to the E_1; half, five-eighths, three-quarters and just less than an E_1 have all been suggested. Two-thirds is perhaps reasonable.

The earliest time given in Table 15.5 is somewhat more conservative than suggested elsewhere, e.g. Wadsworth and Chanmugan (1980). The essential point is that the erythema should have faded completely before a further dose of ultraviolet is given. There is no reason for applying an E_4 dose on skin.

Proportion of body surface irradiated

As ultraviolet provokes an inflammatory reaction in the skin heavy doses involving large areas can cause systemic illness. The usual guidelines for maximum proportion of body surface to be irradiated with UVR are:

- suberythemal or E_1 – whole body
- E_2 – 20%
- E_3 – 4% (about 600 cm^2).

On open wounds larger areas may be safely treated.

PRINCIPLES OF APPLICATION

General UVB application

Theraktin lamps have been traditionally used in physiotherapy departments and are still widely found. They are being replaced gradually with lamps giving more efficient radiation of UVB.

Preparation of patient. A test dose having been completed, the nature and effects of the treatment are explained.

Preparation of apparatus. A suitable plinth is usually kept in position so that the Theraktin tunnel can be placed in a standard position with the tubes about 50 cm (this varies with the model) from the surface of the average patient lying on the plinth.

Setting up. The patient undresses completely, puts on protective ultraviolet goggles and lies down on the plinth with arms and legs straight and a little abducted. It is important not to allow the limbs to shade one another or the trunk. The head and feet protrude from the tunnel and thus receive a somewhat lower dose. The tunnel is then lowered and the correct distance from patient to tubes is measured. The position of the patient with respect to the tunnel must be repeatable from one treatment to the next. If the patient starts in prone lying with the palms facing upwards the position of the head must be made comfortable, often turned to one side.

Instructions and warnings. The patient is warned to keep still and not to touch the tunnel or lamps.

Application. The lamp is switched on for the appropriate time for the required dose. After this time the lamp is switched off and the patient turns over, this time with the palms facing downwards and the head turned to the same side, to give an equivalent dose to the opposite side of the face. The lamps are again switched on for the required time and then off, and the treatment is completed.

Table 15.6 Regression of general UVB treatments

If no treatments have been given for:	Dose
Up to 4 days	Usual progression
5–7 days	Repeat previous dose
8–13 days	Use the dose given at 4 treatments before this one
14–20 days	Use the dose given at 8 treatments before this one
21–27 days	Use the dose given at 12 treatments before this one
28 days or more	Use the original dose

Practical point

If desired, a suitable cloth can be used to cover the genitalia and removed by the patient as treatment begins. Wearing underwear is inefficient since it is best to expose as large an area of skin as possible. If it is considered desirable for the patient to wear a pair of briefs they must be the same pair at each treatment, otherwise a previously untreated region of skin becomes exposed late in the course so that the patient suffers perhaps an E_2 in a very inconvenient site!

Progression.   Treatment may be given each day for an E_0 for the whole body, or half the body (i.e. one side only) daily with an E_1, or the whole body with an E_1 on alternate days. At each treatment the dose is increased by prolonging the time of treatment. Increasing by exactly 12.5% (one-eighth) at each treatment to repeat a suberythemal dose would be absurdly pedantic; it is sensible to increase to convenient fractions of a minute.

If an erythema occurs after treatment the dose has obviously been greater than suberythemal and should be reduced. If it is a mild erythema not progressing the dose is usually adequate. If for any reason the regular treatments are missed for a time some of the protective pigmentation and thickening is lost and a difficult judgement must be made about the appropriate dose to use. It is best to presume all protective effect is lost over 4 weeks. Table 15.6 offers suggested guidance only, as people vary widely in their response.

It is evident that progression cannot be continued indefinitely since the protective changes will reach their maximum at some stage. Protection has been achieved such that the E_1 (or MED) is many times the original E_1 but most UVB treatment regimens are given to raise the E_1 to between 3 and 5 times the original. The extent to which the dose can be progressed will depend primarily on the skin type, which is genetically determined. As any possible carcinogenic effects are dependent on age and annual ultraviolet exposure (see above) and since the only reasonable measure of exposure is the MED or E_1 (Diffey, 1989), it seems sensible to limit the progression of treatment in terms of multiples of the E_1 rather than an arbitrary length of course in weeks or a maximum dosage in minutes: 4-week courses and 20-min maximum applications have been recommended by some.

PUVA treatment

The use of psoralens to sensitize patients to UVA, principally for the treatment of psoriasis, was described above. It is also used for some other conditions, such as atopic eczema, vitiligo and prophylactically for polymorphic light eruptions (British

Photodermatology Group, 1994). Some PUVA units are like the Theraktin tunnel – the patient is treated lying; others are in vertical cabinets in which the patient stands. Patients are given 8-methoxypsoralen by mouth and exposed to the UVA some 2–3 h later. They are given grey or green glasses to wear while sensitized, i.e. from the time of taking the tablets until 8 h afterwards. They are also warned not to expose themselves to the sun for at least 8 h from ingestion (Fusco *et al.*, 1980).

If there is only a small area of psoriasis or a resistant area, a topical preparation of 8-methoxypsoralen can be applied. The concentration of the drug in the skin is much higher than that with tablets so the dose of UVA is much lower (Klaber, 1980).

A test dose is usually given to determine the patient's sensitivity and subsequently a whole-body dose of UVA is applied. This can either be sufficient to produce a mild erythema at about 3 days (the erythema due to UVA appears much later than that due to UVB) or suberythemal. Treatment may be given twice a week, progressively increasing the dose at weekly intervals for several weeks. The UVA dosage is measured in J/cm^2 and increases of $0.5–1 J/cm^2$ are a usual progression. The principle of basing the dosage on the response of the patient and progressing the dose is the same as for UVB, the difference being that the response to UVA is slower than to UVB.

After 2 or 3 weeks of PUVA treatment marked pigmentation can develop. UVA stimulates the production of melanin, but the melanosomes are not transferred to the more superficial layers of the epidermis, as with UVB. This, plus the fact that UVA does not result in a thicker stratum corneum, explains why exposure to UVA results in minimum or no protection against UVB (Black *et al.*, 1985; Stewart, 1987). It is important for physiotherapists to recognize this since patients who are deeply tanned by PUVA or from commercial sunbeds may not be as well protected as their colour might suggest.

There are some undesirable effects resulting from prolonged UVA treatment, notably skin changes similar to ageing of the skin after high doses, which recover after treatment is completed. UVA radiation is also carcinogenic to some extent, so it is recommended that the number of treatments be limited. There is also the possibility of inducing cataracts, which are associated with high doses.

The comparative benefits of UVB and PUVA have been investigated in a number of studies, e.g. Kenicer *et al.* (1981). It seems that UVB and low-dose PUVA are successful and very similar in their effect on psoriasis and that high-dose PUVA is best used on selected patients who have not improved with UVB or low-dose PUVA. Van Weelden *et al.* (1980) suggest that UVB is not only as good as UVA but safer and more economical.

Some regimens for both UVB and PUVA continue as maintenance, that is a moderate dose applied at weekly, fortnightly or monthly intervals in an attempt to prevent the recurrence of psoriasis. The value of this method is difficult to quantify and now most feel that treatment should not be prolonged unless there is good evidence that cessation leads to further development of psoriasis.

Local UVB application with an air-cooled Alpine sunlamp

The majority of treatments with the Alpine sunlamp will be local – treating a defined area rather than general treatment of the whole body – although the lamp can be used for whole-body treatment using a sectional technique.

Preparation of patient. The nature of the treatment and especially the skin reaction should be fully explained to the patient as well as the necessity of keeping as still as possible during setting up and application of treatment. The patient, and in particular the part to be treated, is conveniently and comfortably positioned and supported. The dosage will have been determined by doing a test, as already described.

Preparation of apparatus. The lamp must be switched on some 5 min before it is to be used to allow the UV output to become stabilized. During this time it must be positioned so as to avoid irradiating patient or therapist.

Preparation of the part to be treated. The part to be treated is exposed and cleaned to remove surface grease, either by washing or by using alcohol wipes. It is important not to irradiate more than the maximum skin surface for a given dose, as described above.

All areas of the patient that could be exposed to radiation when the lamp is positioned and that are not to be treated are protected with clothing or suitable screening material (see above).

Setting up. The part to be treated is then covered with a separate sheet of sufficient thickness and the lamp is positioned so that radiation will strike the area at right angles and irradiate the whole area intended for treatment. The distance between the burner of the lamp and the skin is carefully measured; the usual distance is 50 cm. This is more safely measured, from the physiotherapist's point of view, either from the rim of the reflector to the central point of the area to be treated or using a measuring stick. In these cases the distances measured will be 45 and 40 cm respectively (Fig. 15.7). It is critically important to record this correctly and without ambiguity as an accidental reduction in distance between test dose and treatment or between subsequent treatments could lead to a much greater dose than intended (see the inverse square law; Chapter 11).

Application and termination. Accurate and precise timing of irradiation is also essential. After irradiation is completed the part is either immediately rescreened or the lamp switched off if not required further.

Progression. If the part is to be treated several times the dose will need to be increased (see Table 15.5). It is important that the

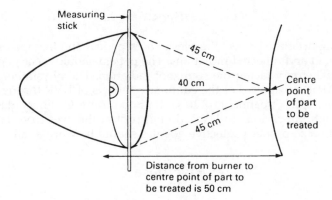

Measuring stick

45 cm

40 cm

Centre point of part to be treated

45 cm

Distance from burner to centre point of part to be treated is 50 cm

Fig. 15.7 Measuring distances from the Alpine sunlamp.

same area is treated on each occasion since the application of the higher dose to previously unexposed skin will lead to an excessive reaction. This problem is solved in many situations due to the curved shape of the body. Radiations applied to the whole surface of a limb or the rounded back will gradually reduce in intensity around the curve (see cosine law and Fig. 11.4, Chapter 11). Thus there is no sharp demarcation with untreated skin and small changes of position of the lamp will have little effect.

Records of UVR treatment

It is important to keep adequate records of all treatments but for ultraviolet treatments the information must be particularly precise and complete both for safety and in order to give adequate treatment. For all ultraviolet treatments the following should always be recorded:

- *date* – it is essential to know the exact date of a given treatment for calculating progression etc.
- *lamp* used – the particular lamp should be clearly identified
- *distance* at which treatment is applied; this must be unequivocal
- exact *area treated* – and precisely where and how untreated regions were screened; the position of the patient should be noted in the case of the Theraktin
- *time* for which the treatment was applied
- *reaction* obtained; this should be recorded at the subsequent attendance.

Other information may also be needed, such as any change in the condition (the size of the ulcer, perhaps, or the condition of the psoriatic patches etc.).

DANGERS

Since the results of ultraviolet treatment are not immediately evident, as there is no sensation and visible erythema appears only later, mistakes can easily occur.

Practical point
In flat areas such as the upper back, it is possible to produce the same gradual shading effect by moving the screening slightly during treatment; thus after, say, a quarter of the treatment time the cover is rolled down 2 or 3 cm; after half the time a further 3 cm; after three-quarters of the time it is completely removed. The result is a gradual change over the area of skin at the edge of the treatment area which is both safer for subsequent treatments and cosmetically more acceptable. The alternative is to screen the skin to the same exact line each time, which of necessity has to be a fixed point. This becomes easier if the line is subsequently marked by pigmentation.

Eyes

It is important to protect the eyes of both patient and therapist from scattered and reflected radiations. The patient should wear goggles even when not facing the source of radiation. The physiotherapist should also be aware of the cumulative effects of UVR throughout the day, e.g. six treatments of 10 s = 1 min exposure. Ordinary glasses, although impervious to UVR, do not protect the eyes from lateral radiation so proper protective goggles should be worn at all times.

Overdose

- *Too long an exposure*. It is essential to use an accurate timing device and for periods over about 1 min to have a timer with an audible warning.
- *Too close to the lamp*. This will occur either because of inaccurate measurement or because the patient moves. Patients have been known to move closer to the lamp in the hope of receiving more effective treatment. A failure of the therapist to recognize the implications of the inverse square law is possibly the most frequent cause of excessive exposure when positioning the lamp, e.g. if an E_1 at 50 cm is 2 min, at 10 cm, just beyond the rim of the reflector, an E_1 is obtained in under 5 s.
- *Previously protected skin* being irradiated at subsequent treatments. This can be caused by alterations in screening, different clothes, a haircut or even removal of a watch strap.
- *Sensitizers*, e.g. change of drugs.
- *Change of lamp*.

Ozone

Because ozone is formed it is important to ensure adequate ventilation in the area.

CONTRAINDICATIONS

- acute skin conditions – acute eczema, dermatitis and an existing ultraviolet erythema.
- skin damage due to ionizing radiations – deep X-ray therapy.
- systemic lupus erythematosus can be triggered or exacerbated.
- photoallergy – allergic reaction to UVR.
- acute febrile illness – whole-body treatment should be avoided.
- recent skin grafts.

HELIOTHERAPY

Heliotherapy is treatment by natural sunlight and has been used since Greek and Roman times. Early in this century heliotherapy was widely used for the treatment of tuberculosis.

A more recent form of heliotherapy involves the treatment of psoriasis at the Dead Sea in Israel. It is considered that the lower UVB spectrum of the sun in this region, which is well below sea level, may allow patients to receive more ultraviolet without burning; that is, the spectrum contains relatively more UVA. Some local minerals are also considered to contribute. There are claims that this is a highly effective treatment for psoriasis.

It is well known that sunburn – due to solar UVB – is only likely to occur in the summer in temperate zones. The UVB component of solar radiation is particularly dependent on the angle of the sun to the surface of the earth, thus although visible and UVA radiations increase in summer, the UVB increases proportionally much more. In fact the UVB is about 100 times more intense in summer than in winter (Diffey, 1982b). This large change occurs very slowly and it is reasonable to presume that human skin is biologically adapted to adjust to slow change.

SUNBEDS

The use of UVA-emitting sunbeds for cosmetic tanning has increased enormously in the past few years. Such sunbeds are of various types but are usually panels containing a number of fluorescent tubes giving UVA and visible radiations. An individual may lie under, and sometimes on, such a panel of tubes and it is claimed that pigmentation without erythema will occur: 'tanning without burning'. Those who already have some pigmentation tend to pigment further but for others the effect may not be marked (Rivers *et al.*, 1989). It is also important to be aware that the pigmentation induced is not a very efficient protection against later applications of UVB from the sun. There have also been found to be a high level of acute temporary adverse effects – like irritation – as well as some possibly serious disturbances of the cell-mediated immunity system of the skin (Hawk, 1983; Rivers *et al.*, 1989).

IONOZONE THERAPY

This involves the production of ionized water vapour. The steam is produced by heating water in a tank in the body of the machine. It is passed over an ultraviolet lamp and emitted as ionized water with some ozone and oxygen. This gentle jet is applied to open wounds such as ulcers and pressure sores, and to the upper respiratory tract.

The effects are said to include a sedatory effect on nerve endings which leads to pain relief; increased blood flow affecting metabolic processes of the skin; and a bacteriocidal effect (Dolphin and Walker, 1979).

Application

Once the distilled water has been heated sufficiently to produce vapour from the nozzle of the machine the ultraviolet is turned on (it is not emitted from the machine). The nozzle is directed at the wound from a distance of 35–50 cm. The surrounding skin is protected with plastic sheeting to prevent it becoming wet. Treatment is given for 10–30 min once a day or less if the wound is clean. The moisture which accumulates in the wound should be removed before a dressing is applied.

The application should not be too close to the patient in case the surrounding skin is heat-damaged.

No controlled trials seem to have been published but a survey of 200 patients treated by this modality found that 168 had their lesions completely healed (Dolphin and Walker, 1979).

REFERENCES

Acland K. M., Leslie T. A., Dowd P. M. (1995). The use of ultraviolet in the management of psoriasis. *Br. J. Therapy Rehabil.*, **2**, 426–9.

Black G., Matzinger E., Gange R. W. (1985). Lack of photoprotection against UVB-induced erythema by immediate pigmentation induced by 382 nm radiation. *J. Invest. Dermatol.*, **85**, 448–9.

British Photodermatology Group. (1994). Guidelines for PUVA. *Br. J. Dermatol.*, **130**, 240–55.

Burger A., Jordaad M. J., Schombee G. E. (1985). The bacteriocidal effect of ultraviolet light on infected pressure sores. *South Afr. J. Physiother.*, **41**, 55–7.

Burton J. L. (1979). *Essentials of Dermatology.* Churchill Livingstone.

Cerio R., Low J. L. (1987). Successful treatment by general ultraviolet radiation of pruritus due to biliary cirrhosis. *Physiotherapy*, **73**, 89.

Cerio R., Murphy G. M., Sladen G. E., MacDonald D. M. (1987). A combination of phototherapy and cholestyramine for the relief of pruritus in primary biliary cirrhosis. *Br. J. Dermatol.*, **116**, 267–8.

Corless D., Gupta S., Switala S. (1978). Response of plasma 25-hydroxyvitamin D to ultraviolet irradiation in long-stay geriatric patients. *Lancet*, **ii**, 649–51.

Cox N. H., Williams S. J. (1985). Lowered ultraviolet minimal erythema dose in hemiplegia. *Postgrad. Med. J.*, **61**, 575–7.

Croucher J. S., Oliver E. (1979). *Statistics: an Introduction.* Australia: McGraw-Hill.

De Leo V. A., Horlick H., Hanson H. *et al.* (1984). Ultraviolet radiation induces changes in membrane metabolism of human keratinocytes in culture. *J. Invest. Dermatol.*, **83**, 323–6.

Diffey B. L. (1982a). The consistency of studies of ultraviolet erythema in normal human skin. *Phys. Med. Biol.*, **27**, 715–20.

Diffey B. L. (1982b). *Ultraviolet Radiation in Medicine.* Medical physics handbooks 11. Bristol: Adam Hilger.

Diffey B. L. (1989). Ultraviolet radiation and skin cancer. *Physiotherapy*, **75**, 615–16.

Diffey B. L. (1994).The physics of ultraviolet phototherapy. The Chartered Society of Physiotherapy and the Institute of Physical Sciences in Medicine; *Electrotherapy: A Multi-disciplinary Conference.* Manchester, 12–13 April 1994.

Diffey B. L., Oakley A. M. (1987). The onset of ultraviolet erythema. *Br. J. Dermatol.*, **116**, 183–7.

Diffey B., Oliver R. (1981). An ultraviolet radiation monitor for routine use in physiotherapy. *Physiotherapy*, **67**, 64–6.

Dodd H. J., Sarkany I., Gaylarde P. M. (1989). Short term benefit and long term failure of ultraviolet light in the treatment of venous leg ulcers. *Br. J. Dermatol.*, **120**, 809–18.

Dolphin S., Walker M. (1979). Healing accelerated by ionozone therapy. *Physiotherapy*, **65**, 81–2.

English J. (1965). Recent advances in ultraviolet irradiation: photosensitivity tests. *Physiotherapy*, **51**, 156–8.

Evans P. (1980). The healing process at cellular level: a review. *Physiotherapy*, **66**, 256–9.

Farr P. M., Diffey B. L. (1984). Quantitative studies on cutaneous erythema induced by ultraviolet radiation. *Br. J. Dermatol.*, **111**, 673–82.

Farr P. M., Diffey B. L. (1985). The erythemal response of human skin to ultraviolet radiation. *Br. J. Dermatol.*, **113**, 65–76.

Fears T. R., Scotto J., Schneiderman M. A. (1977). Mathematical models of age and ultraviolet effects on the incidence of skin cancer among whites in the United States. *Am. J. Dermatol.*, **114**, 479–84.

Forster A., Palastanga N. (1985). *Clayton's Electrotherapy: Theory and Practice.* Eastbourne: Baillière Tindall.

Fusco R. J., Jordan P. A., Kelley A., Samuel M. (1980). PUVA therapy for psoriasis. *Physiotherapy*, **66**, 39–40.

Gilchrist B. A., Rowe J. W., Brown R. S. *et al.* (1977). Relief of uremic pruritus with ultraviolet phototherapy. *N. Z. J. Med.*, **297**, 136–8.

Goats G. C. (1988). Appropriate use of the inverse square law. *Physiotherapy*, **74**, 8.

Griffin J. E., Karselis T. C. (1988). *Physical Agents for Physical Therapists*, 3rd edn. Springfield: Charles C. Thomas.

Gupta A. K., Ellis C. N., Tellner D. C. *et al.* (1989). Double-blind placebo controlled study to evaluate the efficacy of fish oil and low dose UVB in the treatment of psoriasis. *Br. J. Dermatol.*, **120**, 801–7.

Hawk J. L. M. (1983). Sunbeds. *Br. Med. J.*, **286**, 329.

High A. S., High J. P. (1983). Treatment of infected skin wounds using ultraviolet radiation – an in vitro study, 2. *Physiotherapy*, **69**, 359–60.

Ingram J. T. (1954). The significance and management of psoriasis. *Br. Med. J.*, 823–8.

Kenicer K. J. A., Lakshmipathi T., Addoh A. *et al.* (1981). An assessment of the effect of photochemotherapy (PUVA) and UV-B phototherapy in the treatment of psoriasis. *Br. J. Dermatol.*, **105**, 629–39.

Klaber M. R. (1980). Ultraviolet light for psoriasis. *Physiotherapy*, **66**, 36–8.

Krause R., Bühring M., Hopfenmüller W., Holick M. F., Sharma A. M. (1998). Ultraviolet B and blood pressure. *Res. Letts, Lancet*, **352**, 709–10.

Le Vine M. J., White H. A. D., Parrish J. A. (1979). Components of the Goeckerman regimen. *J. Invest. Dermatol.*, **73**, 170.

Licht S. (1983). History of ultraviolet therapy. In K. Stillwell (ed.), *Therapeutic Electricity and Ultraviolet Radiation*, 3rd edn. London: Williams & Wilkins.

Low J. L. (1986). Quantifying the erythema due to UVR. *Physiotherapy*, **72**, 60–4.

National Radiological Protection Board. (1977). *Protection Against Ultraviolet Radiation in the Work Place*. Didcot: Her Majesty's Stationery Office.

Nonaka S., Kaidley K. H., Kligman A. M. (1984). Photoprotective adaptation – some quantitative aspects. *Arch. Dermatol.*, **120**, 609–13.

Olson R. L., Gaylor J., Everett M. A. (1973). Skin colour, melanin and erythema. *Arch. Dermatol.*, **108**, 541–4.

Olson R. L., Sayre R. M., Everett M. A. (1965). The effect of field size on ultraviolet MED. *J. Invest. Dermatol.*, **68**, 516–18.

Olson R. L., Sayre R. M., Everett M. A. (1966). Effect of anatomic location and time on ultraviolet erythema. *Arch. Dermatol.*, **93**, 211–15.

Parrish J. A., Jaenicke K. F. (1981). Action spectrum of phototherapy for psoriasis. *J. Invest. Dermatol.*, **76**, 359–62.

Räsänen L., Reunala T., Lehto M. *et al.* (1989). Immediate decrease in antigen-presenting function and delayed enhancement of interleukin-I production in human epidermal cells after in vivo UVB radiation. *Br. J. Dermatol.*, **120**, 589–96.

Rivers J. K., Norris P. G., Murphy G. M. *et al.* (1989). UVA sunbeds: tanning, photoprotection, acute adverse effects and immunological changes. *Br. J. Dermatol.*, **120**, 767–77.

Robson J., Diffey B. (1990). Textiles and sun protection. *Photodermatol. Photoimmunol. Photomed.*, **7**, 32–4.

Sayre R. M., Olson R. L., Everett M. A. (1966). Qualitative studies on erythema. *J. Invest. Dermatol.*, **46**, 240–4.

Scott B. O. (1983). Clinical uses of ultraviolet radiation. In *Therapeutic Electricity and Ultraviolet Radiation*, 3rd edn (Stillwell G. K., ed.) Baltimore: Williams & Wilkins. pp. 228–61.

Shono S., Imura M., Ota M. *et al.* (1985). The relationship of skin colour, UVB induced erythema and melangenesis. *J. Invest. Dermatol.*, **84**, 265–7.

Stewart D. S. (1987). Indoor tanning: the nurse's role in preventing skin damage. *Cancer Nurs.*, **10**, 93–9.

Van Weelden H., Young E., Van der Leun J. C. (1980). Therapy of psoriasis: comparison of photochemotherapy and several variants of phototherapy. *Br. J. Dermatol.*, **103**, 9.

Wadsworth H., Chanmugan A. P. P. (1980). *Electrophysical Agents in Physiotherapy*. Marrickville, NSW, Australia: Science Press.

Williams P. L., Warwick R., Dyson M., Bannister L. (eds) (1989). *Grays Anatomy*, 37th edn. Edinburgh: Longman.

Wolff K., Gschnait F., Honigsmann H. *et al.* (1977). Phototesting and dosimetry for photochemotherapy. *Br. J. Dermatol.*, **96**, 1–10.

Wood K., Reed A. (1990). A study of the intensity of ultraviolet radiations transmitted through a variety of screening materials. *Physiotherapy*, **76**, 720–4.

Yaar M., Gilchrest B. A. (1990). Cellular and molecular mechanisms of cutaneous aging. *J. Dermatol. Surg. Oncol.*, **16**, 915–22.

Yoshikawa T., Rae V., Bruins-Slot W. *et al.* (1990). Susceptibility to effects of UVB radiation on induction of contact hypersensitivity as a risk factor for skin cancer in humans. *J. Invest. Dermatol.*, **95**, 530–6.

Appendix

NATURE OF AN ELECTRIC CURRENT

An electric current is a flow of electric charges. Electrons, protons and ions are the charges involved, although other subatomic particles may carry charges. Conductors are materials in which the outer shell electrons are free to move between constituent atoms. Normally this movement is random but if a voltage (an electric pressure) is applied to the material electrons will move away from the negative towards the positive charge. Although the motion of electrons is very rapid the movement of electrons from atom to atom (the electron drift) is quite slow. This is a conduction current and it is how charges move in metals and carbon and hence in electrical apparatus. Current is a rate of flow, that is a quantity of electrons per unit time. A rather large number of electrons (6.25×10^{18}) is the unit of quantity called a coulomb and when this quantity passes a point in 1 s the rate of flow, or current intensity, is called 1 ampere.

It is important to recognize that random electron movement occurs constantly at normal temperatures and that the electric current is superimposed on this. It is analogous to the arrivals channel of a large international airport; aircraft deliver passengers who pass through passport control, customs etc. and eventually leave by car, bus or train. Looked at over a time period of, say, a day the number of passengers leaving the airport is the same as the number arriving – the rate of flow may be expressed as so many thousand passengers per day – yet individual passengers have followed different pathways and spent different lengths of time at the airport. Some have been delayed by customs, some have had to wait for friends to meet them, some have gone to the restaurant for a meal and so forth, while others have passed through as quickly as they could. On a normal working day the airport is full of people as a conductor is full of electrons.

In a conductor it is only the electrons that move because the atoms are firmly held in crystalline structures which are typical of metal (and metalloid) solids; it is therefore called a conduction current. In fluids, liquids and gases, the atoms and molecules are free to move and therefore can take part in the flow of charges if they become charged. When an atom gains or loses an electron – hence it becomes negatively or positively charged – it is called an ion. Electrolytes are solutions containing ions. Body fluids are electrolytes and current can pass by the movement of these ions. Positive ions move towards the negative pole, the source of additional electrons, while negative ions move to the positive pole where electrons are being removed. Thus there is a two-way motion of ions which constitutes the current, called a convection current.

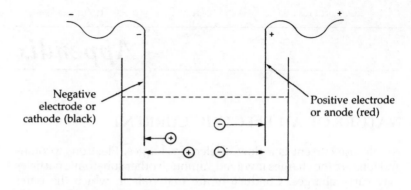

Fig. A1

In any given conductor, current intensity will simply depend on the electric pressure or electric force, known as the voltage. It is ultimately due to the attraction of electrons for protons, that is the electric force of the atom. This is measured in volts and is known, descriptively, as an electromotive force. The difficulty electrons have in moving within a solid conductor, or ions have in moving in an electrolyte, will also determine the rate of flow and this is described as the resistance, measured in ohms. Thus a conductor with a greater resistance will allow a smaller flow of electrons. These concepts are expressed in Ohm's law which states that the current intensity (I) in amperes is directly proportional to the electromotive force (E) in volts and inversely proportional to the resistance (R) in ohms. $I = E/R$ thus $A = V/\Omega$. This is analogous to the flow of water from a tap which depends on the pressure driving it (height of the tank) and the resistance offered by the tap (how far it is turned on).

ELECTROLYSIS

Electrolytes are solutions containing ions. When crystalline substances dissolve in water some separation into ions always occurs. If an electric field is applied by means of a pair of metal electrodes the ions will move through the solution, as shown in Figure A1. Thus positive ions move towards the negative electrode or cathode and are sometimes, rather confusingly, called cations. Negative ions move to the positive electrode or anode, hence these may be called anions. When the ions reach the metal plate or electrode they lose their charge. Positive ions gain an electron from the negatively charged metal plate and the negative ions give up their extra electron to the positive plate. The current in the solution is transmitted as ions (charges) moving in both directions. This is called a convection current. As the ions are neutralized electrically to form atoms they will act chemically. Ions 'used up' in this way are replaced in the solution by further dissociation to maintain the supply of charges. The chemical interactions that can occur at the electrodes are often complex and can involve the metal of these electrodes, so that metal may sometimes be removed from one plate and deposited on the other.

Sodium chloride solutions are utilized in transmitting current to and from the tissues for treatment purposes and will be considered, but similar effects occur where other salts, acids or bases are involved. The sodium chloride and water molecules dissociate into sodium and chlorine ions, and hydrogen and hydroxyl ions respectively:

$$NaCl \rightarrow Na^+ + Cl^-$$

$$H_2O \rightarrow H^+ + OH^-$$

The positive ions move to the negative electrode, the cathode, where they receive electrons. The negative ions move to the positive electrode, the anode, where they give up electrons.

At the cathode:

$$H^+ + e = H$$
$$2H = H_2$$

Hydrogen gas is given off. The hydrogen ion concentration falls (the pH value rises), therefore the reaction is alkaline:

$$Na^+ + e = Na$$
$$2Na + 2H_2O = 2NaOH + H_2$$

At the anode:

$$Cl^- - e = Cl$$
$$2Cl_2 + 2H_2O = 4HCl + O_2$$

Hydrochloric acid is formed and oxygen gas given off:

$$OH^- - e = OH$$
$$4OH = 2H_2O + O_2$$

These effects of altered pH and release of oxygen and hydrogen will occur whatever the salt, acid or base in solution with inert electrodes. The amount of gas produced is small in therapeutic situations and tends to remain dissolved in the water. However, if the current density is made high – say by passing a large current between two wires placed in a bowl of water – gas bubbles can be seen. These are especially evident at the cathode because of the larger quantity of hydrogen produced; in fact this can be used to determine the polarity as can the acidity/alkalinity tested with litmus paper.

DESCRIPTION OF WAVES

In order to characterize any wave several features must be described. The frequency, that is the number of complete cycles in a second, given in hertz (Hz), has already been noted. Hertz is the unit of frequency. It is:

$$\frac{\text{The number of items}}{\text{Seconds}}$$

These 'items' could be pulses (electrical or cardiac), waves, nerve impulses etc. Since this is simply a number, having no units, the SI unit for Hz is $\frac{1}{s}$ or s^{-1}.

The time taken for a complete cycle is known as the period. This describes the relation of the wave motion to time. The distance through which the wave motion repeats itself – the distance from, say, one wave peak to the next – is called the wavelength and is often denoted by λ (lambda). In the case of longitudinal waves passing in a medium it is the distance from, say, the central point of one compression of molecules to the next. This describes the motion in relation to distance (Fig. 6.1).

This can be understood by considering the familiar experience of standing knee-deep in the sea. A photograph taken looking out to sea would show a series of waves spaced apart, that is the height of the surface of the sea varies with distance at a single instant of time. The cold seawater regularly falling to the ankles and rising, breathtakingly, up the thighs makes the observer vividly aware of the variation over time in one place.

It is obvious that the velocity at which the wave passes through the material will depend on the frequency and wavelength: either a higher frequency or a greater wavelength, or both, will lead to a greater velocity. For any given velocity the wave could travel with either a high frequency and small wavelength or a low frequency and long wavelength. The fundamental equation for wave motion is thus expressed as:

$$\text{Velocity} = \text{frequency} \times \text{wavelength}$$
$$V = f\lambda$$
$$ms^{-1} = s^{-1}m$$

This relationship is obvious when it is realized that the speed of travel of any cyclical motion depends on the length of the cycle and the number of repetitions per unit time. Consider a 5-year-old boy walking hand in hand with his father; both travel at the same velocity, covering the same distance in the same time; the boy takes many small steps (of high frequency, short length) while the father takes fewer longer strides (of low frequency, large length).

The amplitude is the magnitude of the wave. It can be described as the distance from the mean position that a particle is made to move by the wave.

ENERGY AND POWER

Frequent reference is made to energy and power in this text, so it may be helpful to look at their relationship.

The concept of energy is not easily explained, because it only becomes evident when one form of energy is converted to another, such as when electrical energy is converted to heat energy in the wire of an infrared lamp, or in the tissues during the application of shortwave diathermy. Perhaps even more evident is the action of some mechanical force, such as a pull or push on a solid piece of matter, causing it to move.

Energy can be considered in two forms; kinetic energy, by virtue of motion, and potential energy, which is a stored form by virtue of structure, weight, charge, position etc.

The unit of energy is the joule (J); it represents the ability to do work. Work is also measured in joules. Thus 1 joule is the energy that results, or the work done, when a force of 1 newton acts through a distance of 1 metre:

$$E = Fd$$
$$J = Nm$$

In many practical situations the important factor is the rate of energy conversion or work done, i.e. the number of joules per second or watts:

$$1 J/s = 1 W$$

This rate of energy use is called power.

Alternatively, if we want to work out how much energy has been delivered, we multiply watts by seconds:

$$1 J = 1 Ws$$

For example: 1 watt hour = 3600 J. Because this is a small quantity, kilojoules (kJ) and kilowatt hours (kWh) are often used.

If an ultrasound transducer is delivering 5 W, it means that electrical energy is being converted to sonic energy at a rate of 5 joules every second.

Often it is more helpful to know the amount of power per unit area. This is called power density and is measured in W/cm^2. With ultrasound, this value is often called intensity, and for lasers and light is termed brilliance or irradiance. In the same way it is sometimes convenient to describe energy density (J/cm^2).

Whatever conversions occur, the principle of conservation of energy applies, which states that energy can neither be created nor destroyed. Unfortunately the use of energy is a costly business!

Index

A delta fibres, 90–1, 92
  cold application response, 258–9, 262
  pain control, 94, 95
Absorption:
  electromagnetic radiations, 320, 324
  infrared radiations, 345
  laser radiations, 364–5
  microwave diathermy, 329–31
  sonic energy, 180, 181
Accommodation, 72
Accommodation pulses, 59–60
Achilles tendon injury, 82
Acne vulgaris, 392
Acoustic streaming, 25
  ultrasound, 185
Actinic radiation, 377
Actinotherapy, 377
Action potential, 8–9, 10
  skeletal muscle cells, 13
Active transport, 5, 6
Acupuncture, 95
Acupuncture points, 118
  laser therapy application, 367
  TENS electrode placement, 114
Adrenaline:
  inflammatory response, 18, 19
  thermoregulation, 224, 226
Allergic rhinitis, 45
Alpine sunlamp, 380–1
  application, 406–7
Alternating currents, 63–4
  diadynamic, 63–4
  sinusoidal, 63
Angiogenesis:
  healing, 20
  ultrasound stimulation, 187
Ankle sprain, 303
Antibiotics:
  iontophoresis, 43
  ultraviolet sensitization, 401
Antidromic propagation, 9
Anti-inflammatory drugs, iontophoretic application, 43–4
Apparatus preparation, 28
Arndt–Schultz law, 302, 365
Arteriosclerosis, 249, 272
Autonomic nervous system responses, 102
Axonotmesis, 143, 144, 147

Back pain, 301, 303, 366
Balance control biofeedback, 164
Bell's palsy, 147
Benzydamine hydrochloride, 204
Biofeedback, 157–70
  application techniques, 161–2, 166–7
  control of muscle activity/movement, 159–65
  effectiveness, 167–8
  electromyographic, 145, 159–63
    evaluation, 168–70
  feedback loop principle, 158, 159
  mechanism, 167
  purposes, 158–9
  stress-related conditions, 165–7
Bipolar water baths, 107
Blepharoplasty recovery, 305–6
Blood clotting, 17
Blood flow, *see* Vascular changes
Blood pressure:
  cold therapy response, 272
  infrared radiations response, 354
Blood viscosity, 229
Body temperature, 218
  core–surface gradients, 219, 220
  see also Thermoregulation
Bone:
  remodelling, 102
  strain-generated potentials, 14, 37
Bony union, 25
  low-frequency magnetic fields, 308
  ultrasound, 187, 189
Bradykinin, 18
Brown adipose tissue, 224, 227, 261
Buerger's disease (thromboangiitis obliterans), 249, 272
Burns, 127, 128, 237–8
  direct current, 31
  heat therapies (hot water), 249
  immediate treatment, 238, 261
  infrared radiations, 353
  microwave diathermy, 334, 336
  pulsed shortwave, 305
  shortwave diathermy, 294–6
Bursitis, 43, 366

C fibres, 90, 91
  cold application response, 258, 262
  pain control, 94, 95
  thermal perception, 221

Calcium (Ca^{2+}), intra/extracellular fluid, 7, 8
Calcium (Ca^{2+}) pump, 7
  laser radiation effects, 365
  ultrasound effects, 186–7
Calorie, 213
Capacitance, cell membrane, 6–7
Capacitive resistance of tissues, 105
Cardiac arrhythmias, 165
Cardiac disease, 272
Cardiac pacemakers, treatment contraindications:
  microwave diathermy, 337, 339
  pulsed shortwave, 305
  shortwave diathermy, 296
Causalgia, 303
Cavitation, 185
Cell membrane, 3–4
  capacitance, 7
  electrical charge, 6–7
  pulsed shortwave actions, 300
  resting potential, 7
  transport processes, 4–5, 6
  ultrasound effects, 184, 186–7
Cell signalling, 12–13
Cellular electrical charge, 2, 3–7
Cerebral palsy, 82
Chemical cold packs, 268
Chloride (Cl$^-$), intra/extracellular movement, 7, 8
Chondromalacia patellae, 81
Chromophores, 364
Chronaxie, 150
Chronic pain, 92, 93
Coherent electromagnetic radiations, 320
Cold, 217
  adaptive behaviour, 225–6
  nerve conduction inhibition, 230
Cold induced vasodilation (CIVD), 257
Cold packs, 267–9
  commercial products, 268
  ice, 267–8
Cold stress responses, 227, 260–1
Cold therapy, 23, 255–74
  application methods, 266–70
    cold packs, 267–9
    cold-compression units, 269
    evaporating sprays, 269–70
    ice massage, 269
    ice towels, 269
    local immersion, 267
    technique, 266–7
  contraindications, 271–4
    pathological cold sensitivity, 271–2
  heat treatment comparison, 270–1
  physiological changes, 256–60
    blood pressure response, 272
    cutaneous blood flow, 257
    metabolic rate, 258, 261
    motor system, 259

    muscle blood flow, 258
    pain receptor responses, 260
    peripheral nervous system, 258–9
    thermoreceptor responses, 258, 260
  safety, 271
  therapeutic uses, 261–5
  tissue temperature changes, 255–6
Cold urticaria, 272
Cold-compression units, 269
Collagen:
  healing process, 20–1, 187
  remodelling process, 21, 187–8
  temperature-related changes, 229
  ultrasound effects, 187–8
Colour therapy, 351
Conduction, 23, 216, 217
  body temperature regulation, 219
  cold therapy tissue temperatures, 255
  therapeutic heat application, 236
  see also Superficial heating therapies
Connective tissue:
  cellular electrical charge, 14–15
  remodelling, 15, 21
Constant current, *see* Direct current
Continuous shortwave diathermy, 307
Contractures, 21, 82
  heat therapy, 234
Contrast baths, 247–8
Convection, 216, 217
  body temperature regulation, 216, 219
  forced, 216–17, 219, 242
  heat movement through tissues, 242
  therapeutic heat application, 236
Copper iontophoresis, 45
Core body temperature, 218, 219
Corticosteroids, 18
  phonophoresis, 204
Cosine law, 322
Counter-current heat exchange, 220–1
Counter-irritation, 230
Cryoglobinaemia, 272
Cryotherapy, *see* Cold therapy
Current, *see* Electric current
Cutaneous blood flow, 220, 224–5
  cold therapy response, 257, 260–1
  electrical stimulation response, 100
  see also Vascular changes; Vasodilation
Cyclotherm systems, 251
Cystic fibrosis, 227
Cytochromes, 365
Cytokines, 18

Denervated muscle stimulation, 88–90
Dental surgery healing, 189
Depolarization, 9, 10
Dermatitis, acute, 150

Dexamethasone, 44
Diadynamic currents, 63–4, 121
  therapeutic effects, 121
Diapedesis, 19
Diathermy, 24, 25, 54
  see also Longwave diathermy; Microwave
    diathermy; Shortwave diathermy
Diffusion, 5, 6
Diode lasers, 361–3
Dipole rotation, 280, 329
Direct current, 23, 30–49
  application principles, 45–7
  contraindications, 40
  current density, 31
  current production, 34–5, 38–9
  dangers, 49
  dosage, 48
  electrotonus, 36
  healing acceleration, 36–40, 70
    mechanisms, 39
  historical aspects, 30
  hyperaemia, 35–6
  iontophoresis, *see* Iontophoresis
  pain relief, 36
  patient preparation, 45–6
  procedure, 39–40
  sensory stimulation, 35
  stimulation characteristics, 31, 54, 58
  therapeutic uses, 35–9
  time–amplitude relationship, 55
  tissue destruction, 40–1
  transmission, 31
Displacement currents, 282
Dithranol, 391, 401
Double insulation, 130
Drug-induced ultraviolet sensitization, 401
Dry air (heated air) treatment, 250
Dupuytren's contracture, 189
Dystonic conditions, 161

Ear chondritis, 43
Eczema, 150
  PUVA treatment, 404
  ultraviolet radiation treatment, 392–3
Eddy currents, 280, 287
Electric current, 277, 413–14
  amplitude, 56
  density, 31, 33
  intensity, 56
  modulation, 56
  phase, 54, 56
  pulse, 54, 56, 57
    biphasic, 57
    unidirectional, 56
  types, 58–66
  waveform, 54, 56, 57

Electric heating pads, 251
Electric shock, 127
  first-aid treatment, 129
  macroshock, 128
  mains-type current, 128–30
  microshock, 128
  therapeutic currents, 130–1
Electrical apparatus safety, 129–30
Electrical charge, 1–3
  cellular regions, 3–4
  connective tissue cells, 14–15
  muscle cells, 13–14
  therapeutic effects, 24–6
Electrical gradients in development/regeneration, 15
Electrical stimulation application, 103–10
  contraindications, 132
  diadynamic currents, 121
  electroacupuncture, 118
  electrode polarity, 107
  electrode position, 106
  electrode systems, 103–4
  electrode–tissue interface, 103
  faradic-type currents, 110–14
  H-wave therapy, 117
  high-voltage pulsed galvanic stimulation (HVPGS),
    119–20
  interferential currents, 123–7
  precautions, 131–2
  rebox, 121–2
  Russian currents, 122–3
  safety, 110, 127–32
  sinusoidal currents, 120–1
  skin surface preparation, 108
  transcutaneous nerve stimulation, *see*
    Transcutaneous nerve stimulation
  transcutaneous spinal electroanaesthesia (TSE),
    118–19
  water baths, 107
Electrical stimulation, neuromuscular, 24, 53–132
  application principles, *see* Electrical stimulation
    application
  autonomic nervous system effects, 102
  cellular responses, 102–3
  cutaneous blood flow, 100–1
  functional, 83–4
  joint range of motion response, 82–3
  long-term trophic adaptation, 84–6
  muscle fatigue, 87–8
  oedema reduction, 101–2
  pain control, 90
  physiological effects, 77
    denervated muscle, 88–90
    innervated muscle, 78–9, 86–7
    mucle control facilitation, 81–2
    muscle strengthening, 79–81
  principles, 53–8
  pulse characteristics, *see* Pulsed currents

therapeutic uses, 82–8
time–amplitude relationship, 54, 55
tissue resistance, 105–6
Electrical tissue damage, 127, 130–1
Electroacupuncture, 118
    current pulses, 61
Electrocardiogram, 13
Electroconvulsive therapy, 27
Electrode systems:
    carbon rubber electrodes, 104–5
    metal plate electodes, 104–5
Electroencephalography, 13
Electrolysis, 414–15
    direct current application, 31
Electromagnetic energy, 276–8
Electromagnetic fields, 276–311
    frequency, 277–8
    safety, 308–11
    wavelengths, 277
Electromagnetic radiation, 277, 315–26
    amplitude, 317
    characteristics, 315–18
    coherence, 320
    frequency, 316, 317, 318
    interactions with matter, 320–6
        absorption, 320, 324
        penetration, 324
        reflection, 320–3
        refraction, 321, 323–4
        scattering, 320, 324–5
        transmission, 320
    inverse square law, 319
    phase difference, 319–20
    rectilinear propagation, 319
    velocity, 316
    wavelength, 316, 317, 318
Electromagnetic spectrum, 317–18
Electromyographic biofeedback, 145, 159–63
    application technique, 161–2
    evaluation, 168–70
    therapeutic uses, 160–2
Electromyography, 13, 141, 143–5
Electron orbit distortion, 281–2, 329
Electrons, 2
    energy levels, 317, 318, 357–9, 378
Electrophysiological evaluation, 141–56
    electromyography, 141, 143–5
    evoked potentials, 153, 154
        central nervous system, 155–6
    muscle contraction observations, 146–7
    nerve conduction velocity studies, 153–4
    reflex testing, 155
    strength–duration (S–D) testing, 148–52
Electrostatic forces, 277
Electrotonus, 36
Embryonic development, 15
Endothelial cells, 20

Energy:
    application methods, 22–4
    conversions, 215
    power relationship, 416–17
Epicondylitis, 44
Epilepsy, biofeedback, 166
Episiotomy scar treatment, 189
Epithelialization, 22
Ethylmorphine hydrochloride, 45
Evaporating sprays, 269–70
Evaporative heat loss, 216, 219, 225
Evoked potentials, 141, 153, 154
    central nervous system, 155–6
Extracellular fluid, 7
Eye safety:
    infrared radiations, 354
    laser radiations, 373
    microwave diathermy, 337, 339
    shortwave diathermy, 297
    ultraviolet radiation, 388–9, 408

Facial nerve assessment, 147
Facilitated diffusion, 5, 6
Faradic-type current muscle stimulation, 112–3
    application technique, 110, 112–3
    motor points, 111, 112
    oedema reduction, 113–14
    patient preparation, 110
Faradic-type pulsed current, 60
Feedback:
    negative, 157–8
    positive, 157–8
Feedback loop, 158, 159
Fever, 226–7
Fibroblasts, 21
    direct current responses, 39
    healing, 20
    ultrasound stimulation, 187
Fluidotherapy, 250–1
Fluorescent lamps, 379–80
Frostbite, 271
Functional breathing disorder, biofeedback, 163
Functional electrical stimulation, 83–4
    spasticity, 84
    splinting replacement, 83–4
Fungal infection:
    heat therapy, 232, 235
    hydrotherapy contraindications, 150
    infrared radiation treatment, 232, 349–50
Fuses, 130

Galium aluminium arsenide (GaAlA) lasers, 362
Galvanism, *see* Direct current
Gamma radiation, 318
Gases, 212, 214

Glycopyrronium bromide, 42, 47, 48
Goeckerman regimen, 391
Granulation tissue, 20, 21
    ultrasound effects, 187
Grotthus's law, 320
Growth stimulation, 68
    neurons, 25
    skin, ultraviolet response, 387–8
Guidelines for treatment, 27–8
Guillain–Barr, syndrome, 143

H reflex, 155
H-wave current pulses, 61, 62
H-wave therapy, 117
Hair removal, 40–1
Half-value depth 180–1, 323, 345–8
Hand injuries, 235
Healing, 16–22, 102
    epithelialization, 22
    inflammation, 17–19, 20
    initial injury response, 16–17
    proliferation, 20–1
    remodelling, 21–2
    time scale, 21, 22
    ultrasound effects, 186–8
        acute inflammation stage, 186–7
        proliferative (granulation) stage, 187
        remodelling stage, 187–8
    ultrasound imaging, 206
Healing promotion, 25
    diadynamic currents, 121
    direct current, 36–40, 70
    H-wave therapy, 117
    heat therapy, 232
    high-voltage pulsed galvanic stimulation (HVPGS), 119
    infrared radiations, 349, 352
    laser therapy, 365–6, 368
    magnetic fields, 307
    microwave diathermy, 334
    pulsed shortwave effects, 302–3
    red light, 351
    transcutaneous nerve stimulation, 39
Heat energy, 212–18
    change of state of matter, 214–15
    chemical reactions acceleration, 215
    electromagnetic radiations, 215, 317, 318
    energy conversions, 215
    expansion effects, 214
    first law of thermodynamics, 213
    microstructure of matter, 212–13
    pulsed shortwave, 301, 302
    quantity measurement, 213–14
    Seebeck effect, 215
    shortwave diathermy, 280–2
    temperature (level) measurement, 213

thermionic emission, 215
    transfer, 216–17
Heat stroke, 227
Heat syncope, 227
Heat therapy, 212–39
    burns, 237–8
    cold therapy comparison, 270–1
    conduction heating, *see* Superficial heating therapies
    deep heating, 238, 239
    extent of tissue heating, 236–7
    physiological effects, 228–31
        collagenous tissue, 229
        erythema, 230
        metabolic activity, 228–9
        nerve stimulation, 229
        tissue fluid exchange, 231
        vasodilation, 230–1
        viscosity, 229
    reflex heating, 237
    shortwave diathermy, *see* Shortwave diathermy
    subcutaneous fat influences, 242
    superficial heating, 238, 239
    therapeutic effects, 232–6
    thermal sensation assessment, 238
Heated air treatment, 250
Heliotherapy, 377, 408–9
Helium–neon lasers, 361
Hemiplegia, 82, 83, 84
    electromyographic biofeedback, 160
    ultraviolet sensitization, 402
Herpes simplex lesions, 204
High-frequency currents, 66
High-voltage galvanic stimulation (HVGS), 62
High-voltage pulsed galvanic stimulation (HVPGS),
        38, 39, 40, 62, 121
    current pulses, 62
    therapeutic uses, 119–20
Histamine, 17, 18, 187, 348, 384
Histamine diphosphate, 43, 45
Hormones, 12
Hot climate adaptive behaviour, 226
Hyaluronidase, 45
Hydrocollator hot packs, 242, 246–7, 252
Hydrocortisone, 204
Hydrogen (HS+s), intra/extracellular movement, 7, 8
Hydrotherapy, 248–50
    contraindications, 249–50
    whirlpool baths, 248–9
Hyperhidrosis, idiopathic, 42–3, 47, 48
Hypertension:
    biofeedback, 165
    cold therapy contraindications, 272
    ultraviolet radiation treatment, 394
Hypertrophic scars, 39
Hypothalamic temperature-regulating centres, 226, 260
Hypothermia, 227
Hysterical paralysis, 82

Ice application, *see* Cold therapy
Ice burn, 271
Ice massage, 269
Ice packs, 267–8
Ice towels, 269
Implants:
    microwave diathermy contraindications, 337
    shortwave diathermy contraindications, 296, 298
    slow-release hormone capsules, 297
    ultrasound contraindications, 201–2
Incontinence control:
    biofeedback, 164
    electrical stimulation, 82
    interferential currents, 127
Indiba treatment, 280
Inductothermy, *see* Shortwave diathermy application
Infection:
    heat therapy, 232
    pulsed shortwave, 302
    ultraviolet radiation, 393
Inflammation, chronic, 264
Inflammatory exudate, 18
Inflammatory mediators, 18
    pain, 18–19
Inflammatory response, 17–19, 20
    cellular responses, 19
    cold application effects, 261–2
    mediators, 18
    nervous system involvement, 19
    pain, 18–19
    ultrasound effects, 186–7
    ultraviolet-associated erythema, 384
    vascular changes, 17–18
Information for patient, 27, 28
Infrared radiations, 24, 317, 318, 341–50
    absorption, 345
    application, 352–3
    burns, 353
    characteristics, 341–2
    classification, 341
    contraindications, 354
    penetration depth, 345–8
    physiological effects, 348–9
    production, 342
    safety, 353–4
    therapeutic sources, 342–4
        emission, 344
        luminous generators (radiant heat), 344, 351
        non-luminous lamps, 342–3, 351
        power, 344
    therapeutic uses, 232, 235, 349–50
    wavelengths, 341
Ingram (Leeds) regimen, 391
Interferential currents, 66, 123–7
    current control settings, 123, 124–5
    current distribution, 123, 124
    electrode application, 125–6

pain control, 99–100
    precautions, 126
    therapeutic effects, 23, 126–7
    ultrasound combination therapy, 206–7
Interpulse interval, 56, 57
Intracellular fluid, 7
Inverse square law, 319
    ultraviolet lamp dosage, 397
Ion transfer, *see* Iontophoresis
Ionic movements, 2
Ionizing radiation, 317
Ionozone therapy, 409–10
Ions, intracellular fluid, 7
Iontophoresis, 25, 31
    anti-inflammatory drugs application, 43–4
    antibiotics application, 43
    current density, 33
    dangers, 49
    dosage, 48
    duration of treatment, 33
    idiopathic hyperhidrosis, 42–3
    local anaesthesia, 41–2
    mechanism, 32–4
    neurogenic pain, 44
    therapeutic uses, 41–5

Joint angle biofeedback, 164
Joint disease, 264
Joint effusions, 264–5
Joint range of movement:
    electrical stimulation, 82–3
    heat therapy, 234–5
    high-voltage pulsed galvanic stimulation (HVPGS), 120
Joint stiffness, 229, 235

Keloid scars, 39
Kenny packs, 247
Keratinization, 382–3
Kilohertz frequency devices, 306, 307
Kinetic energy, 212, 213, 280
    heat transfer, 216
Kinins, 18, 384
Knee effusion, 252
Knee injury, 82
Kromayer lamp, 381

Langerhans cells, 384
Lasers, 24, 320, 356–73
    application technique, 368–9
        treatment area, 371
        treatment progression, 371
    classification, 363
    cluster probes, 363

coherence, 356, 358
collimation, 357
  divergence angle, 364
contraindications, 373
dosage, 369–71, 372
  pulsed output, 370–1
  wavelength, 370
energy density, 363, 370
energy measurement, 363–4
eye protection, 372–3
monochromaticity, 356
nerve conduction rate, 367–8
power density, 363, 364
principle, 357–9
safety, 372–3
therapeutic efficacy, 368
therapeutic uses, 365–8
tissue effects, 364–5
  absorption, 364–5
  penetration, 364
trigger/acupuncture point application, 367
types, 357, 360–3
Latent heat, 214
Lateral humeral epicondylitis, 188
Leukotrienes, 18
Lewis 'hunting reaction', 257
Ligament sprains, 305
Limb regeneration, 15
Liquids, 212, 215
Local anaesthesia, iontophoresis, 41–2
Longwave diathermy, 280
Low-frequency stimulation, 58
  tissue effects, 68, 70
Low-frequncy magnetic fields, 308
Low-intensity laser therapy (LILT), 365
Low-power pulsed high-frequency energy, 305–6, 307
Low-reactive level laser therapy (LLLT), 365

Macrophages:
  healing, 20
  inflammatory response, 19, 187
  laser radiation responses, 365, 366
  ultrasound stimulation, 187
Magnetic fields, 307–9
  low-frequency, 308
  static, 307–8
Magnetic therapies, 276
Magnetron, 328
Margination, 17, 19
Mast cell degranulation, 18, 187
Medium frequency current, 64–5
  direct, 31
  interferential, 65
  Rebox-type, 64
  'Russian', 64

Medium-pressure mercury arc lamp, *see* Alpine sunlamp
Melanin, 383
Melanocytes, 383, 384
  ultraviolet radiation response, 383, 387
Mercury vapour lamp, 378
Metabolic activity:
  cold application response, 258, 261
  infrared radiation response, 348
  temperature-related changes, 228–9
Micromassage, 186
Microwave diathermy, 24, 327–39
  absorption patterns, 329–31
    tissue morphology effects, 331, 332
  application, 334–5
  characteristics, 327–8
  contraindications, 339
  dosage, 335–6
  emitter, 328, 329
    contact, 332–3, 334
    shape, 332
  frequencies, 327
  heating effect, 328, 329, 331, 333, 334
  physiological effects, 329–33
    tissue penetration, 329, 331
  production, 328–9
  reflection, 331, 332
  refraction, 331, 332
  safety, 336–9
    exposure standards, 338–9
  therapeutic uses, 334
  wavelengths, 327
Microwave dosage:
  specific absorption rate (SAR), 336
Microwaves, 317
Migraine, biofeedback, 166
Monocytes, 19
Motor fibres, 68
  classification, 69
  electrical stimulation, 73, 74, 77
Motor nerve conduction velocity, 153–4
Motor skills, cold application response, 259
Motor unit, 77–8, 144, 145
  action (spike) potentials, 13–14
Movement practice, biofeedback, 165
Mud packs (peloids), 247
Muscle blood flow:
  cold application, 258
  electrical stimulation, 85–7
Muscle contraction, 78
  body heat production, 224, 226
  observation, 146–7
    nerve continuity, 146–7
    tendon integrity, 146
  stimulation, 68
Muscle control facilitation, 81–2
Muscle fatigue, 87–8

Muscle fibres:
  electrical charge, 13–14
  types, 77–8
    recruitment order, 78
Muscle metabolism, 86–7
Muscle spasm:
  cold application, 262
  heat therapy, 230, 234
  high-voltage pulsed galvanic stimulation (HVPGS),
    120
  infrared radiations, 350
Muscle stimulating currents, 23, 54, 55, 56
  high-voltage pulsed galvanic stimulation (HVPGS),
    120
  interferential currents, 127
  ultrasound combination therapy, 206–7
  see also Electrical stimulation, neuromuscular
Muscle strengthening:
  cold application, 259, 263–4
  electrical stimulation, 79–81
Muscle training programmes, biofeedback, 161, 164
Myelin sheath, 11
Myofibroblasts, 20
Myositis ossificans, 44

Neck pain, 305
Neonatal jaundice, 350
Nernst equation, 7
Nerve conduction, 11–12
Nerve conduction velocity, 153–4
  cold application response, 230, 258, 259
  heat therapy response, 230
Nerve continuity assessment, 146–7
Nerve impulse, 8–12
  all-or-none response, 70, 71
  depolarization, 9, 10
  electrical nerve stimulation, 54, 70–1, 77
    rheobase, 71, 72
  information transfer, 12
  propagation speed, 11–12
  refractory period, 10, 11
  repolarization, 9, 10
  threshold, 9, 72
Nerve regeneration, pulsed shortwave, 302
Neurapraxia, 142, 147
Neurogenic pain, 93
  iontophoresis, 44
  laser therapy, 367
  pulsed shortwave treatment, 303–4
Neurometer, 118
Neuromuscular electrical stimulation (NMES), *see*
    Electrical stimulation, neuromuscular
Neurons:
  cell membrane capacitance, 9
  growth stimulation, 25
  resting membrane potential, 7–8
    direct current effects, 36

Neurotmesis, 143, 144
Neurotransmitters, 12
Neutrophils, 17, 19
Nociceptors:
  cold application responses, 260
  heat therapy responses, 230
  pain pathways, 91
  physiology, 90–1
  stimulation, 73, 74, 77
Nodes of Ranvier, 11
Non-steroidal anti-inflammatory drugs, 18, 44
  phonophoresis, 204

Obesity, 297
Oedema formation, 25
  inflammatory response, 18
Oedema reduction:
  cold application, 264–5
  diadynamic currents, 121
  electrical stimulation, 100–1
  faradic-type current muscle stimulation, 113–14
  H-wave therapy, 117
  heat therapy, 235
  high-voltage pulsed galvanic stimulation (HVPGS),
    120
  infrared radiations, 350
  sinusoidal currents, 120
Ohmic resistance of tissues, 105
Organelle charges, 7
Orthodromic propagation, 9, 70
Osteoarthritis, 366
  cold application, 264
  pulsed shortwave, 303
Osteoporotic pain, 303
Ozone, 408

Pain, 90–5
  acute, 91
  alteration in perception, 93–4
  assessment, 114
  chemical mediators, 18–19
  chronic, 92, 93
  definitions, 90
  gate control theory, 90, 94
  inflammatory response, 18–19, 25
  neurogenic, 93
  nociceptors, 90–1
  pathways, 91–3
  psychogenic, 93
  referred, 93
  skin thermoreceptors, 221, 230
  somatogenic, 92–3
Pain control, 68, 94–7
  cold application, 262
  diadynamic currents, 122

direct current application, 36
electrical stimulation, 90
H-wave therapy, 117
heat therapy, 230, 232–3
  superficial heating, 252–3
high-voltage pulsed galvanic stimulation (HVPGS), 119
infrared radiations, 350
interferential currents, 126–7
laser therapy, 366–8
magnetic fields, 307
pulsed shortwave, 303–4
therapeutic ultrasound, 189
transcutaneous nerve stimulation, *see* Transcutaneous nerve stimulation
Paraffin wax baths, 244–6
  application methods, 244–5
  contraindications, 246
  mode of action, 245–6
Paranasal sinusitis, 303
Paraplegia, 84
Paronychia, 150, 232, 235, 349
Patient anxiety, 131
Penetration depth, 180–1, 324, 345–8
Penicillin, 204
Perineal post-natal pain, 189
Peripheral nerve, 68
  conduction studies, 12
  fibre types, 68, 69, 70
Peripheral nerve pathology, 141–3, 144
  recovering injuries electromyographic biofeedback, 161
Perthes disease, 308
Phagocytosis, 5
  inflammatory response, 19
Phantom limb pain, 303–4
Phonophoresis, 202–6
  application, 204–5
  contraindications, 205–6
  drug penetration, 203
  drugs transmitted, 204, 205
  mode of action, 203
Photobiomodulation, 365, 377
Photobiostimulation, 365
  see also Lasers
Photochemotherapy, 391–2
Photodermatoses, 394
Photodiodes, 382
Photons, 317, 318
  absorption/emission, 358–9
  excitation, 359
  mercury vapour lamp emission, 378
  stimulated emission, 359
Phototherapy, 377
Piezoelectric effects, 14
  bone stress-generated potentials, 37
  pulsed shortwave actions, 301

Piezoelectric transducers, 174–5
Pinocytosis (endocytosis), 5
Placebo effect, 25–6, 97
Plantar fasciitis, 189
Plasmin, 18
Platelet activating factor, 18
Poldine methylsulphate, 42
Polymorphic light eruptions, 404
Polymorphonuclear leucocytes, 17, 19
Polyneuritis, 143
Postherpetic pain, 367
Posture control biofeedback, 163
Potassium (KS+s) channels, 9
Potassium (KS+s), intra/extracellular fluid, 7, 8
Poultices, 232
Power, energy relationship, 416–17
Pregnancy, exposure contraindications:
  laser therapy, 373
  microwave diathermy, 338, 339
  shortwave diathermy, 297–8
Preparation of patient, 27
Pressure application, 22
Pressure sores:
  cold application, 265
  direct current, 38
  prophylactic heat therapy, 235
  pulsed shortwave, 303
  ultraviolet radiation, 393
PRICE, 261
Prostaglandins, 18, 19
Pruritus, 204
  ultraviolet radiation treatment, 394–5
Psoralens, 391–2, 401
  see also PUVA treatment
Psoriasis, 204
  heliotherapy, 409
  infrared heating, 235, 350
  ultraviolet radiation treatment, 390–2
    Goeckerman regimen, 391
    Ingram (Leeds) regimen, 391
    photochemotherapy, 391–2
Psychogenic pain, 93
Psychological well-being, ultraviolet radiation treatment, 395
Pulse frequency, 56, 57
  refractory periods, 75–6
Pulse generators, 66–8
  amplifying circuit, 67
  modulating circuit, 67
  oscillating circuit, 67
  power source, 67
Pulse interval, 56
Pulse (phase) charge calculation, 56
Pulsed currents, 58–62, 65
  long duration, 59–60
    accommodation pulses, 59–60
    rectangular wave pulses, 59

nerve stimulation, 70–4, 77
  motor fibres, 73, 74, 77
  nociceptors, 73, 74
  pulse application to tissue, 73, 74
  rate of rise of pulse, 71–2
  refractory periods, 74–6
  sensory fibres, 73, 74, 77
penetration through tissues, 77
short duration, 60–2
  electroacupuncture, 61
  faradic-type pulses, 60
  H-wave, 61, 62
  high-voltage galvanic/pulsed galvanic
    stimulation (HVGS; HVPGS), 62
  transcutaneous nerve stimulation, 60–1, 62
Pulsed high-frequency electromagnetic energy, *see*
    Pulsed shortwave
Pulsed shortwave, 276, 299–305, 307
  application, 303
  contraindications, 304
  dosage, 304–5
  infection, 303
  pain control, 303–4
  physiological effects, 302–3
  production, 299–300
  therapeutic mechanisms, 299–302
  therapeutic uses, 303–4
PUVA (psoralen plus UVA) therapy, 391–2
  application, 404–5

Quantum, 317

Radiation, 216–17, 377
  body temperature regulation, 219
Radiowaves, 317–18
Raynaud's phenomenon, 271–2
  biofeedback, 165
Rebox currents, 64, 121–2
Records, 28
Rectangular wave pulses, 59
Referred pain, 93
Reflection of electromagnetic radiation, 320–3
  cosine law, 322
  microwave diathermy, 331, 332
  parallel radiations on curved surfaces, 322, 323
Reflex sympathetic dystrophies, 235
Reflex testing, 155
Refraction, 321, 323–4
  microwave diathermy, 331, 332
Refractory period, 10, 11
  pulsed current stimulation, 74–6
Regeneration, 22
  electrical gradients, 15
  nerve, pulsed shortwave, 303
Relaxation biofeedback, 165–7

Remodelling, 21–2
  ultrasound effects, 187–8
Repolarization, 9, 10
Resting membrane potential, 7
  neurons, 7–8
Rheobase current, 71, 72
  strength–duration testing, 148, 151
Rheumatoid arthritis, 44, 234, 366, 367, 368
  cold application response, 264
Rotator cuff tendinitis, 308
Ruby lasers, 360–1
Russian currents, 64, 122–3
Ryodu-Raku, 118

Scanning lasers, 364
Salicylates phonophoresis, 204
Saltatory conduction, 11
Scar tissue, 21, 82
  heat therapy, 234, 235
  therapeutic ultrasound, 187, 189
Scattered electromagnetic radiation, 34–325
  laser radiation, 364
Scleroderma, 204
Scoliosis, 83
Seasonal affective disorder, 350
Sebaceous glands, 384
Sedative effects, 234
Seebeck effect, 215
Sensory fibres, 68
  classification, 69
  conduction velocity, 154
  stimulation, 54, 55, 56, 73, 74, 77
Serotonin (5-hydroxytryptamine), 18
Shivering, 223–4, 261
Shortwave diathermy, 23–4, 276, 277
  application technique, *see* Shortwave diathermy
    application
  contraindications, 298–9
  frequencies, 278
  operator exposure
    operator distance, 297
    pregnancy outcome, 297–8
  oscillator circuit, 278–9
  production, 278–80
  resonator circuit, 279
  safety, 294–8
    eye treatment, 297
  therapeutic effects, 282
  tissue heating effects, 280
    dipole rotation, 280
    molecular distortion, 281, 282
    vibration of ions, 280, 281
  wavelenths, 278
Shortwave diathermy application, 280, 283–90
  capacitive (capacitor field) method, 280, 283, 290,
    291

contraplanar technique, 291
coplanar technique, 286, 291
cross-fire technique, 291, 292
electrode placement, 284, 285, 291
electrode size, 284
tissue heating pattern, 283–6
tissue variables, 286
dosage, 293–4
inductive method (inductothermy), 280, 283, 290
cable application, 291, 292
tissue heating pattern, 287–9
technique, 290–3
Silica gel cold packs, 268
Silver iontophoresis, 43
Sinusoidal currents, 58, 63, 120–1
application, 121–2
effects, 120
Size comparisons, 2
Skin, 382–4
epidermal structure, 382
growth promotion, 387–8
keratinization, 382–3
Langerhans cells, 384
pigmentation, 383–4
prolonged ultraviolet radiation exposure, 389
sebaceous glands, 384
sweating, 219, 225
thermoreceptors, 221–3
thermoregulation, 224–5
vasoconstriction/vasodilation, 220, 224–5
cold therapy, 257
electrical stimulation, 100
vitamin D production, 388
Skin battery, 14
Skin cancer, 389
Skin disease, 235
Skin infection, 393
Skin temperature biofeedback, 157, 158
application technique, 166–7
Snow blindness, 388
Sodium (NaS+s) channels, 9
Sodium (NaS+s), intra/extracellular fluid, 7, 8
Sodium diclofenac, 44
Sodium salicylate, 44
Sodium–potassium (NaS+s–KS+s) pump, 7, 8
neuron cell membrane, 9
Soft tissue injury:
direct current, 36
immediate cold application, 261–2
therapeutic ultrasound, 189
Solids, 212, 215
Somatogenic pain, 92–3
Sonic waves, 173–4
Sound, 23, 172
waves, 173–4
Space average temporal averaged dose, 193
Space average temporal peak dose, 193

Spasticity, 82, 83, 84
cold application, 262–3
electromyographic biofeedback, 160–1
Specific heat, 213–14
Spinal cord injury, 160
Spinoreticular–thalamic tract, 92
Spinothalamic tract, 91
Sports injury:
pulsed shortwave, 303
therapeutic ultrasound, 189
Static magnetic fields, 307
Strain-generated potentials, 14, 15
Strength–duration (S–D) testing, 147–52
chronaxie, 150
interpretation, 149
pulse ratio, 150
reliability, 150–2
rheobase, 148, 151
technique, 149
Stress fractures, 189
Substance P, 19, 91
Sudeck's atrophy, 303
Sunbeds, 409
Sunburn, 384
ultraviolet radiation prophylactic treatment, 394
Superficial heating therapies, 241–53
contrast baths, 247–8
cyclotherm systems, 251
electric heating pads, 251
fluidotherapy, 250–1
heated air treatment, 250
hydrocollator packs, 246–7
hydrotherapy, 248–50
Kenny packs, 247
mud packs (peloids), 247
pain control, 252–3
paraffin wax baths, 244–6
tissue effects, 252
tissue temperature rises, 241–3
Superluminous diodes (SLDs), 362
Supraspinatus tendinitis, 367
Surged (ramped) current, 56
Sweating, 219, 220, 225
idiopathic hyperhidrosis, 42–3, 47, 48
infrared radiations, 348, 354
salt/water loss replacement, 227, 354
Synthetic materials, disadvantages, 296–7

Tanning response, 383–4, 395
Temperature, 213
Tendinitis, 43
Tendon integrity assessment, 146
Tension headache, 166
Testicular exposure, microwave diathermy contraindications, 337–8, 339
Tetanic contraction, 75

Thalamus, 92
Theraktin lamps, 403
Therapeutic ultrasound, *see* Ultrasound
Thermal sensation assessment, 238
Thermionic emission, 215
Thermistor, 218
Thermography, 218
Thermometers, 213, 217–18
Thermoreceptors, skin, 221–3
  cold application response, 258, 260
  sensitivity assessment, 223
  subjective sensation, 223
Thermoregulation, 218–28
  babies, 227
  behavioural regulation, 225–6
  central regulation, 226–7
  counter-current heat exchange, 220–1
  elderly people, 227, 274
  gender differences, 220, 221
  mechanisms, 219–20
    heat gain, 219
    heat loss, 219, 220, 227
    sweating, 219, 225, 227, 228
  metabolic control, 223–4
  subcutaneous fat influences, 220
  thermoreceptors, 221–3
  vasomotor control, 220, 224–5
Thromboangiitis obliterans (Buerger's disease), 249,
    272
Tinea pedis, 45, 150
Tissue damage, 16–17, 24
  direct current, 40–1
Tissue fluid viscosity, 229
Transcutaneous nerve stimulation (TENS), 23, 54, 55
  acupuncture points application, 118
  brief intense, 115
  burst, 115, 116
  contraindications, 117–18
  conventional, 114
  current parameters, 115–17, 117
  current pulses, 60–1, 62
  electrical stimulation, 101, 113–16, 117
  electrode fixation, 116
  electrode placement, 114–15, 117
  healing acceleration, 39
  high-intensity, low-frequency (acupuncture-like),
    114–15
  modulated, 115–6
  pain control, 55, 94–7
    duration of pain relief, 99
    TENS parameters, 98–9
    therapeutic effectiveness, 97–8
  pre-treatment pain assessment, 113
  spasticity, 83
  see also H-wave therapy
Transcutaneous spinal electroanaesthesia (TSE),
    118–19

Transmitted electromagnetic radiation, 320
Traumatic injury, immediate cold application, 261
Trigeminal neuralgia, 367
Trigger points, 118
  laser therapy application, 367
TENS electrode placement, 114
Trophic electrotherapy, 25, 85
Trophic stimulation, 84–6
Tumour regression, 39
Type I (slow twitch) muscle fibres, 77
Type II (fast twitch) muscle fibres, 78

Ulcer healing:
  iontophoretic antibiotics application, 43, 45
  laser therapy, 366
  therapeutic ultrasound, 189
Ulnar nerve assessment, 146
Ultrasound, 23, 172–207
  absorption of sonic energy, 180, 181
  application techniques, *see* Ultrasound application
  cell membrane transport effects, 184, 186–7
  combination therapy, 206–7
  contraindications, 200–2
    implants, 201–2
  frequencies, 172, 173, 206
  half-value depth, 180–1
  imaging, 206
  longwave, 206
  non-thermal effects, 184, 185–6
    acoustic streaming, 185
    cavitation, 185
    micromassage, 186
    standing waves, 179, 185
  phonophoresis, *see* Phonophoresis
  production, 174–5
  pulsed, 183
    treatment applications, 183–4
  safety, 200
  scattering of energy, 181
  sonic waves, 173–4
  therapeutic mechanisms, 186
  therapeutic uses, 188–90
    efficacy, 188–9
  thermal effects, 184
  tissue acoustic impedence, 181, 182
  tissue attenuation, 181–3
  tissue healing influences, 186–8
  tissue heating, 182–3, 184
  transmission, 175–6
    beam characteristics, 175–8
    media interface effects, 178–9
  wavelengths, 173, 174, 175–6
Ultrasound application, 190–5
  couplant, 190, 191
    solid gel, 194–5
  direct contact, 190, 191–2

technique, 192–3
dosage parameters, 195–9
continuous/pulsed mode, 196
duration, 198
frequency, 196–7
intensity, 197–8
treatment repetition, 198
open wounds, 194–5
treatment head movement, 191, 192–3
water bag, 190, 194
water bath, 190, 193–4
Ultrasound generators, 174–5
beam intensity, 176–8
pulsed ultrasound, 183
Ultrasound transmission:
Beam non-uniformity ratio (BNR), 176
Fresnel zone or near field, 176
Frauhofer zone or far field, 176
Ultraviolet lamps, 377–82
distance from skin, 396–7
output, 396
Ultraviolet radiation, 24, 317, 318, 376–410
acute eye irritation, 388–9
application, 403–7
characteristics, 376–7
classification, 377
contraindications, 408
dosage, 395–402
biological response, 397–8
progression, 402, 404, 406–7
quantity of energy, 396–7
response assessment, 398–9
test doses, 399–401
erythema, 385–7
action spectrum, 387, 390–1
practical assessment, 399
eye protection, 408
heliotherapy, 408–9
immunosuppressive effects, 388
ionozone therapy, 409–10
measurement, 382
melanocyte stimulation (pigmentation response),
383, 387
overdose, 408
physiological effects, 384–90
practical classification, 398
production, 377–82
fluorescent lamps, 379–80
Kromayer lamp, 381
medium-pressure mercury arc lamp (Alpine
sunlamp), 380–1
mercury vapour lamps, 378
prolonged skin exposure, 389
safety, 407–8
sensitization, 401–2
skin growth stimulation, 387–8
sunbeds, 409

tanning response, 383–4, 385, 395
therapeutic uses, 390–5
treatment records, 407
vitamin D production response, 388
wavelengths, 377, 387
Unipolar water baths, 107

Van't Hoff's law, 215, 258
Vascular changes:
cold therapy, 257, 258, 260–1
electrical stimulation, 85–7, 100
inflammatory response, 17–18
therapeutic ultrasound, 189
see also Vasodilation
Vasodilation:
cold application, 257
heat therapy, 230–1, 252
infrared radiation, 348
reflex heating, 237
see also Vascular changes
Vasospasm, 271–2
Vibration, 22–3, 172
Vinca alkaloids, 44
Viscosity, temperature-related changes, 229
Visible radiations, 317, 318, 341
physiological effects, 351
reflection, 321
therapeutic uses, 350, 351
Visual analogue scale, 114
Vitamin D deficiency, 394
Vitamin D production, 388
Vitiligo:
PUVA treatment, 404
ultraviolet radiation, 393–4
Voltage-gated sodium (NaS+s) channels, 9

Wallerian degeneration, 143, 144
Warts, 40
Water baths:
cold therapy, 267
electrical stimulation, 108
Waves characterization, 415–16
frequency, 415–16
period, 416
wavelength, 416
Weakened muscle, electrical stimulation response,
80–1
Weight-bearing biofeedback, 164
Wheal and flare response, 19
Whirlpool baths, 248–9

X-rays, 317, 318
Xanthinol nicotinate, 43

Zinc iontophoresis, 45